BASIC & APPLIED CONCEPTS *of*

BLOOD BANKING and TRANSFUSION PRACTICES

Third Edition

BASIC & APPLIED CONCEPTS *of* BLOOD BANKING and TRANSFUSION PRACTICES

Third Edition

Kathy D. Blaney, MS, BB(ASCP)SBB
Tissue Typing Laboratory
Florida Hospital
Orlando, Florida;
LifeSouth Community Blood Centers
Gainesville, Florida

Paula R. Howard, MS, MPH, MT(ASCP)SBB
Community Blood Centers of Florida
A Division of OneBlood, Inc.
Lauderhill, Florida

ELSEVIER
MOSBY

3251 Riverport Lane
St. Louis, Missouri 63043

Notices

Knowledge and best practice in this field are constantly changing. As new research and experience
broaden our understanding, changes in research methods, professional practices, or medical
treatment may become necessary.

Practitioners and researchers must always rely on their own experience and knowledge in
evaluating and using any information, methods, compounds, or experiments described herein. In
using such information or methods they should be mindful of their own safety and the safety of
others, including parties for whom they have a professional responsibility.

With respect to any drug or pharmaceutical products identified, readers are advised to check the
most current information provided (i) on procedures featured or (ii) by the manufacturer of each
product to be administered, to verify the recommended dose or formula, the method and duration
of administration, and contraindications. It is the responsibility of practitioners, relying on their
own experience and knowledge of their patients, to make diagnoses, to determine dosages and the
best treatment for each individual patient, and to take all appropriate safety precautions.

To the fullest extent of the law, neither the Publisher nor the authors, contributors, or editors
assume any liability for any injury and/or damage to persons or property as a matter of products
liability, negligence or otherwise, or from any use or operation of any methods, products,
instructions, or ideas contained in the material herein.

Working together to grow
libraries in developing countries

www.elsevier.com | www.bookaid.org | www.sabre.org

ELSEVIER   BOOK AID International   Sabre Foundation

This book is dedicated to my family, **Tommy** *and* **Sean**, *for their support.*
And to all the students and professionals
I have worked with throughout my career in
immunohematology.
KDB

This third edition is dedicated in loving memorium to my parents,
William and Olga Juda,
who encouraged my individuality and desire for continuous learning
and to my partner,
Jack,
for his perpetual belief and support of my professional goals.
And as always to all of my
former CLS students
who energized my personal joy of learning and
inspired my desire for excellence in teaching.
PRH

Reviewers

Charlotte Bates, MEd, MT(ASCP)
Instructor
Medical Laboratory Science Department
Armstrong Atlantic State University
Savannah, Georgia

Dorothy A. Bergeron, MS, CLS(NCA)
Associate Professor and Program Director
Clinical Laboratory Science Program
Department of Medical Laboratory Science
University of Massachusetts Dartmouth
North Dartmouth, Massachusetts

Kim Boyd, MS, MT(AMT)
Assistant Professor
Medical Laboratory Technology Program
Amarillo College
Amarillo, Texas

Cara Calvo, MS, MT(ASCP)SH
Program Director and Lecturer
Medical Technology Program
Department of Laboratory Medicine
University of Washington
Seattle, Washington

Linda Collins, MS, MT(ASCP)
Instructor
Delaware Technical and Community College
Georgetown, Delaware

Terry Kotrla, MS, MT(ASCP)BB
Department Chair and Professor
Medical Laboratory Technology Program
Austin Community College
Austin, Texas

Max P. Marschner, MBA, MT(ASCP)SBB, CHS
Manager, Tissue Typing Lab
Florida Hospital Medical Center
Orlando, Florida

Nicole S. Pekarek, MAT, MT(ASCP)
Instructor
Clinical Laboratory Science Instructor
Winston-Salem State University
Winston-Salem, North Carolina

Ellen F. Romani, MHSA, MT(ASCP)DLM, BB
Department Chair
Medical Laboratory Technology Program
Spartanburg Community College
Spartanburg, South Carolina

Judith A Seidel, MT(ASCP)SBB
Clinical Instructor, Immunohematology
Clinical Laboratory Science Program
Indiana University Health
Indianapolis, Indiana

Melissa Volny, MT(ASCP)SBB, MBA
Coordinator of Transfusion Services
Centegra Health System
McHenry, Illinois;
Elgin Community College
Elgin, Illinois

Preface

Basic & Applied Concepts of Blood Banking and Transfusion Practices was developed for students in 2- or 4-year medical laboratory science programs, laboratory professionals undergoing retraining, and other health care professionals who desire knowledge in routine blood banking practices. Basic didactic concepts are introduced, and the practical application of these theories to modern transfusion and blood bank settings is emphasized.

The third edition includes updates to the ever-changing field of blood banking. Donor criteria and testing have been updated to include the current donor restrictions, infectious disease testing methods, and current requirements for viral marker testing. A new chapter was added to address automation for the transfusion service. The section on molecular techniques applying to blood banking was expanded, accompanied by an expanded section on HLA. The chapter on blood components and therapy includes a description of new products such as leukoreduced components and red cell apheresis.

This textbook provides important features to assist both the student and the instructor. Each chapter features:

- Chapter outlines listing the important elements in the chapter
- Learning objectives for use by both the student and the instructor
- Study questions for self-assessment
- Key words with definitions on the same page
- Chapter summaries, in varying formats, to provide a succinct overview of the chapter's important points
- Critical thinking exercises to illustrate the practical applications to the clinical environment
- Illustrations and tables designed to reinforce and summarize the most important information found in the chapter

The third edition's presentation of topics was reorganized to improve the overall flow of the information. We also included additional details on some topics more appropriate for the 4-year medical laboratory science programs.

The third edition also has an accompanying Evolve website where the ancillaries are highlighted. For students, the ancillaries include additional case studies and access to the laboratory manual. The instructor ancillaries include an image collection that features figures found in the text, an extensive collection of test bank questions as well as answers to the critical thinking exercises, and PowerPoint presentations for each chapter that include illustrations appearing in this text.

We are very appreciative of the editors at Elsevier for their patience and professionalism in the manuscript review and publication process for this third edition. We are proud of the final product, which is user friendly to students and instructors.

Kathy D. Blaney
Paula R. Howard

Contents

IMMUNOLOGY: Basic Principles and Applications in the Blood Bank

CHAPTER OUTLINE

LEARNING OBJECTIVES

On completion of this chapter, the reader should be able to:

1. Define the following terms in relation to red cells and transfusion: antigen, immunogen, epitopes, and antigenic determinants.
2. Describe the characteristics of antigens that are located on red cells, white cells, and platelets.
3. Diagram the basic structure of an IgG molecule and label the following components: heavy and light chains, Fab, and Fc regions, variable region, hinge region, antigen-binding site, and macrophage-binding site.
4. Compare and contrast IgM and IgG antibodies with regard to structure, function, and detection by agglutination reactions.
5. Distinguish the primary and secondary immune response with regard to immunoglobulin class, immune cells involved, level of response, response time, and antibody affinity.
6. Apply the properties that influence the binding of an antigen and antibody to agglutination tests to achieve optimal results.
7. List the variables in the agglutination test that affect sensitization and lattice formation.
8. Accurately grade and interpret observed agglutination reactions using the agglutination grading scale for antigen-antibody reactions performed in test tubes.
9. Compare the classical and alternative pathways of complement activation.
10. Outline the biological effects mediated by complement proteins in the clearance of red cells.
11. Recognize hemolysis in an agglutination reaction and explain the significance.
12. Outline how the immune system responds to antigen stimulation through transfusion and pregnancy. Explain the factors that cause variations in these in vivo responses.
13. Using the principles of tissue matching, select the best potential graft given the HLA typing and antibody specificities.
14. Predict the probable HLA typing results in a family study performed for graft selection.

15. Compare and contrast the class I and II MHC complexes with regard to antigens, their associated immune cells, and their role in immunity.

16. Explain the role of HLA testing in platelet transfusion support, organ transplants, and hematopoietic progenitor cell transplants.

17. Define graft-versus-host disease (GVHD) and select methods of prevention in transfusion and transplantation.

18. Outline the serologic test methods used in HLA typing and antibody identification.

Immunohematology: study of blood group antigens and antibodies.

The science of **immunohematology** embodies the study of blood group antigens and antibodies. Immunohematology is closely related to the field of immunology because it involves the immune response to the transfusion of cellular elements. Red cells (erythrocytes), white cells (leukocytes), and platelets are cellular components that can potentially initiate immune responses after transfusion. To enhance the reader's understanding of the physiology involved in this immune response, this text begins with an overview of the immune system with an emphasis on the clinical and serologic nature of antibodies and antigens.

SECTION 1
CHARACTERISTICS ASSOCIATED WITH ANTIGEN-ANTIBODY REACTIONS

GENERAL PROPERTIES OF ANTIGENS

Antigen: foreign molecules that bind specifically to an antibody or a T-cell receptor.

Allogeneic: cells or tissue from a genetically different individual.

Autologous: cells or tissue from self.

Hapten: small-molecular-weight particle that requires a carrier molecule to be recognized by the immune system.

B lymphocytes (B cells): lymphocytes that mature in the bone marrow, differentiate into plasma cells when stimulated by an antigen, and produce antibodies.

T lymphocytes (T cells): lymphocytes that mature in the thymus and produce cytokines to activate the immune cells including the B cell.

Cytokines: secreted proteins that regulate the activity of other cells by binding to specific receptors. They can increase or decrease cell proliferation, antibody production, and inflammation reactions.

Memory B cells: B cells produced after the first exposure that remain in the circulation and can recognize and respond to an antigen faster.

Plasma cells: antibody-producing B cells that have reached the end of their differentiating pathway.

An **antigen** is a molecule that binds to an antibody or T-cell receptor. This binding can occur within the body (in vivo) or in a laboratory test (in vitro). In chemical terms, antigens are large-molecular-weight proteins (including conjugated proteins such as glycoproteins, lipoproteins, and nucleoproteins) and polysaccharides (including lipopolysaccharides). These protein and polysaccharide antigens may be located on the surfaces of cell membranes or may be an integral portion of the cell membrane. Antigens are located on viruses, bacteria, fungi, protozoa, blood cells, organs, and tissues.

Transfused red cells contain antigens that may be recognized as foreign to the individual receiving the blood. These antigens are called **allogeneic** because they are unfamiliar to the individual being transfused but are derived from the same species. These foreign antigens may elicit an immune response in the recipient. The body's immune system normally recognizes and tolerates self-antigens. These antigens are termed **autologous** because they originate from the individual. However, the failure to tolerate self-antigens may cause an immune response against cells or tissue from self. This immune response to self may result in various forms of autoimmune disease. In terms of transfusion, an allogeneic transfusion involves the exposure to antigens that are different from the individual receiving a transfusion, whereas an autologous transfusion involves antigens that originated in the recipient.

The concept of an antigen having sufficient size to induce an immune response contrasts with a **hapten,** which is a small-molecular-weight particle that requires a carrier molecule to initiate the immune response. Haptens may include medications such as penicillin and are sometimes referred to as partial antigens.

The immune response to foreign or potentially pathogenic antigens involves a complex interaction between several types of leukocytes. In the transfusion setting, immune response is primarily humoral, involving mainly **B lymphocytes (B cells).** Following a transfusion, the recipient's B cells may "recognize" these foreign red cell antigens through B-cell receptors (Fig. 1-1). This recognition causes the B cells to present the antigen to the **T lymphocytes (T cells).** After presentation, the T-cell **cytokines** signal the B cells to be transformed into plasma cells that produce antibodies with the same specificity as the original B-cell receptors. These antibodies are glycoprotein molecules that continue to circulate and specifically recognize and bind to the foreign antigen that originally created the response. **Memory B cells** are also made at this time. If there is a reexposure at a later date, the memory B cells can respond quickly and change into antibody-producing **plasma cells;** memory B cells do not require presentation to the T cell to be activated. Memory B cells allow a fast response to an antigen, an important principle used in vaccination.

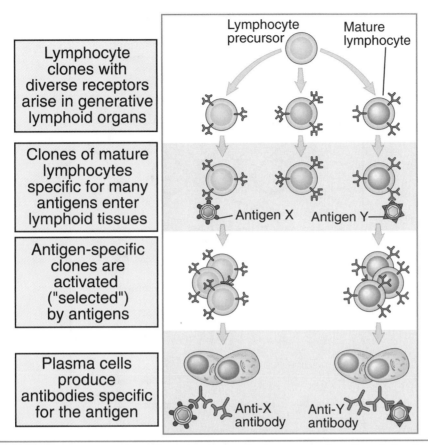

Fig. 1-1   B-cell response to an antigen. Mature lymphocytes develop receptors for antigens before they encounter the antigen. The antigen stimulates the lymphocyte that has the receptor with the best fit. These lymphocytes are signaled to produce a B-cell clone, which differentiates into plasma cells that produce an antibody with a single specificity. (From Abbas AK, Lichtman AH: *Basic immunology,* ed 3, Philadelphia, 2011, Saunders.)

Many different antibodies to foreign antigens can be produced in the immune response, each binding to a different antigen on the surface. For example, red cells have many different antigens on their surface. When red cells from one donor are transfused to a patient, several different antibodies may be produced in the immune response to the transfused red cells. The different **antigenic determinants,** also called **epitopes,** on a red cell can elicit the production of different antibodies. Each B cell has a unique specificity, which is "selected" by the antigenic determinant to expand into a **clone** of identical plasma cells making antibodies with the same specificity as the original B-cell receptor.

The term antigen is often inappropriately used as a synonym for an immunogen. An **immunogen** is an antigen that is capable of eliciting an immune response in the body. The immune system's ability to recognize an antigen and respond to it varies among individuals and can even vary within an individual at a given time. Several important characteristics of a molecule contribute to its degree of immunogenicity (Table 1-1). For example, different biological materials have varying degrees of immunogenicity. Protein molecules are the most immunogenic, followed by **carbohydrates** and **lipids,** which tend to be immunologically inert. In addition, complex compounds, such as a protein-carbohydrate combination, are more immunogenic than simpler molecules. Antigens on red cells, white cells, and platelets vary in their ability to elicit an immune response.

GENERAL PROPERTIES OF ANTIBODIES

Molecular Structure

Antibody molecules are glycoproteins composed of four polypeptide chains joined together by disulfide bonds (Fig. 1-2). The terms **antibody** and **immunoglobulin** (Ig) are often used

---

Antigens that exhibit the greatest degree of foreignness from the host elicit the strongest immune response.

Antigenic determinants: sites on an antigen that are recognized and bound by a particular antibody or T-cell receptor (also called epitopes).

Epitopes: single antigenic determinants; functionally, they are the parts of the antigen that combine with the antibody.

Clone: family of cells or organisms having genetically identical constitution.

Immunogen: antigen in its role of eliciting an immune response.

Carbohydrates: simple sugars, such as monosaccharides and starches (polysaccharides).

Lipids: fatty acids and glycerol compounds.

An immunogen is an antigen that provokes the immune response. Not all antigens are immunogens.

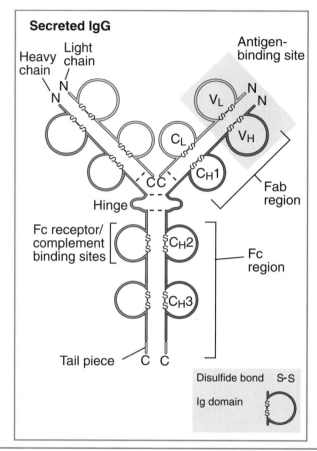

Fig. 1-2 Basic structure of an IgG molecule. Antigen binds to the variable region of the heavy and light chains. The variable region (VL and VH) is part of Fab (fragment, antigen-binding). The opposite end, composed of the heavy chain, is constant for each type of immunoglobulin. It is called the Fc (fragment, crystallizable) region, which determines the antibody function. The Fc region contains the complement binding region and the cell activation region. (Modified from Abbas AK, Lichtman AH: *Basic immunology*, ed 3, Philadelphia, 2011, Saunders.)

TABLE 1-1	Factors Contributing to Immunogenicity: Properties of the Antigen
Chemical composition and complexity of the antigen	Proteins are the best immunogens, followed by complex carbohydrates
Degree of foreignness	Immunogen must be identified as nonself; the greater the difference from self, the greater likelihood of eliciting an immune response
Size	Molecules with a molecular weight >10,000 D are better immunogens
Dosage and antigen density	Number of red cells introduced and the amount of antigen that they carry contribute to the likelihood of an immune response
Route of administration	Manner in which the antigenic stimulus is introduced; intramuscular or intravenous injections are generally better routes for eliciting an immune response

Antibody: glycoprotein (immunoglobulin) that recognizes a particular epitope on an antigen and facilitates clearance of that antigen.

Immunoglobulin: antibody; glycoprotein secreted by plasma cells that binds to specific epitopes on antigenic substances.

Heavy chains: larger polypeptides of an antibody molecule composed of a variable and constant region; five major classes of heavy chains determine the isotype of an antibody.

Light chains: smaller polypeptides of an antibody molecule composed of a variable and constant region; two major types of light chains exist in humans (kappa and lambda).

synonymously. Five classifications of antibodies are designated as IgG, IgA, IgM, IgD, and IgE. The five classes are differentiated on the basis of certain physical, chemical, and biological characteristics. Each antibody molecule has two identical **heavy chains** and two identical **light chains** joined by disulfide bond (S-S) bridges. These molecular bridges provide flexibility to the molecule to change its three-dimensional shape.

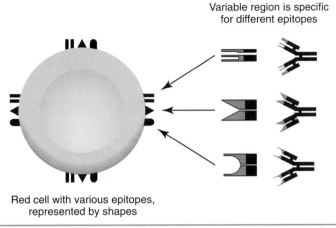

Variable region is specific
for different epitopes

Red cell with various epitopes,
represented by shapes

Fig. 1-3   Variable region of an immunoglobulin. The specificity of an antibody is determined by the unique variable region that "fits" antigenic determinants or epitopes.

> Each immunoglobulin molecule consists of two identical heavy chains and two identical light chains (either kappa or lambda).

The five distinctive heavy-chain molecules distinguish the class or **isotype**. Each heavy chain imparts characteristic features, which permit them to have unique biological functions. For example, the IgA family, which possesses alpha heavy chains, is the only antibody class capable of residing in mucosal linings. IgE antibodies can activate mast cells causing immediate hypersensitivity reactions. IgD is an antigen receptor on the naive B cell.[1] The immunoglobulins most involved in transfusion medicine are IgM and IgG, and these are discussed in more detail subsequently. There are two types of light chains: **kappa chains** and **lambda chains**. Antibodies possess either two kappa or two lambda chains but never one of each.

Each heavy-chain and light-chain molecule also contains **variable regions** and **constant regions** (or domains). The constant regions of the heavy-chain domain impart the unique antibody class functions, such as the activation of complement or the attachment to certain cells. The variable regions of both the heavy chains and the light chains are concerned with antigen binding and constitute the area of the antibody that contains **idiotope** (the idiotypic portion). This area is the binding site or pocket into which the antigen fits (Fig. 1-3). T-cell receptors also have specific antigen-binding receptors referred to as the idiotope. The **hinge region** of the antibody molecule imparts flexibility to the molecule for combination with the antigen.

Fab and Fc Regions

Early experiments to identify antibody structure and function used enzymes to cleave the immunoglobulin molecule. Enzymes such as pepsin and papain can divide the immunoglobulin molecule to produce two fragments known as Fab (fragment, antigen-binding) and Fc (fragment, crystallizable). Fab contains the portion of the molecule that binds to the antigenic determinant. Fc consists of the remainder of the constant domains of the two heavy chains linked by disulfide bonds (see Fig. 1-2). Certain immune cells, such as macrophages and neutrophils, possess receptors for the Fc region of an immunoglobulin. These immune cells are able to bind the Fc portion of antibodies that are attached to red cells or pathogens and assist in their removal by phagocytosis. This mechanism is one way that antibodies facilitate the removal of potential harmful antigens (Fig. 1-4). In transfusion medicine, the antibodies attached to red cell antigens can signal clearance in the liver and spleen, a process called **extravascular hemolysis**.

COMPARISON OF IgM AND IgG ANTIBODIES

Because IgM and IgG antibodies have the most significance in immunohematology, the following discussion focuses on these two immunoglobulins. Table 1-2 summarizes important features of IgM and IgG antibodies.

Isotype: one of five types of immunoglobulins determined by the heavy chain: IgM, IgG, IgA, IgE, and IgD.

Kappa chains: one of the two types of light chains that make up an immunoglobulin.

Lambda chains: one of the two types of light chains that make up an immunoglobulin.

Variable regions: amino-terminal portions of immunoglobulins and T-cell receptor chains that are highly variable and responsible for the antigenic specificity of these molecules.

Constant regions: nonvariable portions of the heavy and light chains of an immunoglobulin.

Idiotope: variable part of an antibody or T-cell receptor; the antigen-binding site.

Hinge region: portion of the immunoglobulin heavy chains between the Fc and Fab region; provides flexibility to the molecule to allow two antigen-binding sites to function independently.

Extravascular hemolysis: red cell destruction by phagocytes residing in the liver and spleen usually facilitated by IgG opsonization.

Fig. 1-4   Antibody attaches to the Fc receptor on a macrophage to signal clearance. The variable portion of the immunoglobulin attaches to the antigen on the red cell, while the macrophage attaches to the Fc portion. The red cell is transported to the spleen and liver for clearance. (Modified from Abbas AK, Lichtman AH: *Basic immunology*, ed 3, Philadelphia, 2011, Saunders.)

TABLE 1-2   Comparison of IgM and IgG

CHARACTERISTIC	IgM	IgG
Heavy-chain composition	Mu (μ)	Gamma (γ)
Light-chain composition	Kappa (κ) or lambda (λ)	Kappa (κ) or lambda (λ)
J chain	Yes	No
Molecular weight (D)	900,000	150,000
Valence	10	2
Total serum concentration (%)	10	70-75
Serum half-life (days)	5	23
Crosses the placenta	No	Yes
Activation of classical pathway of complement	Yes; very efficient	Yes; not as efficient
Clearance of red cells	Intravascular	Extravascular
Detection in laboratory tests	Immediate-spin	Antiglobulin test

From Abbas AK, Lichtman AH: *Basic immunology*, ed 3, Philadelphia, 2011, Saunders.

The visible agglutination of antigen-positive red cells with IgM antibodies in vitro is also referred to as immediate-spin or direct agglutination.

Valency: number of epitopes per molecule of antigen.

IgM Antibodies

When the B cells initially respond to a foreign antigen, they produce IgM antibodies first. The IgM molecule consists of five basic immunoglobulin units containing two mu heavy chains and two light chains held together by a joining chain (J chain) (Fig. 1-5). Classified as a large pentamer structurally, one IgM molecule contains 10 potential antigen-combining sites or has a **valency** of 10. Because of their large structure and high valency, these molecules are capable of visible agglutination of antigen-positive red cells suspended in saline. The agglutination of red cell antigens by IgM antibodies is also referred to as immediate-spin and direct agglutination. IgM antibodies constitute about 10% of the total serum immunoglobulin concentration.[1]

An important functional feature associated with IgM antibodies is the ability to activate the classical pathway of complement with great efficiency. Only one IgM molecule

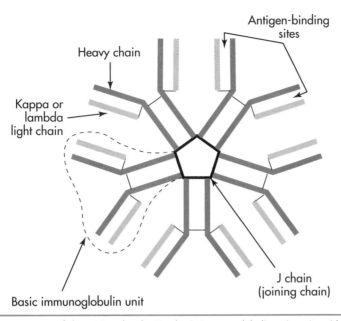

Fig. 1-5 Pentamer structure of the IgM molecule. Five basic immunoglobulin units exist with 10 antigen-binding sites.

is required for the initiation of the classical pathway in complement activation. Complete activation of the classical pathway of complement results in hemolysis of the red cells and intravascular destruction (**intravascular hemolysis**). Antibodies of the ABO blood group system are typically IgM and can cause rapid hemolysis of red cells if an incompatible unit of blood is transfused. The complement system is discussed later in this chapter.

Intravascular hemolysis: red cell lyses occurring within the blood vessels usually by IgM activation of complement.

IgG Antibodies

The IgG antibody molecule consists of a four-chain unit with two gamma heavy chains and two light chains, either kappa or lambda in structure. This form of an immunoglobulin molecule is known as a monomer. IgG antibodies constitute about 70% to 75% of the total immunoglobulin concentration in serum.[1] The molecule is **bivalent**; it possesses two antigen-combining sites. Because of the relatively small size and bivalent structure of the molecule, most IgG antibodies are not effective in producing a visible agglutinate with antigen-positive red cells suspended in saline. The antigen-antibody complexes can be viewed with the use of the antiglobulin test discussed in Chapter 2.

Bivalent: having a combining power of two.

Fc receptors on placental cells allow the transfer of IgG antibodies across the placenta during pregnancy. This transfer of IgG antibodies from the mother to the fetus protects newborns from infections. The mother's IgG antibodies may also cause destruction of fetal red cells in a condition called **hemolytic disease of the fetus and newborn** (HDFN). This condition occurs if the mother makes an antibody to red cell antigens from exposure through transfusions or prior pregnancies. If the fetus has the corresponding antigen, the IgG antibodies target the red cells for destruction. Laboratory testing to detect this process is discussed in subsequent chapters.

Hemolytic disease of the fetus and newborn: condition caused by destruction of fetal or neonatal red cells by maternal antibodies.

Four IgG subclasses (IgG1, IgG2, IgG3, and IgG4) exist as a result of minor variations in the gamma heavy chains. The amino acid differences in these heavy chains affect the biological activity of the molecule. Subclasses IgG1 and IgG3 are most effective in activating the complement system.[2] Because of their immunoglobulin structure, two molecules of IgG are necessary to initiate the classical pathway of complement activation.

The antiglobulin test method is necessary to detect antigen-antibody complexes involving IgG antibodies in vitro.

PRIMARY AND SECONDARY IMMUNE RESPONSE

Immunologic response after exposure to an antigen is influenced by the host's previous history with the foreign material. There are two types of immune responses: primary and secondary. The **primary immune response** is elicited on first exposure to the foreign

Primary immune response: immune response induced by initial exposure to the antigen.

antigen. The primary response is characterized by a lag phase of approximately 5 to 10 days and is influenced by the characteristics of the antigen and immune system of the host. Host properties that can contribute to the antigen response include the following:

- Age
- Route of administration
- Genetic makeup
- Overall health—stress, fatigue, disease
- Medications (immunosuppressive)

Lag phases may extend for longer periods. During this period, no detectable circulating antibody levels exist within the host. After this lag period, antibody concentrations increase and sustain a plateau before a decline in detectable antibody levels. IgM antibodies are produced first, followed by the production of IgG antibodies. The specificity of the original IgM molecule (determined by the variable region) is the same as the specificity of the IgG molecule seen later in the immune response. As a result of a process of gene rearrangement in the B cell, the affinity of the antibody produced after each exposure increases. This process is called **affinity maturation,** and it is the reason why antibodies often produce a stronger reaction in laboratory tests if the patient has had repeated exposure to the antigen.

The second contact with the identical antigen initiates a **secondary immune response,** or **anamnestic response,** within 1 to 3 days of exposure. Because of the significant production of memory B cells from the initial exposure, the concentrations of circulating antibody are much higher and sustained for a much longer period. Antibody levels are many times higher because of the larger number of plasma cells. IgM antibodies are also generated in the secondary immune response. However, the principal antibody produced is of the IgG class (Fig. 1-6). In the clinical setting, detecting a higher level of the IgM form of an antibody may indicate an acute or early exposure to a pathogen, whereas finding an increase in the IgG form of an antibody of the same specificity may indicate a chronic or late infection.

ANTIGEN-ANTIBODY REACTIONS

Properties That Influence Binding

The binding of an antigen and antibody follows the law of mass action and is a reversible process. This union complies with the principles of a chemical reaction that has reached equilibrium. When the antigen and antibody combine, an antigen-antibody complex or **immune complex** is produced. The amount of antigen-antibody complex formation is determined by the association constant of the reaction. The association constant drives the forward reaction rate, whereas the reverse reaction rate is influenced by the dissociation constant. When the forward reaction rate is faster than the reverse reaction rate, antigen-antibody complex formation is favored. A higher association constant influences greater immune complex formation at equilibrium (Fig. 1-7).

Several properties influence the binding of antigen and antibody. The goodness of fit and the complementary nature of the antibody for its specific epitope contribute to the strength and rate of the reaction. Factors such as the size, shape, and charge of an antigen determine the binding of the antigen to the complementary antibody. This concept of goodness of fit is most easily seen by viewing the antigen-antibody binding as a lock-and-key fit (Fig. 1-8). If the shape of the antigen is altered, the fit of the antigen for the antibody is changed. Likewise, if the charge of the antigen is altered, the binding properties of the antigen and antibody are affected. The strength of binding between a *single* combining site of an antibody and the epitope of an antigen is called the **affinity.**

When the immune complex has been generated, the complex is held together by noncovalent attractive forces, including electrostatic forces (ionic bonding), hydrogen bonding, hydrophobic bonding, and van der Waals forces. The influence of these forces on immune complex stability is described further in Table 1-3. The cumulative effect of these forces maintains the union between the antigen and antibody molecules. **Avidity** is the overall strength of attachment of *several* antigen-antibody reactions and depends on the affinity

Affinity maturation: process of somatic mutations in the immunoglobulin gene causing the formation of variations in the affinity of the antibody to the antigen. B cells with the highest affinity are "selected" for the best fit, and the resulting antibody is stronger.

Secondary immune response: immune response induced after a second exposure to the antigen, which activates the memory lymphocytes for a quicker response.

Anamnestic response: secondary immune response.

Multiple stimulations of the immune system with the same antigen produce antibodies with increased binding strength as a result of affinity maturation.

Immune complex: complex of one or more antibody molecules bound to an antigen.

Affinity: strength of the binding between a single antibody and an epitope of an antigen.

Avidity: overall strength of reaction between several epitopes and antibodies; depends on the affinity of the antibody, valency, and noncovalent attractive forces.

Fig. 1-6 **Primary and secondary immune responses.** The initial exposure to an antigen elicits the formation of IgM, followed by IgG antibodies and memory B cells. The second response to the same antigen causes much greater production of IgG antibodies and less IgM antibody secretion. (From Abbas AK, Lichtman AH: *Basic immunology,* ed 3, Philadelphia, 2011, Saunders.)

The table below corresponds to panel B of the figure:

	Primary response	Secondary response
Lag after immunization	Usually 5-10 days	Usually 1-3 days
Peak response	Smaller	Larger
Antibody isotype	Usually IgM>IgG	Relative increase in IgG and, under certain situations, in IgA or IgE (heavy chain isotype switching)
Antibody affinity	Lower average affinity, more variable	Higher average affinity (affinity maturation)

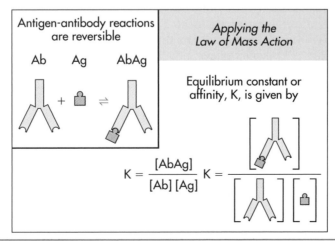

Fig. 1-7 **Kinetics of antigen-antibody reactions.** The ratio of the forward and reverse reaction rates gives the equilibrium constant. *Ab,* antibody; *Ag,* antigen.

Antigen-antibody reactions are reversible

Ab   Ag   AbAg

Applying the Law of Mass Action

Equilibrium constant or affinity, K, is given by

$$K = \frac{[AbAg]}{[Ab][Ag]}$$

Fig. 1-8 Good fit. A good fit between the antigenic determinant and the binding site of the antibody molecule results in high attraction. In a poor fit, the forces of attraction are low.

TABLE 1-3	Forces Binding Antigen to Antibody
Electrostatic forces (ionic bonding)	Attraction between two molecules on the basis of opposite charge; a positively charged region of a molecule is attracted to the negatively charged region of another molecule
Hydrogen bonding	Attraction of two negatively charged groups (X–) for a H+ atom
Hydrophobic bonding	Weak bonds formed as a result of the exclusion of water from the antigen-antibody complex
van der Waals forces	Attraction between the electron cloud (–) of one atom and the protons (+) within the nucleus of another atom

of the antibody, valency of the antigen, and noncovalent attractive forces. The goal of laboratory testing procedures in the blood bank is to create optimal conditions for antigen-antibody binding to facilitate the detection and identification of antibodies and antigens.

SECTION 2

CHARACTERISTICS ASSOCIATED WITH RED CELL ANTIGEN-ANTIBODY REACTIONS

Before discussing red cell antigens and antibodies, the reader must have a solid knowledge of the location of these concepts. When a blood sample undergoes centrifugation, the denser red cells travel to the bottom of the tube. The liquid portion of the sample is known as plasma (if an anticoagulant was added) or serum (no anticoagulant added and sample is allowed to clot).

- Red cell *antigens* are located on the red cells. They are part of the cell membrane or protrude from the cell membrane.
- Red cell *antibodies* are molecules in the plasma or serum (Fig. 1-9).

RED CELL ANTIGENS

Researchers have defined 30 blood group systems with more than 250 unique red cell antigens.[3] A blood group system is composed of antigens that have been grouped according to the inheritance patterns of many blood group genes. Every individual possesses a unique set of red cell antigens. Because of a diversity of blood group gene inheritance patterns, certain racial populations may possess a greater prevalence of specific red cell antigens.

Scientific research has determined the biochemical characteristics of many red cell antigens and their relationship to the red cell membrane. In biochemical terms, these antigens may take the form of proteins, proteins coupled with carbohydrate molecules

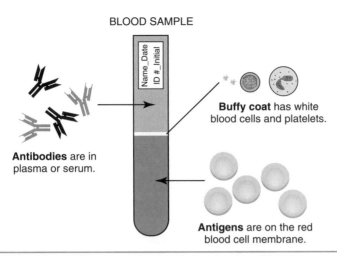

Fig. 1-9 Blood sample with red cell antigen and antibody locations identified. The serum or plasma contains the antibody, whereas the red cell membrane contains the antigen. (Modified from Immunobase, Bio-Rad Laboratories, Inc., Hercules, CA.)

Fig. 1-10 Illustration of multiple epitopes. The red cell has multiple epitopes or antigenic determinants. The unique configuration of the antigenic determinant allows recognition by a corresponding antibody molecule. (From Reid ME, Lomas-Francis C: *The blood group antigen facts book*, ed 2, San Diego, 2004, Elsevier Academic Press.)

(glycoproteins), or carbohydrates coupled with lipids (glycolipids). Generally, the red cell antigens protrude from the surface of the red cell membrane in three-dimensional configurations (Fig. 1-10). Because of this orientation on the surface of the red cell, the antigens are accessible to antibody molecules for **agglutination** reactions. Agglutination using red cells is called hemagglutination. Determination of the specificity of the red cell antigen or antibody in most routine blood banking procedures is performed by hemagglutination tests that can be done in a tube, in a microplate, or in a microtube filled with gel particles (the gel test). Solid-phase testing is an alternative method that uses red cell adherence to a solid support rather than hemagglutination. Chapters 2 and 9 discuss these methods and the reagents used in these laboratory tests.

Some red cell antigens are more immunogenic than others and must be matched to the patient receiving a transfusion. For example, the D antigen within the Rh blood group system is highly immunogenic compared with other red cell antigens. The possibility of stimulating anti-D antibody production is high in an individual lacking D antigens who is transfused with red cells possessing D antigens. Patients who lack the D antigen should receive components containing red cells that also lack the D antigen.

Glycoproteins: compounds containing carbohydrate and protein molecules.

Glycolipids: compounds containing carbohydrate and lipid molecules.

Agglutination: visible clumping of particulate antigens caused by interaction with a specific antibody.

RED CELL ANTIBODIES

The most significant immunoglobulins in transfusion medicine are IgG and IgM. Most clinically important antibodies react at body temperature (37° C), are IgG, and can cause immune destruction of transfused red cells possessing the corresponding antigen. The destruction of the red cells can cause transfusion reactions, anemia, and HDFN.

IgM antibodies react best at room temperature (20° C to 22° C) or lower (to 4° C) and are usually not implicated in the destruction of transfused red cells. The antibodies to ABO antigens are an important exception to this rule. Antibodies to ABO antigens are of the IgM class and react in vitro at room temperature and in vivo at body temperature. A transfusion of the wrong ABO blood group (antigen) would effectively activate the complement system and cause hemolysis of the transfused cells.

> IgG antibodies react best at 37° C, and IgM antibodies react best at room temperature or lower (in vitro).

IMMUNOHEMATOLOGY: ANTIGEN-ANTIBODY REACTIONS IN VIVO

Transfusion, Pregnancy, and the Immune Response

During transfusion and pregnancy, a patient is exposed to many potentially foreign antigens on red cells, white cells, and platelets that possess varying degrees of immunogenicity. Because of this exposure to foreign antigens, a patient's immune system may become activated or "sensitized" with the resultant production of circulating antibodies. The antibodies produced in response to transfusion and pregnancy are classified as **alloantibodies.**

The **antibody screen test** is performed on the patient before transfusion to detect any existing red cell alloantibodies. If a red cell alloantibody is detected, a test is performed to identify the specificity of the antibody. Once the specificity is identified, donor units lacking the red cell antigen are selected for transfusion. Detecting and identifying antibodies in the patient before transfusion is important to avoid the formation of antigen-antibody complexes **in vivo** (within the patient's body), which would lessen the survival of the transfused cells.

Immunization may also occur during pregnancy as fetal blood cells may enter the maternal circulation at delivery. Alloantibody production may be observed as an immune response to red cell, white blood cell, or platelet antigens of fetal origin. Women are routinely screened during the first trimester of pregnancy for the presence of red cell alloantibodies that can destroy fetal red cells before or after delivery. The red cell destruction may lead to clinical complications of anemia and high levels of bilirubin in the fetus or newborn.

Alloantibodies: antibodies with specificities other than self; stimulated by transfusion or pregnancy.

Antibody screen test: test to determine the presence of alloantibodies.

In vivo: referring to a reaction within the body.

Complement Proteins

The **complement system** is a group of serum proteins that have numerous biological roles related to antigen clearance, cell lysis, and vasodilation (Fig. 1-11). These proteins normally circulate in an inactive or proenzyme state. On activation, they are converted into active enzymes that enhance the immunologic processes.

Nine components of the complement family are designated C1 through C9. When activation occurs by an antibody in the classical pathway, the C1q, C1r, C1s complex splits C4 and C2 proteins into two parts. Each protein is converted into protein fragments and given the distinction a or b (e.g., C4 is converted to C4a and C4b). The smaller fragment is designated a, and the larger one is designated b. Typically, the larger b fragment binds to the cell, and the smaller a fragment enhances the inflammatory response. From the splitting of C4 and C2, C4b and C2a fragments join to form C3 convertase, which splits C3 into C3a and C3b. The C3 convertase joins with C3b to form C5 convertase, which splits C5. The final formation of a **membrane attack complex** causes lysis of various cells (**hemolysis** of red cells), bacteria, and viruses by disrupting the cell membrane. The direct attachment of the membrane attack complex, consisting of the complement proteins C5 to C9, to the cell surface produces holes in the cell membrane and osmotic lysis. If the membrane attack complex becomes attached to transfused red cells, hemolysis occurs with a subsequent release of free hemoglobin into the circulation.

Complement system: group of serum proteins that participate in an enzymatic cascade, ultimately generating the membrane attack complex that causes lysis of cellular elements.

Membrane attack complex: C5 to C9 proteins of the complement system that mediate cell lysis in the target cell.

Hemolysis: lysis or rupture of erythrocytes.

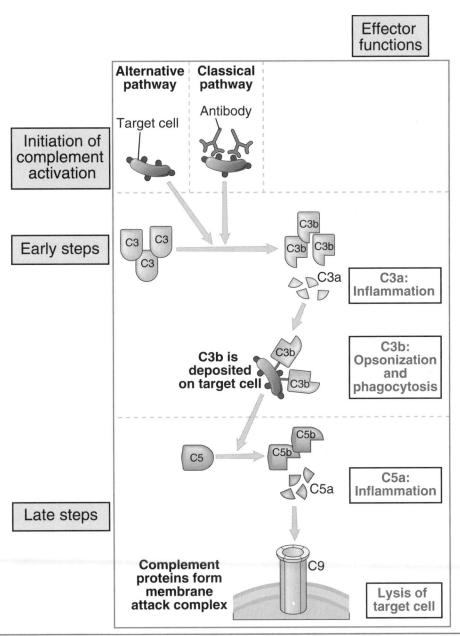

Fig. 1-11   Comparison of the classical and alternative complement systems. The classical pathway is initiated by an antigen-antibody reaction. The alternative pathway is initiated by the membrane property of a microorganism. Following the split of the C3 component, the two pathways are identical. Three major biological activities of the complement system are opsonization, lysis of target cells, and stimulation of inflammatory mediators.[4] (Modified from Abbas AK, Lichtman AH: *Basic immunology*, ed 3, Philadelphia, 2011, Saunders.)

The early steps in the activation of the complement proteins can occur in either of two pathways:

- The **classical pathway** is activated by the presence of an antibody bound to an antigen. Red cell destruction that may result from antibody-coated red cells is caused by the activation of this pathway.

- The **alternative pathway** does not require a specific antibody for activation. Foreign cell-surface constituents, such as bacteria, viruses, and foreign proteins or carbohydrates, initiate it.

Regardless of the activation mode, the final steps involved in cell lysis are common to both pathways. In addition, the consequences of complement activation, which serves as an important amplifier of the immune system, are common to both pathways. The

Classical pathway: activation of complement that is initiated by antigen-antibody complexes.

Alternative pathway: activation of complement that is initiated by foreign cell-surface constituents.

TABLE 1-4	Biological Effects Mediated by Complement Proteins
Opsonization	Clear immune complexes Enhance phagocytosis Promote release of enzymes from neutrophils
Anaphylaxis	Increase smooth muscle contraction and inflammation
Lysis	Kill foreign antigens by membrane lysis
Chemotactic	Recruit platelets and phagocytes

Anaphylatoxins: complement split products (C3a, C4a, and C5a) that mediate degranulation of mast cells and basophils, which results in smooth muscle contraction and increased vascular permeability.

Vasoactive amines: products such as histamines released by basophils, mast cells, and platelets that act on the endothelium and smooth muscle of the local vasculature.

Chemotactic: movement of cells in the direction of the antigenic stimulus.

Opsonin: substance (antibody or complement protein) that binds to an antigen and enhances phagocytosis.

Receptors: molecules on the cell surface that have a high affinity for a particular ligand.

Mononuclear phagocyte system: system of mononuclear phagocytic cells, associated with the liver, spleen, and lymph nodes, that clears microbes and damaged cells.

In vitro: reaction in an artificial environment, such as in a test tube, microplate, or column.

Sensitization: binding of antibody or complement components to a red cell.

Lattice formation: combination of antibody and a multivalent antigen to form cross-links and result in visible agglutination.

A positive reaction is indicated by agglutination. A negative reaction is indicated by no agglutination.

peptides generated during the formation of the membrane attack unit have the following additional functions (Table 1-4):

- **Anaphylatoxins** C3a, C4a, and C5a assist in the recruitment of phagocytic cells and the promotion of inflammation. These complement proteins attach to mast cells and promote the release of **vasoactive amines,** which help make blood vessels permeable for fluid and cells to enter the area.
- The C5a protein is **chemotactic** for neutrophils and attracts these cells to the site of injury.
- Complement also functions as an **opsonin,** which is a substance that binds to an antigen to promote phagocytosis. Phagocytic cells are generally inefficient. If the substance is coated with an opsonin, the process of phagocytosis becomes extremely efficient. **Receptors** on the surface of the phagocytic cell have a higher affinity for opsonins. C3b and antibodies are opsonins, which promote the clearance of bacteria and other cells to which the opsonins are attached. A test to determine whether the red cell is coated with complement components is a useful serologic tool when red cell destruction is being investigated. C3b and C4b proteins are made up of a "c" and "d" complex. The C4d and C3d breakdown products can also be detected on red cells.

Clearance of Antigen-Antibody Complexes

Antigen-antibody complexes are removed from the body's circulation through the **mononuclear phagocyte system.**[1] This system acts as a filter to remove microbes and old cells. The system is present in secondary lymphoid organs such as the spleen, lymph nodes, liver, and lungs. The largest lymphoid organ, the spleen, is particularly effective for removing old and damaged red cells from the blood and clearing the body of antigen-antibody complexes. Red cells that have bound IgG or complement components are removed by the spleen.

IMMUNOHEMATOLOGY: ANTIGEN-ANTIBODY REACTIONS IN VITRO

Overview of Agglutination

Antigen-antibody reactions occurring **in vitro** (in laboratory testing) are detected by visible agglutination of red cells or evidence of hemolysis at the completion of testing. The absence of hemagglutination in immunohematologic testing (a negative reaction) implies the lack of antigen-antibody complex formation. A negative reaction is interpreted to mean that the antibody in the test system is not specific for the antigen. A positive reaction indicates that an antigen-antibody immune complex was formed. The specificity of the antibody matched the antigen in the test system. The agglutination test must be performed correctly to reach the correct conclusion regarding the presence or absence of the antigen or antibody.

The next section describes the factors affecting the hemagglutination reaction, which occurs in two stages, referred to as the **sensitization** step and the **lattice formation** step.[4] These concepts are summarized in Table 1-5.

Sensitization Stage or Antibody Binding to Red Cells

In the first stage of red cell agglutination, the antibody binds to an antigen on the red cell membrane. This stage requires an immunologic recognition between the antigen and

TABLE 1-5	Factors Affecting Agglutination	
STAGE	**FACTOR**	**DESCRIPTION**
Sensitization	Temperature	IgG, 37° C; IgM, ≤22° C
	Incubation time	Immediate-spin or following a specific time at 1-8° C, room temperature, or 37° C
	pH	7.0 (physiologic is ideal)
	Ionic strength	Can be adjusted with reagents
Lattice formation	Zeta potential	Distance between cells caused by charged ions
	Zone of equivalence	Antigen and antibody concentrations
	Centrifugation	Time and speed of centrifugation to bring cells close together

antibody. During this recognition stage, antigenic determinants on the red cell combine with the antigen-binding site of the antibody molecule. No visible agglutination is observable at this stage.

The physical joining of an antigen and antibody is essentially a random pairing of the two structures determined largely by chance. Antibody concentration and antigen receptor accessibility and quantity may influence the probability for this collision. An increase in antibody concentration increases the probability of collision events with the corresponding antigen. This concept is referred to as the overall effect of the **serum-to-cell ratio** or concentration of antigen and antibody in immunohematologic tests.

Serum-to-cell ratio: ratio of antigen on the red cell to antibody in the serum.

Increasing the amount of serum placed in the test tube increases the concentration of antibodies available for binding to red cell antigens. When a patient's serum demonstrates weak reactions in agglutination testing, this simple technique may be used to enhance the first stage of the agglutination reaction. Increasing the amount of antigen or red cell concentration does *not* increase the reaction probability.

Factors Influencing First Stage of Agglutination

In addition to the serum-to-cell ratio, certain environmental factors may influence the sensitization and lattice formation in the two stages of agglutination reaction.

Temperature of Reaction

Most antibodies of clinical relevance in transfusion are IgG antibodies reacting at approximately 37° C.[2] By combining the sources of antigen and antibody and incubating them at this temperature, the first stage of the agglutination reaction is enhanced. In contrast, IgM antibodies are more reactive at lower temperatures, generally at room temperature (ambient temperature) or lower.

Incubation Time

Allowing adequate time for the combination of antigen and antibody to attain equilibrium also enhances the first stage of the agglutination reaction. The length of time recommended for optimal antigen-antibody reactivity varies with the test procedure and the reagents used in testing. Some test procedures may indicate a predetermined incubation period performed at variable temperatures, such as 37° C, room temperature, or 1° C to 8° C. Additionally, the test procedures may indicate an **immediate-spin** step that indicates a combination of test reagents and sample with no period of incubation.

Increasing the incubation time may help in weak antibody investigations.

Immediate-spin: interpretation of agglutination reactions immediately after centrifugation and without incubation.

pH

The optimal pH for hemagglutination is around 7.0, which is the physiologic pH range. This pH range is adequate for most of the important red cell antibodies.

Fig. 1-12   Agglutination. Agglutination refers to red cells clumping together as a result of interactions with specific antibodies. (Modified from Immunobase, Bio-Rad Laboratories, Inc., Hercules, CA.)

Fig. 1-13   Effect of the zeta potential on the second stage of agglutination. The zeta potential keeps red cells apart and is less likely to be agglutinated by IgG antibodies. IgM antibodies are more likely to cause direct agglutination. (Modified from Immunobase, Bio-Rad Laboratories, Inc., Hercules, CA.)

Ionic Strength

In an isotonic environment, such as physiologic saline, Na^+ and Cl^- ions are attracted to the oppositely charged groups on antigen and antibody molecules. As a result of this attraction, the combination of antigen and antibody is hindered. If the ionic environment is reduced, this shielding effect is reduced, and the amount of antibody uptake onto the red cell is increased.

> Low-ionic-strength reagents act by increasing the rate of antibody uptake on the cells.

Lattice-Formation Stage or Cell-Cell Interactions

After the red cells have been sensitized with antibody molecules, random collisions between the antibody-coated red cells are necessary to develop cross-linkages for the visualization of red cell clumping or agglutination within the test tube (Fig. 1-12). Visible agglutinates form when red cells are in close proximity to promote the lattice formation of antibody-binding sites to antigenic determinants on adjacent red cells.

Factors Influencing Second Stage of Agglutination

Distance Between Red Cells

> Zeta potential: electrostatic potential measured between the red cell membrane and the slipping plane of the same cell.

The **zeta potential,** or the force of repulsion between red cells in a physiologic saline solution, exerts an influence on the agglutination reaction. Red cells possess a net negative charge on the cell surface in a saline suspension. Cations (positively charged ions) from the saline environment are attracted to these negative charges. A stable cationic cloud surrounds each cell and contributes a force of repulsion between molecules of similar charge. As a consequence of this repulsive force, the red cells remain at a distance from each other. This distance between the cells is proportional to the zeta potential (Fig. 1-13).

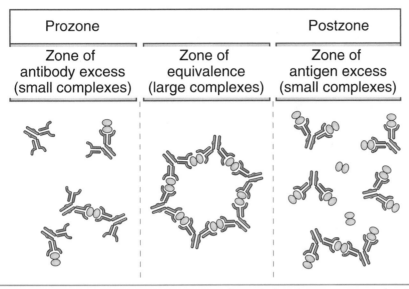

Fig. 1-14 *Zone of equivalence.* Maximum agglutination is observed when the concentrations of antigens and antibodies fall within the zone of equivalence. (Modified from Abbas AK, Lichtman AH, Pillai S: *Cellular and molecular immunology,* ed 7, Philadelphia, 2011, Saunders.)

Because of the larger size, pentamer shape, and multivalent properties of IgM molecules, agglutination is facilitated between adjacent red cells that have IgM attached to them. In contrast, IgG antibody molecules are smaller and less able to span the distance between adjacent red cells generated by the zeta potential. IgG molecules may attach, but visible agglutination might not occur.

Optimal Concentrations of Antigen and Antibody

Maximum amounts of agglutination are observed when the concentrations of antigens (red cells) and antibody (serum) fall within the **zone of equivalence** (Fig. 1-14). When the concentration of antibody exceeds the concentration of antigen, antibody excess (or **prozone**) exists, which decreases the amount of agglutinated red cells. In contrast, **postzone** occurs when the concentration of antigen exceeds the number of antibodies present. The amount of agglutinates formed under these circumstances is also suboptimal and diminished.

Immunohematologic testing is designed to obtain reactions within the zone of equivalence. Commercial antibody preparations are diluted to optimal antibody concentrations for testing. Red cell preparations are diluted to a 2% to 5% suspension in saline for optimal antigen concentrations. The use of red cell suspensions greater than 5% may affect the ability of the test reaction to fall within the zone of equivalence and cause a "false-negative" reaction because of postzone.

Effect of Centrifugation

The time and speed of centrifugation are important factors for the detection of agglutinated red cells. Centrifugation helps to facilitate the formation of a latticed network by forcing the red cells closer together in the test environment. Centrifuges are calibrated to define the optimal speed and time for the best reaction. Overcentrifugation or undercentrifugation and too-high or too-low speeds can cause false-positive or false-negative reactions.

Grading Agglutination Reactions

In immunohematology, antigen-antibody reactions are measured qualitatively. The presence of an antigen-antibody reaction is detected with red cell agglutination, but the concentration of the immune complex is not determined in a quantitative manner. Red cell antigen and antibody reactions may be performed in test tubes, in microplate wells,

Zone of equivalence: number of binding sites of multivalent antigen and antibody are approximately equal.

Prozone: excess antibody causing a false-negative reaction.

Postzone: excess antigen causing a false-negative reaction.

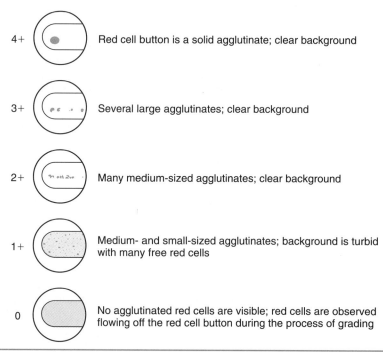

Fig. 1-15   Grading antigen-antibody reactions. Consistency in grading reactions allows for correct interpretation of results in the immunohematology laboratory. (Modified from Gamma Biologicals, Houston.)

and in microtubes filled with gel particles. Because of the qualitative nature of the measurement, the reading and grading of agglutination reactions are subjective.

To standardize this element of subjectivity among personnel performing the testing, a grading system for agglutination reactions has been established. The conventional grading system for tube testing uses a 0 to 4+ scale (Fig. 1-15).

Slight variations in this conventional grading system may be established in individual institutions. Agglutination reactions are read by shaking and tilting the test tubes until the red cell button has been removed from the bottom of the tube. Negative agglutination reactions are interpreted after the red cell button has been completely resuspended. An agglutination viewer lamp with a magnifying mirror is usually used to evaluate the agglutination reactions. Laboratories using a microscopic reading in some testing have criteria established for grading these reactions.

Hemolysis as an Indicator of Antigen-Antibody Reactions

In addition to agglutination as an indicator of an antigen-antibody reaction in the immunohematology laboratory, red cell hemolysis observed in the tube is also an indicator of the reactivity of an antigen and antibody in vitro. If the complement system is activated by an immune complex, hemolysis of the red cells along with agglutination can occur. The final steps in the process of complement activation initiate the membrane attack complex, causing membrane damage. As a consequence of this damage, intracellular fluid is released to the reaction environment. The red cell button is often smaller compared with the red cell button present in other tubes. A pinkish to reddish **supernatant** is observed after the tubes have been centrifuged. For grading a tube with hemolysis, an *H* is traditionally used when this phenomenon is observed. Some red cell antibodies characteristically display hemolysis in vitro, such as antibodies to the Lewis system antigens and anti-Vel, which are discussed in later chapters.[3] It is important to recognize hemolysis as an antigen-antibody reaction. Hemolysis is detected in vitro using fresh serum samples. Serum has active complement proteins. Because anticoagulants bind calcium, which is necessary for complement activation, plasma samples do not demonstrate complement activation.

Supernatant: fluid above cells or particles after centrifugation.

A hemolyzed patient sample is not acceptable for serologic testing in the blood bank because hemolysis is interpreted as a positive reaction.

SECTION 3

HUMAN LEUKOCYTE ANTIGEN (HLA) SYSTEM AND PLATELET IMMUNOLOGY

HUMAN LEUKOCYTE ANTIGENS

Testing Applications in the Clinical Laboratory

Most nucleated cells such as leukocytes and tissue cells possess inherited antigens on the cell surface called human leukocyte antigens (HLA). HLA antigens and the antibodies they elicit are involved in transfusion and transplantation medicine. HLA antibodies, similar to red cell antibodies, result from exposure to foreign antigens during transfusions of blood products and from pregnancy.

These antibodies can cause poor platelet response, or **refractoriness,** in patients requiring platelet transfusions. To improve platelet response, donor platelets that are HLA matched with the recipient may be necessary. HLA antibodies are also responsible for reactions that cause chills and fever in some patients receiving red cell transfusions. In this situation, blood products that are "leukocyte reduced" to avoid HLA antigens and residual cytokines usually prevent further reactions. HLA testing is not routine in the transfusion service or blood bank setting; however, an understanding of its inheritance, nomenclature, and application is important for optimal patient support. Table 1-6 lists applications of HLA testing.

Organ and hematopoietic progenitor cell transplants rely on HLA matching for the best outcome. In addition, HLA testing is used to assess risk factors for disease susceptibility. These tests are not diagnostic for the associated diseases but are used to assess relative risk. A growing application of HLA typing has been in pharmacogenomic applications. Certain HLA antigens are associated with optimal drug therapy regimens for certain diseases.[2]

Inheritance and Nomenclature of HLA

The genes encoding the expression of the HLA antigens are part of the major histocompatibility complex (MHC) gene system located on chromosome 6. Although the MHC system was first recognized and named from experiments in tissue transplantation, it is now known that the role of the MHC is essential in the recognition of self and nonself, the coordination of cellular and humoral immunity, and the immune response to antigens.

The MHC genes are divided into three categories or classes (Fig. 1-16). Class I includes the A, B, and C loci; class II includes the DR, DP, and DQ loci; and class III includes genes coding some complement proteins and cytokines. The genes are closely linked and inherited as a **haplotype.** Each person inherits one haplotype from each parent and both are expressed. This inheritance pattern is illustrated in the example in Fig. 1-17. There are hundreds of possible variations of each gene, called **alleles,** at each locus (Table 1-7). Each antigen expression is identified with a unique number that is determined by either serologic (antigen-antibody reactions) or molecular methods, which are discussed further in Chapter 3. The MHC region is the most **polymorphic** system of genes in humans

Refractoriness: unresponsiveness to platelet transfusions owing to HLA-specific or platelet-specific antibodies or platelet destruction from fever or sepsis. Responsiveness is measured by posttransfusion platelet counts.

Haplotype: set of linked genes inherited together because of their close proximity on a chromosome.

Alleles: different forms of a gene present at a particular chromosomal locus.

Polymorphic: genetic system that expresses several possible alleles at specific loci on a chromosome.

TABLE 1-6	HLA Testing Applications

- Hematopoietic progenitor cell transplants
- Solid-organ transplants
- Platelet selection for refractory patients
- Disease association
  - Ankylosing spondylitis—B27
  - Celiac disease—DQ2
- Optimize certain drug therapy regimens
  - Abacavir sensitivity (for HIV treatment) and B*57:01 allele[9]

HIV, Human immunodeficiency virus.

Fig. 1-16   Major histocompatibility complex (MHC).

MOTHER		FATHER	
A2	A11	A1	A3
B7	B44	B8	B35
Cw7	Cw12	Cw3	Cw5
DR17	DR13	DR4	DR8
DQ2	DQ8	DQ5	DQ7

Potential offspring:

Child 1		Child 2		Child 3		Child 4	
A2	A1	A2	A3	A11	A1	A11	A3
B7	B8	B7	B35	B44	B8	B44	B35
Cw7	Cw3	Cw7	Cw5	Cw12	Cw3	Cw12	Cw5
DR17	DR4	DR17	DR8	DR13	DR4	DR13	DR8
DQ2	DQ5	DQ2	DQ7	DQ8	DQ5	DQ8	DQ7

Fig. 1-17   Example of the inheritance pattern of class I and class II HLA antigens. A complete set of alleles located in each parent's chromosome is inherited as a unit by each child. There is a 25% chance that two children in a family will inherit the same sets and have identical HLA typing.

TABLE 1-7	HLA Nomenclature			
GENETIC LOCUS	ANTIGEN	NUMBER OF ANTIGENS	ALLELE EXAMPLE	NUMBER OF ALLELES
A	A1 to A80	28	A*01:01	1729
B	B7 to B82	50	B*07:02	2329
C	Cw1 to Cw10	10	C*01:02	1291
DR	DR1 to DR18	24	DRB1*01:01	1150
DQ	DQ1 to DQ9	9	DQB1*05:01	160
DP	DP1 to DP6	6	DPB1*01:01	150

http://hla.alleles.org/nomenclature/stats.html. Accessed December 2011.

because of the many possible alleles at each location. The probability that any two individuals will express the same HLA antigens is extremely low.

The naming of the HLA antigens consists of a letter designating the locus, including A, B, C, DR, DQ, and DP, and a number indicating the antigen, for example, A2, B27, Cw7, DR1, DQ5. For the C locus, the "w" is included in the nomenclature to distinguish HLA C-locus antigens from complement components. The HLA nomenclature began when the only test method was the serological lymphocytotoxicity assay. Today, more accurate and specific molecular typing assays are used. As a result of the increased sensitivity of the typing methods and increased knowledge of the glycoprotein structure of the HLA antigens, the number of alleles that can be determined continues to increase, whereas the total number of antigens has remained the same. The World Health

Organization is responsible for standardizing the HLA nomenclature.[5] For example, using the correct nomenclature, as of January 2010, A2 is expressed as A2 for antigen level resolution determined by serologic testing, HLA-A*02 for low-resolution typing, and HLA-A*02:01 if high-resolution testing is performed. Allele-level, high-resolution typing is particularly important for hematopoietic graft survival (discussed later).

Testing and Identification of HLA and Antibodies

Testing to Identify HLA

As described earlier in this chapter, red cell antigens and antibodies are primarily identified by agglutination reactions or hemagglutination test methods. Because of the nature of leukocyte antigens and antibodies, agglutination techniques are not effective. Serologic identification of HLA antigens requires the lymphocytotoxicity test method, which is described subsequently.

Class I antigens are found on the surface of platelets, leukocytes, and most nucleated cells in the body. Mature red cells lack HLA antigens, although reticulocytes express HLA class I antigens. HLA class II antigens are found on the antigen-presenting cells—macrophages, dendritic cells, and B cells. In the circulation, the number of cells expressing class I antigens is greater than the number of cells with class II antigens. Because class II antigens are not found on platelets, it is not necessary to match Class II antigens when HLA-compatible platelets are requested.

In serologic typing methods, a suspension of T or B lymphocytes is added to microtiter plates containing known antibody specificities. After incubation, rabbit complement is added. If the antibody on the plate matches the antigen on the cell, complement is activated, causing cell injury or a positive reaction. Cell damage is detected by the addition of a dye. This injury allows the dye to enter the cell, providing a visual means to distinguish the positive cells from nonreactive cells. Each well is scored while viewing under the microscope, and a pattern of reactivity determines the class I or class II typing.

Serologic typing of the HLA antigens is not always clear because of antibodies that can often react to more than one epitope (cross-reactive). In many cases, specific antibodies have not been developed to recognize the many different HLA antigens that can be expressed. For these reasons, the lymphocytotoxicity test (Fig. 1-18) is being replaced or supplemented with more sensitive and specific molecular methods, which are described in Chapter 3.

Antibody Detection and Identification

ABO compatibility is essential for the success of all solid-organ transplants. Second to ABO compatibility, careful matching of HLA antigens in patients with existing antibodies is important for long-term graft survival for kidney, heart, and lung transplants. Fig. 1-19 shows that the degree of HLA matching for kidney transplants corresponds to the survival of the graft.[6] The soluble nature of HLA antigens in the liver allows for a greater flexibility in the selection of donor tissue for liver transplants, even when preformed antibodies exist. Organ transplant candidates are periodically screened for developing HLA antibodies so that a suitable match can be determined when an organ becomes available.

Negative   Positive

Cells that are positive will take up the dye and stain dark, indicating a positive reaction

Fig. 1-18 Lymphocytotoxicity test for identification of HLA antigens. Complement and a dye are used to determine whether there is antigen-antibody recognition. Complement-mediated cell membrane damage occurs if the antigen and antibody form a complex. The damaged membrane becomes permeable to the dye, which enters the cell, allowing a positive reaction to be observed. Dye exclusion is a negative reaction.

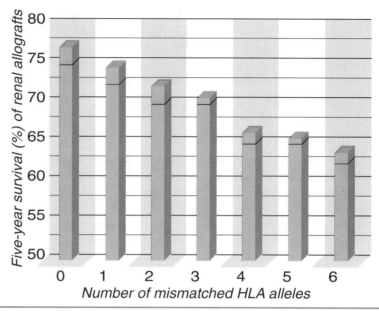

Fig. 1-19   HLA matching correlates with renal graft survival. Matching HLA antigens between the donor and recipient significantly improves renal allograft survival. The data are shown for deceased (cadaver) grafts. (From Abbas AK, Lichtman AH, Pillai S: *Cellular and molecular immunology,* ed 7, Philadelphia, 2011, Saunders.)

Patients can become sensitized to HLA antigens by the following types of exposures to alloantigens[7]:

- *Pregnancies.* About 30% to 50% of women with three or more pregnancies develop HLA antibodies. In some women, the antibodies are present for just a short time (weeks to months), whereas they may persist for many years in other women.
- *Blood transfusions.* About 50% of patients who receive multiple transfusions develop antibodies. Today, most patients who require blood transfusions receive leukocyte-reduced blood, which decreases the chances for a patient to become sensitized.
- *Previous transplant.* About 90% of patients develop HLA antibodies within 2 weeks of a failed graft.

The term panel-reactive antibody (PRA) was developed from serologic tests performed on microtiter trays composed of a panel of common antigens. A higher PRA meant that the recipient had many reactions and was less likely to be compatible with available organs.

With the increase in sensitivity and specificity of newer solid-phase methods, PRA determined by serologic methods has been replaced with a **calculated panel-reactive antibody (CPRA).**[7] This number is based on the antigens that the organ candidate is reactive against, called **unacceptable antigens,** and provides a statistical guide for determining reactivity within the population. The calculation uses a formula and HLA frequencies derived from HLA types found in more than 12,000 donors. This number is used as one assessment in determining a candidate's placement on the waitlist for available organs.

Crossmatching the recipient serum with the T cells and B cells from the potential donor is another important procedure to avoid rejection caused by antibodies to the donor tissue. Crossmatching is possible for kidney and pancreas transplants, when there is sufficient time; however, it is not always possible with heart, lung, and heart/lung transplants. The **mixed lymphocyte culture (MLC),** historically used for crossmatching, has been replaced with immunofluorescent flow cytometric techniques.[8]

HEMATOPOIETIC PROGENITOR CELL TRANSPLANTS

Hematopoietic progenitor cells (HPCs) can be obtained from bone marrow, peripheral blood, and cord blood. Diseases treated with HPCs include but are not limited to

Calculated panel-reactive antibody (CPRA): estimates the percentage of donors that would be incompatible with a transplant candidate, based on the candidate's antibodies to HLA antigens.

Unacceptable antigens: antigens that the potential graft recipient is reacting against; antibodies to these antigens could reduce the graft survival.

Mixed lymphocyte culture (MLC): In vitro reaction of T cells from one individual against MHC antigens on leukocytes from another individual. The technique measures the response of HLA class II differences between donor and recipient cells usually through radioactive measurements of DNA synthesis. This test was historically used for compatibility and D (class II) antigen typing.

congenital immune deficiencies, aplastic anemia, leukemia, lymphoma, and Hodgkin's disease. Close allele-level HLA matching between the donor and the recipient of HPC transplants is important to avoid transplant rejection and graft-versus-host disease (GVHD). Preformed HLA antibodies and ABO compatibility are less important in HPC transplants compared with solid-organ transplants.

Graft-versus-Host Disease

In HPC transplantation, the risk of GVHD increases if HLA matching is not close. Allele-level matching is important for optimal graft survival. GVHD occurs when grafted immunocompetent cells from a donor mount an immune response against the host tissue. Because recipients of HPC transplants are often immunosuppressed to allow for donor cell engraftment, this process is more likely to occur. Clinical symptoms include rash, diarrhea, and jaundice, and GVHD can be fatal if left untreated.

GVHD can also occur in immunocompromised patients receiving blood components from related donors. Irradiation of blood components from first-degree relatives is performed to reduce the risk of transfused leukocytes proliferating in the host. Irradiation prevents the viable leukocytes within the blood component from replicating. Leukocyte reduction of the blood components is insufficient to avoid GVHD because even small amounts of leukocytes can proliferate in a susceptible patient. However, in the case of a bone marrow recipient, irradiation of the progenitor cells is contraindicated because viable stem cells that are able to proliferate are essential. Blood products such as platelets and red cells that are often provided to patients after a bone marrow transplant should be irradiated. Chapter 15 provides a more detailed discussion of transplantation.

PLATELET ANTIGENS

Platelets possess inherited membrane proteins that can also elicit an immune response. Platelet antibodies are less frequently found because there is less antigen variability in the population. Antibodies to platelet antigens are the major cause of **neonatal alloimmune thrombocytopenia** (NAIT), in which maternal **alloantibodies** against antigen inherited from the father can cause fetal platelet destruction. **Posttransfusion purpura** (PTP), in which the platelets of a transfusion recipient are destroyed after transfusion, is caused by platelet antibodies. Platelet antibodies can also decrease the expected increment of platelets after a platelet transfusion.

The most common platelet antibody is directed against HPA-1a antigen, also known as Pl^{A1}. HPA-1a is present on the platelets of about 98% of the population.[2] In cases of NAIT, in which the mother's antibody is directed against the infant's platelet antigen, therapy involves either washed maternal platelets or antigen-negative platelets from a donor who is HPA-1a-negative. Platelet recipients who have become refractory, in addition to HLA matching, can be crossmatched with a test method designed to detect platelet antigen incompatibility.

Neonatal alloimmune thrombocytopenia: antibody destruction of a newborn's platelets caused by antibodies formed from prior pregnancies and directed to paternal antigens.

Alloantibodies: antibodies with specificities other than self; stimulated by transfusion or pregnancy.

Posttransfusion purpura: antibody destruction of platelets after transfusion.

CHAPTER SUMMARY

Characteristics of Antigens
- Antigens are foreign molecules that combine with an antibody or immunoglobulin. The part of the antigen that combines with the antibody is the epitope or antigenic determinant.
- Red cells, white cells, and platelets have numerous antigens that can elicit an immune response after exposure from transfusions, pregnancy, and transplantation.

Characteristics of Antibodies
- The structural components of immunoglobulins consist of heavy chains and light chains, constant regions and variable regions, disulfide bonds, and a hinge region.

- The five types of immunoglobulins—IgM, IgG, IgA, IgD, and IgE—differ in their heavy chain, function, and role in the immune response.
- IgM molecules are pentameric with 10 antigen-binding sites and are most efficient in the activation of complement proteins. IgM is produced first. IgM antibodies are usually detectable by direct or immediate-spin agglutination in tube testing.
- IgG molecules possess two antigen-binding sites and constitute the greatest percentage of the total immunoglobulin concentration in serum. The antiglobulin test is required to detect IgG.

Antigen-Antibody Interactions

- An immune complex is an antibody bound to an antigen. Immune complexes are formed in vivo and are eventually cleared by the body.
- In laboratory testing, immune complexes are formed in vitro to determine the identity of an antigen or antibody or to predict the reaction after transfusion of a blood product. Typically, the antigen is on the red cell, and the antibody is in the patient's serum or plasma or in the reagent.
- Hemagglutination is a two-step process involving the antibody binding to red cells and the formation of lattices between sensitized red cells.
- The fit or the complementary nature of the antibody for its specific epitope determines the strength and rate of the reaction, also called the affinity of the bond.
- The immune complex is held together by attractive forces, including electrostatic forces, hydrogen bonding, hydrophobic bonding, and van der Waals forces.

The HLA System and Platelet Immunology

- Genes encoding the expression of the HLAs are part of the MHC found on chromosome 6 and code for class I (A, B, C), class II (DR, DQ, DP), and class III complement proteins.
- HLA antigens are inherited as a haplotype and are important in recognition of self and nonself, coordination of cellular and humoral immunity, and the immune response to antigens.
- A refractory or poor platelet response to transfused platelets can be caused by antibodies directed against HLA or platelet antigens, and HLA-matched or HLA-compatible platelets may be considered.
- Hematopoietic progenitor cell transplants rely on careful HLA typing to avoid GVHD and transplant rejection.
- GVHD is a serious consequence of transfusion of blood products from donors that have been HLA matched or are related to the recipient and can be avoided by irradiation of the blood product.
- HLA antibody detection and compatibility testing for potential organ recipients are important techniques to avoid graft rejection.

CRITICAL THINKING EXERCISES

EXERCISE 1-1

Draw an IgG molecule and identify the following parts:
a. Antigen-binding site
b. Complement-binding region
c. Macrophage-binding site
d. Variable region
e. Hinge region

EXERCISE 1-2

Two different patients received red cell units during surgery. One patient developed an IgG antibody after transfusion; the other patient did not develop an IgG antibody. What factors contribute to an immune response to transfusion?

EXERCISE 1-3

A specimen was received in the blood bank for antibody identification. Would the patient's serum or red cells be used for this test?

EXERCISE 1-4

A technologist failed to notice that the centrifuge had not properly centrifuged the test tube set up for antibody identification. What would be the potential error in the interpretation of this test?

EXERCISE 1-5

A technologist added extra drops of red cells to the test tube she was using for antibody identification because she was concerned that she had gotten a weak reaction in the initial test. Why is this action not recommended? What could be the potential result of this action?

EXERCISE 1-6

A patient who is not responding to platelet transfusions requires an HLA-matched platelet transfusion. The patient's HLA type is performed and is reported as A2, A11, B8, B35. A donor is called with a compatible type to donate for this patient. Why were the class II antigens not considered for matching?

EXERCISE 1-7

A red cell unit from a donor was received at the transfusion service to be reserved for a directed donation for the donor's sister who was undergoing hip replacement surgery. What must be done before transfusion of this unit to prevent graft-versus-host disease? Why is leukocyte reduction insufficient to prevent this disease?

EXERCISE 1-8

Parents of a kidney transplant candidate were tested for a potential compatible kidney because the candidate demonstrated HLA antibodies. The patient's HLA antigens were typed and found to be A1, A2, B27, B50, DR17, and DR11. Antibodies identified were specific for A3, B18, and DR7 antigens.

   If the mother's HLA typing is A1, A3, B35, B27, DR4, and DR11, and the father's typing is A2, A24, B50, B44, DR11, and DR17, what antigens did the father contribute? List the probable HLA types of the candidate's three siblings. Select the kidney or kidneys with the best match.

EXERCISE 1-9

In the investigation of a patient's serum showing a weak IgM antibody (1+ agglutination reactions), what variables could you change to make the antigen-antibody reactions stronger in vitro?

EXERCISE 1-10

Why do IgM antibodies activate the classical pathway of complement more efficiently than IgG antibodies?

EXERCISE 1-11

Two students performed agglutination tests using the same antigen and antibody. One student observed a 1+ reaction after the immediate-spin reading, whereas the other student observed a 2+ reaction. What variables could cause the differences between these results? When would these differences have a significant impact on testing?

STUDY QUESTIONS

1. Antibodies are produced by:
   a. natural killer cells
   b. T cells
   c. macrophages
   d. plasma cells

2. Which of the following cells expresses HLA class II antigens?
   a. B cells
   b. platelets
   c. erythrocytes
   d. T cells

3. Select the term that describes the unique part of the antigen that is recognized by a corresponding antibody.
   a. immunogen
   b. epitope
   c. avidity
   d. clone

4. _____ molecules are usually not good immunogenic substances.
   a. protein
   b. carbohydrate
   c. lipid
   d. glycoprotein

5. The chemical composition of an antibody is:
   a. protein
   b. lipid
   c. carbohydrate
   d. glycoprotein

6. In a hemagglutination test, the antigen is:
   a. on the red cell membrane
   b. secreted by the red cell
   c. in the red cell nucleus
   d. in the plasma or serum

7. Hemagglutination can be enhanced by increasing:
   a. the temperature higher than 37° C
   b. the incubation time
   c. increasing the antigen concentration
   d. pH greater than 7

8. Molecules that bind to an antigen to increase phagocytosis are:
   a. opsonins
   b. cytokines
   c. haptens
   d. isotypes

9. An epitope is also termed a(n):
   a. binding site
   b. allotype
   c. antigenic determinant
   d. immunogen

10. Agglutination reactions characterized by many small agglutinates in a background of free cells would be graded in tube testing as:
    a. 1+
    b. 2+
    c. 3+
    d. 4+

11. An order for blood products for a recent recipient of a bone marrow graft was received in the transfusion service. Because these patients are especially susceptible to GVHD from a transfusion, which blood product would best prevent GVHD?
    a. leukocyte reduction of the unit
    b. washing the unit with normal saline
    c. irradiation of the blood product
    d. providing HLA-matched blood products

12. Complement activation can result in:
    a. cell lysis
    b. enhanced cell clearance
    c. neutrophil activation
    d. generation of vasoactive amines
    e. all of the above

13. The mixed lymphocyte culture (MLC) is an older technique in the HLA laboratory used to determine:
    a. HLA-A antigens
    b. HLA-C antigens
    c. HLA antibody identification
    d. HLA-D antigens and compatibility

For questions 14 through 25, match the characteristic with the correct immunoglobulin class.

Characteristic	Class
14. contains 10 antigen-binding sites	a. IgA
15. produced early in an immune response	b. IgG
16. found in mucosal linings	c. IgM
17. able to cross the placenta	d. IgE
18. highest plasma/serum concentration	
19. pentamer shape	
20. activates the complement cascade most efficiently	
21. can initiate allergic reactions	
22. associated with intravascular cell destruction	
23. detected with the antiglobulin test	
24. detected in the immediate-spin phase of the agglutination test	
25. reacts best at room temperature	

REFERENCES

1. Stevens CD: *Clinical immunology and serology*, ed 2, Philadelphia, 2003, FA Davis.
2. Brecher ME: *Technical manual*, ed 17, Bethesda, MD, 2011, AABB.
3. Reid ME, Lomas-Francis C: *The blood group antigen facts book*, ed 3, London, 2004, Elsevier.
4. Abbas AK, Lichtman AH: *Basic immunology*, ed 3, Philadelphia, 2011, Saunders.
5. *HLA nomenclature*. http://hla.alleles.org. Accessed December 2011.
6. Abbas AK, Lichtman AH, Pillai S: *Cellular and molecular immunology*, ed 7, Philadelphia, 2011, Saunders.
7. Organ Procurement and transplant network; http://optn.transplant.hrsa.gov/. Accessed December 2011.
8. Rodey GE: *HLA beyond tears*, ed 2, Durango, CO, 2000, Denovo.
9. Mallal S, Phillips E, Carosi G, et al: HLA-B*5701 screening for hypersensitivity to abacavir, *N Engl J Med* 358:568, 2008.

2

BLOOD BANKING REAGENTS:
Overview and Applications

CHAPTER OUTLINE

LEARNING OBJECTIVES

On completion of this chapter, the reader should be able to:

1. Describe the basic principles of routine testing in the immunohematology laboratory.
2. Identify sources of antigen and antibody used in testing.
3. List several routine tests performed in the immunohematology laboratory.
4. Describe the relationship of potency and specificity to blood banking reagents.
5. Compare and contrast polyclonal and monoclonal antibodies.
6. Describe the reagents available for ABO typing.
7. Describe the reagents available for D typing.
8. Define the low-protein reagent control and describe its purpose.
9. Describe the different types and purposes of reagent red cells.
10. Describe the basic principles of antiglobulin testing.
11. Distinguish between direct and indirect antiglobulin tests.
12. Identify the indications for implementing direct and indirect antiglobulin tests.
13. Discuss the different sources of possible errors in the performance of antiglobulin testing.
14. Compare and contrast the composition and appropriate uses of polyspecific and monospecific antiglobulin reagents.
15. Discuss the role of potentiators in routine testing.
16. Describe and differentiate the mechanism of action for the following potentiators: low-ionic-strength saline, bovine serum albumin, polyethylene glycol, and proteolytic enzymes.
17. Define and identify common lectins used in blood banking.
18. Compare and contrast the principles of gel technology, microplate techniques, and solid-phase red cell adherence techniques.
19. Analyze quality control data for performance criteria and acceptability.
20. Research product inserts and quality control procedures for product requirements.
21. Apply critical thinking skills to solve issues associated with reagent performance.

This chapter demonstrates how the basic principles of antigen-antibody (Ag-Ab) reactions in vitro are applied in the immunohematology laboratory. Basic laboratory procedures and the major reagents used in the testing of patient and donor samples are discussed. A section on gel technology and solid-phase red cell adherence is included to introduce technologies used in the detection of Ag-Ab reactions that are different from traditional tube testing.

SECTION 1
INTRODUCTION TO ROUTINE TESTING IN IMMUNOHEMATOLOGY

The basic procedures in immunohematology are derived from the principle of placing a source of antigen and a source of antibody into a testing environment to detect an Ag-Ab reaction (Fig. 2-1). The evidence for the formation of an Ag-Ab reaction in-vitro has traditionally been the visualization of agglutinates or the presence of hemolysis within the test tube. Alternative techniques for the detection of Ag-Ab reactions are available based on detection systems using gel and solid-phase adherence technology. These methods all share common denominators: a source of antigen and a source of antibody added to a testing environment.

Selection of the appropriate source of either antigen or antibody for inclusion in the procedure depends on the purpose or intent of the test. Is testing directed toward detecting the presence or absence of a particular red cell antigen? Or is testing directed toward detecting the presence or absence of a particular red cell antibody? In either situation, no matter what variable is unknown in testing, a known source is used for the other variable. If the unknown variable is the antigen, the unknown antigen source combines with a known source of antibody to enable Ag-Ab reactions. In the procedure to detect the presence of the B antigen on a patient's red cells, the red cells are combined with a commercial source of antibody, anti-B reagent. If the B antigen is present on the red cells, agglutination is observed in the test tube. If the B antigen is absent on the red cells, no agglutination is observed in the test tube (Fig. 2-2).

> For antigen testing, antigens are on the red cell; antibodies are in the antisera (commercial antibodies).

SOURCES OF ANTIGEN FOR TESTING

Sources of antigen for immunohematologic testing include reagent red cells or red cells from patient or donor blood samples. Reagent red cells are commercially prepared cell suspensions. The manufacturer of reagent red cells has previously identified many of the red cell antigens. Therefore these reagent red cells provide known sources of red cell antigens. By using a known antigen, an unknown antibody can be detected or identified based on a positive or negative reaction.

When using red cell suspensions from a patient's sample, the red cell antigens are the unknown factor. The patient's red cells are tested with a known antibody to determine

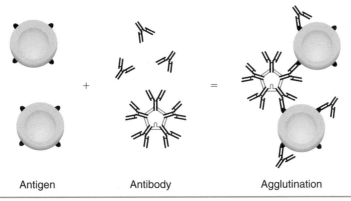

Antigen   Antibody   Agglutination

Fig. 2-1 **Routine testing in the immunohematology laboratory.** Sources of antigen from red cells and sources of antibody from serum are added. A positive result is the Ag-Ab reaction shown as agglutination. (Modified from Immunobase, Bio-Rad Laboratories, Inc., Hercules, CA.)

Testing patient RBCs for B antigen with reagent anti-B

Reagent Anti-B   Patient RBCs

Fig. 2-2 **Example of a routine test.** Patient red cells are tested for the presence of B antigen with a commercial antibody reagent, anti-B. The presence of agglutination indicates that the patient's red cells contain B antigens. (Modified from Immunobase, Bio-Rad Laboratories, Inc., Hercules, CA.)

TABLE 2-1	Sources of Antigen and Antibody in Agglutination Reactions for Blood Bank Tests	
TESTING FOR	**KNOWN SOURCE**	**UNKNOWN SOURCE**
Antigen	Reagent red cells	Patient or donor red cells
Antibody	Commercial antisera (anti-A, anti-B)	Patient or donor serum/plasma

the antigen identity. When a known antibody is used, the unknown antigens on the patient's red cells can be detected, based on agglutination reaction. If antigen is present, agglutination is visible. If antigen is absent, no agglutination is visible (see Fig. 2-2).

SOURCES OF ANTIBODY FOR TESTING

Sources of antibody for immunohematologic testing include commercial antisera or serum or plasma from the patient. Commercial antisera contain known red cell antibodies and are used to identify unknown antigens.

Antibodies may also be present in the serum or plasma of blood samples from patients or donors. Similar to patient antigens, the antibodies made by patients are usually unknown. Patient serum or plasma samples are tested for the presence of red cell antibodies using a known antigen source for identification or detection (Table 2-1).

ROUTINE TESTING PROCEDURES IN THE IMMUNOHEMATOLOGY LABORATORY

Several universal procedures in immunohematology apply these principles in the testing of patient samples before transfusion with blood products containing red cells or in the testing of donor samples. Table 2-2 lists the sources of antigen and antibody in these procedures.
- ABO and D typing for the detection of the A, B, and D antigens
- ABO serum/plasma testing for the detection of ABO antibodies, anti-A and anti-B
- Determination of the presence or absence of red cell antigens from other blood group systems in patient and donor samples (e.g., testing a donor unit for the E antigen of the Rh blood group system)
- Antibody screen (antibody detection) for the detection of preformed antibodies to red cell antigens as a result of previous exposure to red cells through transfusion and pregnancy
- **Antibody identification** for determination of the red cell antibody specificity after detection with the antibody screen

Antibody identification: procedure that determines the identity of a red cell antibody detected in the antibody screen by reacting serum with commercial panel cells.

TABLE 2-2	Routine Procedures in the Immunohematology Laboratory		
PROCEDURE	**PURPOSE**	**SOURCE OF ANTIGEN**	**SOURCE OF ANTIBODY**
ABO/D typing (forward grouping)	Detects A, B, and D antigens	Patient's red cells	Commercial anti-A, anti-B, and anti-D
ABO serum testing (reverse grouping)	Detects ABO antibodies	Reverse grouping cells (A_1 and B)	Patient's serum or plasma
Antibody screen	Detects antibodies with specificity to red cell antigens	Screening cells	Patient's serum or plasma
Antibody identification	Identifies specificity of red cell antibodies	Panel cells	Patient's serum or plasma
Crossmatch	Determines serologic compatibility between donor and patient before transfusion	Donor's red cells	Patient's serum or plasma

- **Crossmatch** for the serologic check of the donor unit and patient compatibility before transfusion

Crossmatch: procedure that combines donor's red cells and patient's serum to determine the serologic compatibility between donor and patient.

SECTION 2

INTRODUCTION TO BLOOD BANKING REAGENTS

As introduced in the previous section, reagent red cells and commercial antibodies are routinely used in the blood bank to detect Ag-Ab reactions. These reagents are the tools of blood banking, allowing the provision of safe and viable blood products. Technologists using these tools require a technical knowledge of correct reagent use and the limitations of each reagent to interpret the results from patient and donor testing rapidly. A discussion of the composition, sources, uses, and limitations of reagents is presented following an overview of the regulatory aspects of reagent manufacturing.

Reagents categories include:
- Reagent red cells: known red cell antigens
- Antisera: known red cell antibodies
- Antiglobulin reagents: anti-IgG or anti-C3d or combination of anti-IgG and anti-C3d
- Potentiators to enhance antibodies

REGULATION OF REAGENT MANUFACTURE

Commercial antisera and reagent red cell products are licensed by the Center for Biologics Evaluation and Research of the U.S. **Food and Drug Administration (FDA).** The publication, *Code of Federal Regulations,* outlines the FDA criteria for the licensure of reagents in conjunction with other regulations for the manufacture of blood and blood components.[1]

The FDA has established minimum standards relating to product **specificity** and **potency** for use in blood banks and transfusion services before a license is assigned to a commercial reagent. Specificity reflects the unique recognition of the antigenic determinant and its corresponding antibody molecule. For example, commercial anti-D reacts with red cells possessing D antigens and does not react with red cells lacking D antigens. Potency addresses the strength of the Ag-Ab reaction. For example, commercial anti-A reagents are manufactured to agglutinate strongly (3+ to 4+) with red cells possessing the A antigen.

When a manufacturer has shown that a product has met the FDA specificity and potency requirements, the reagent is assigned a product license number that is displayed on the product's label. Each product is also labeled with a manufacturer's expiration date. According to FDA regulations, routine blood banking reagents cannot be used in testing after the expiration date. Exceptions to this rule can be made for rare antisera and red cells if the reagent has acceptable quality control results. If reagents are produced for

Food and Drug Administration (FDA): U.S. agency responsible for the regulation of the blood banking industry and other manufacturers of products consumed by humans.

Code of Federal Regulations: FDA publication outlining the legal requirements of blood banking facilities.

Specificity: unique recognition of an antigenic determinant and its corresponding antibody molecule.

Potency: strength of an Ag-Ab reaction.

in-house use (within the facility), a license is not required. In this situation, the FDA requirements for specificity and potency must also be met and documented.

Each manufacturer provides a package or product insert to the consumer that describes in detail the reagent, intended use, summary, principle, procedure for proper use, the specific performance characteristics, and the limitations of the reagent. Laboratory **standard operating procedures** (SOPs) are written to reflect the procedures outlined in these product inserts. As new lots of reagents are received in the blood bank, the product inserts must be reviewed for any procedural changes. Any revisions must be incorporated into the SOPs before introduction of the reagent in routine testing. The total compliance with the manufacturer's directions cannot be overemphasized because that document details the appropriate procedures and recommends the appropriate reagent controls for accurate interpretation of test results.

REAGENT QUALITY CONTROL

Quality control is the term assigned to technical procedures designed to determine whether the analytical testing phase is working properly. Quality control includes checks on blood banking reagents and equipment before their use in tests on patient or donor samples. Requirements for quality control are obtained from regulations, accreditation standards, manufacturers' product inserts, and state and local requirements. Using these requirements, each laboratory establishes quality control protocols for the validation and documentation of reagent and equipment function. The quality control of reagents is performed daily on commercial reagent red cells and antisera. These reagents are tested to determine whether they meet preset acceptable performance criteria.

Components of a quality control program for blood banking reagents include the following[2]:
1. *Statement of criteria for acceptable reagent performance.*
   Requirements for the acceptable performance of a reagent are outlined in the facility's SOP. Typically, the potency of the agglutination reaction defines the acceptability of the reagent performance when challenged with the corresponding red cell antigen. For example, anti-A is tested against reagent red cells known to possess the A antigen. When the anti-A reagent and group A red cells are combined, a 3+ to 4+ reaction is expected for optimal reagent performance. When anti-A is reacted with group B red cells, no agglutination is expected. If agglutination results are less than 3+ in strength with group A red cells (e.g., 2+ or less), the potency of the anti-A reagent may be deteriorating. The loss of agglutination strength over time is an indicator of a loss of potency, and the ability to detect A antigens in patient samples is potentially compromised.
2. *Documentation of reagent use.*
   Reagents are tested, and the results of quality control testing are recorded and reviewed. Records of quality control testing must be maintained, including results, interpretations, date of testing, and identity of personnel performing the testing.
3. *Corrective actions for lack of performance.*
   Appropriate corrective actions for reagents that do not meet the performance requirements must be outlined in the SOP.

SECTION 3
COMMERCIAL ANTIBODY REAGENTS

POLYCLONAL VERSUS MONOCLONAL ANTIBODY PRODUCTS

An ideal reagent antibody product contains a concentrated suspension of highly specific, well-characterized, uniformly reactive immunoglobulin molecules. Commercially prepared antibody reagents can be either polyclonal antibody–based or monoclonal antibody–based products. If multiple clones of B cells secrete antibodies in an immunologic response to a foreign antigen, the antiserum produced is called polyclonal. If the antibody is the product of a single clone of B cells, the reagent produced is called monoclonal.

Polyclonal Antibody Reagents

Until the more recent introduction of monoclonal antibody–based blood banking reagents, commercial antisera were derived from polyclonal sources as a result of the immunization of animals and humans with purified antigens. Time-consuming separation techniques were used to produce the polyclonal antisera.

In the polyclonal immune response, B cells secrete antibodies that are specific for the multiple epitopes of the injected antigen. A heterogeneous population of antibodies is made recognizing different epitopes on a single antigen. Examples of **polyclonal antiserum** produced for blood bank testing are known as antihuman globulin (AHG) reagents. These products contain multiple antibody specificities directed toward different antigens in the immunization injection or toward different parts of a purified antigen injected for an immune response.

Polyclonal antiserum: made from several different clones of B cells that secrete antibodies of different specificities.

Polyclonal antihuman IgG serum is produced by immunizing rabbits with purified human IgG molecules. The rabbits respond by the activation of multiple B-cell clones. Each B-cell clone produces an antibody directed at a specific epitope of the IgG molecule. The combination of the multiple B-cell clones secreting many antibodies in the rabbit serum makes a polyclonal antibody reagent (Fig. 2-3).

Monoclonal Antibody Reagents

In contrast to polyclonal antisera, **monoclonal antibody** production creates an immortal clone that manufactures antibodies of a defined specificity (Fig. 2-4). Monoclonal antibodies are manufactured in vitro using hybridoma technology. Monoclonal antibodies are the products of a single clone of B cells. Mice are immunized with antigen; the spleens are harvested and fused with an abnormal cell from a mouse that has myeloma producing hybrid cells. These hybrid cells (**hybridomas**) are cultured, grow rapidly, and are screened for the production of antibody. Each hybridoma is descended from a single B-cell clone. All cells of the hybridoma cell line make the same antibody molecule, called a monoclonal antibody. In contrast to polyclonal antibodies, monoclonal antibodies recognize one specific epitope of the immunized antigen.

Monoclonal antibody: made from single clones of B cells that secrete antibodies of the same specificity.

Hybridomas: hybrid cells formed by the fusion of myeloma cells and antibody-producing cells; used in the production of monoclonal antibodies.

Monoclonal antibody–based reagents were introduced into the blood bank to replace polyclonal-based reagents because of necessity and desirability. Examples of FDA-approved monoclonal antibodies include anti-A, anti-B, anti-A,B, anti-D, anti-C, anti-E, anti-c, anti-e, anti-IgG, anti-C3b, anti-C3d, and other blood group system antibodies.[3]

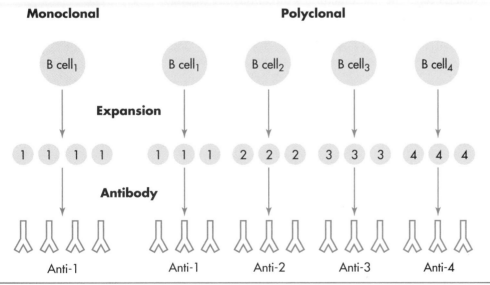

Fig. 2-3 Comparison of polyclonal and monoclonal immune responses. Polyclonal immune responses: After exposure to the antigen, multiple clones of B cells are activated by the immune response to secrete antibodies of different specificities. In response, the antigen, anti-1, anti-2, anti-3, and anti-4 were secreted by different B-cell clones. Monoclonal immune responses: A single clone of B cells is active by the immune response and secretes an antibody with one specificity (anti-1).

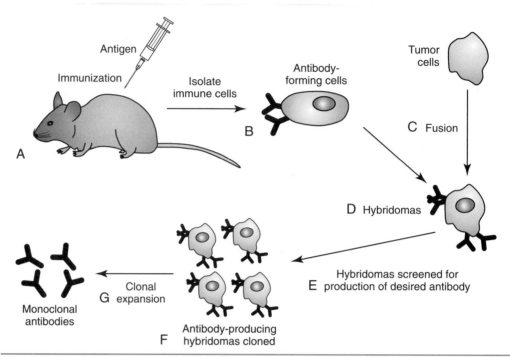

Fig. 2-4   Monoclonal antibody production. Monoclonal antibodies are the products of a single clone of B cells. **A,** Mice are immunized with antigen. **B,** The spleens are harvested for immune cells. **C,** The antibody-forming cells are fused with a tumor cell from a mouse in a process called fusion. **D,** Hybrid cells (hybridomas) are formed, cultured, and grow rapidly. **E,** The hybridomas are screened for the production of desired antibody. **F,** Each hybridoma is descended from a single B-cell clone. **G,** The hybridoma cell line is expanded and makes the same antibody molecule. (Modified from Immucor, Norcross, GA.)

Monoclonal antibody reagents have the advantage of producing large quantities of the desired antibody with lot-to-lot consistency of a single specificity.[4]

Monoclonal antibody–based reagents are correctly used in serologic testing by following these guidelines:
- Careful review of the manufacturers' product inserts for proper use and product limitations
- Adherence to the manufacturer's directions for testing
- Recognition of the relevant characteristics of the hybridoma clone

Monoclonal antibodies may vary in the recognition of a red cell antigen because red cells might not express every antigenic determinant. Some monoclonal antibody reagents are blends of more than one monoclonal antibody to allow for better antigen recognition.
- Review of the manufacturer's formulation

Protein concentrations in the formulation of products produced by different manufacturers may vary. Most of these monoclonal antibody reagents possess a low concentration (3% to 8%) of protein.

Monoclonal and Polyclonal Antibody Reagents

Monoclonal and polyclonal antibodies are also blended to produce reagents with specific advantages in blood bank testing. Antiglobulin reagents, discussed later in this chapter, can be a combination of rabbit polyclonal antibodies and a murine (mouse) monoclonal antibody.

The differences between monoclonal and polyclonal antibody–based reagents are summarized in Table 2-3.

REAGENTS FOR ABO ANTIGEN TYPING

Anti-A and anti-B commercial reagents are used to determine whether an individual's red cells possess the A or B antigens of the ABO blood group system. Donor or patient red

TABLE 2-3   Summary of Monoclonal and Polyclonal Antibody Products

MONOCLONAL ANTIBODY	POLYCLONAL ANTIBODY
Secreted by a single clone of antibody-producing B cells	Secreted by several different clones of antibody-producing B cells
One immunoglobulin class (IgG or IgM)	Mixture of IgM and IgG antibodies
Unique specificity for a particular epitope	Mixture of antibodies that may be directed at different epitopes of the same antigen

TABLE 2-4   ABO Red Cell Testing (ABO Forward Grouping)

ABO BLOOD GROUP ANTIGENS	REACTION WITH ANTI-A	REACTION WITH ANTI-B	ANTIGENS DEFINED
A	+	0	A
B	0	+	B
AB	+	+	AB
O	0	0	O

+, Agglutination; 0, no agglutination.

cells (unknown antigen) are combined with commercial antisera (known antibodies) and observed for the presence or absence of agglutination. Agglutination indicates the presence of antigen; no agglutination indicates the absence of antigen on the red cells tested (Table 2-4).

Based on the testing results, an ABO blood type is assigned to the patient or donor. Four major blood types in the ABO blood group system exist: A, B, AB, and O. Group A individuals possess the A antigen and lack the B antigen. Group B individuals possess the B antigen and lack the A antigen. Group AB individuals possess both the A and B antigens. Group O individuals lack both the A and B antigens. The procedure to determine ABO blood group system assignment has been referred to as ABO grouping, ABO forward grouping, front typing, and ABO red cell testing. The *Technical Manual* of the **AABB** (formerly the American Association of Blood Banks) refers to the act of typing, or determining the ABO of an individual's red cells as a type rather than a group.[5] This textbook adopts the AABB terminology and refers to the determination of an individual's ABO *type (phenotype),* not an ABO *group.* Many other references still retain the terminology of ABO grouping. The FDA name for these reagents remains "ABO grouping reagents."

The first ABO red cell typing reagents were derived from pooled human plasma sources. The polyclonal antibodies were obtained from individuals who were stimulated with A or B blood group substances to produce antibodies of high titer. Today manufacturers use monoclonal antibodies to formulate ABO typing reagents. Reagent manufacturers cite many benefits to the adoption of murine monoclonal reagents, including the recognition of weaker A and B antigens, the removal of contaminating antibodies, cost-effectiveness, and the availability of a reagent source not dependent on human sources.[6]

The murine monoclonal antibody ABO typing reagents are tested to meet FDA potency and specificity requirements before licensure. The antibodies are suspended in a diluent that usually does not exceed a 6% bovine albumin concentration and is considered a low-protein medium. The commercial anti-A and anti-B red cell typing reagents are formulated to demonstrate strong agglutination reactions (3+ to 4+) for most antigen-positive red cells. Testing is performed in **immediate-spin phases.** Manufacturers recommend that testing be confirmed by checking for expected **ABO antibodies** using reagent red cells. Anti-A always contains a blue dye, whereas anti-B contains a yellow dye. These dyes were added to reduce potential errors in testing. A summary of ABO typing reagents is presented in Fig. 2-5.

Technical Manual: publication of the AABB that provides a reference to current acceptable practices in blood banking.

AABB: professional organization that accredits and provides educational and technical guidance to blood banks and transfusion services.

Immediate-spin phases: source antigen and source antibody used in immunohematologic testing are combined, immediately centrifuged, and observed for agglutination.

ABO antibodies: anti-A, anti-B, and anti-A,B; patients possess the ABO antibody to the ABO antigen lacking on their red cells (e.g., group A individuals possess anti-B).

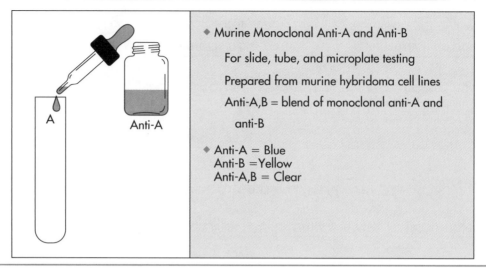

Fig. 2-5 Summary of ABO reagents. Blood banks are using monoclonal antibodies for ABO reagents in routine testing. (Modified from Immucor, Norcross, GA.)

TABLE 2-5	Typing for D Antigen with Patient or Donor Red Cells	
D ANTIGEN	**REACTION WITH ANTI-D**	**REACTION WITH REAGENT CONTROL**
D-positive	+	0
D-negative	0	0
Cannot interpret typing	+	+

+, Agglutination; 0, no agglutination.

ABO typing reagents are labeled with the antibody specificity and a phrase that specifies how the product can be used. For instance, a bottle of anti-A may contain the phrase "for slide, tube, and microplate testing." This statement specifies the test method in which the product may be used according to its FDA licensure. The detailed methods are provided in the product insert, along with the unique characteristics of each product.

REAGENTS FOR D ANTIGEN TYPING

Of the antigens within the Rh blood group system, the D antigen is the most important in routine blood banking. The D antigen has been linked to adverse consequences in patients, including hemolytic transfusion reactions and hemolytic disease of the fetus and newborn (HDFN). Because of its increased immunogenicity as a blood group antigen, D antigen typing of all patient and donor samples is required by the AABB *Standards for Blood Banks and Transfusion Services.*[7] This requirement enables the distinction of D-positive and D-negative individuals.

In the D typing procedure, commercial anti-D is combined with patient or donor red cells. Agglutination indicates the presence of the D antigen on the red cells tested (e.g., D-positive), and no agglutination in these tests indicates absence of the D antigen (e.g., D-negative). A negative reagent control ensures that a **false-positive result** is not present (Table 2-5).

Historically, reagents for D typing have been obtained from various sources. The reagents were divided into two categories: high-protein and low-protein reagents. High-protein reagents of human polyclonal origin were first used for most routine D typing. Low-protein reagents formulated with monoclonal anti-D antibodies or monoclonal and polyclonal antibody blends have replaced these high-protein reagents. Similar to ABO typing reagents, D typing reagents are labeled with the antibody specificity and a phrase that specifies how it can be used. This statement specifies the test method in which the

Standards for Blood Banks and Transfusion Services: publication of the AABB that outlines the minimal standards of practice in areas relating to transfusion medicine.

False-positive result: test result that incorrectly indicates a positive reaction (the presence of agglutination or hemolysis); no antigen-antibody reaction occurred.

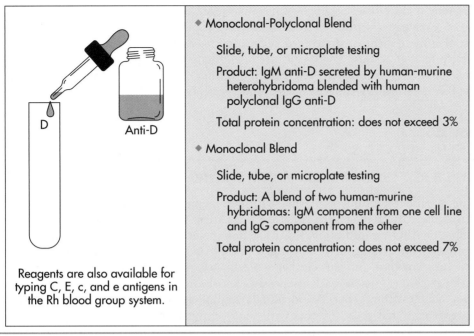

Fig. 2-6 Summary of reagents for D-antigen phenotyping. Blood banks are using monoclonal antibodies or blends of polyclonal and monoclonal antibodies for D reagent in routine testing. (Modified from Immucor, Norcross, GA.)

product may be used according to its FDA licensure. The detailed methods and the unique characteristics of each product are provided in the product insert (Fig. 2-6). In addition to D typing, similar products are available for the phenotyping of other antigens within the Rh blood group system, such as C, E, c, and e.

Monoclonal anti-D reagents possess a low-protein diluent formulation similar in protein concentration to the diluent of the ABO reagents (approximately 6% bovine albumin). Monoclonal anti-D reagents are derived from human-murine heterohybridoma sources, are IgM, and are often formulated with several different clones to ensure reactivity with the D antigen. Some manufacturers blend monoclonal (IgM) and polyclonal antibodies (IgG) to allow the detection of weak D antigen with the same reagent. The low-protein diluent does not promote the false-positive agglutination associated with the use of high-protein D typing reagents. These reagents do not require a separate Rh control test.

Discrepancies in D antigen phenotyping have occurred in patients as a consequence of different monoclonal antibody clone anti-D formulations used in reagent manufacture. Monoclonal antibody formulations for anti-D can vary in the ability to detect partial D antigen and weak D phenotypes. Transfusion service laboratories and blood banks may use different anti-D monoclonal antibody reagents. D typing discrepancies can be observed depending on the commercial source of anti-D. An understanding of the manufacturer's clone formulations and reagent limitations is important in the resolution of these discrepancies.

LOW-PROTEIN REAGENT CONTROL

A reagent control is used to ensure that the typing results were interpreted correctly. The control should show no agglutination (a negative result). The ABO and D typing reagents are formulated with protein concentrations similar to human serum (approximately 6% bovine albumin). At this low-protein concentration, spontaneous agglutination of red cells occurs less frequently than with reagents formulated using higher concentrations of protein. Spontaneous agglutination of red cells can cause a false-positive result in typing. False-positive test results can occur if strong cold **autoantibodies** or protein abnormalities

Autoantibodies: antibodies to self-antigens.

are present in the blood specimen. A negative result using ABO low-protein reagents can serve as a reagent control. An additional reagent control in ABO and D typing is not essential if the patient or donor red cells show no agglutination with anti-A, anti-B, or anti-D in red cell testing. If red cells are agglutinated with anti-A, anti-B, and anti-D, a reagent control is required to interpret the results. The reagent control should be performed as described by the reagent manufacturer (Table 2-6).

SECTION 4
REAGENT RED CELLS

A₁ AND B RED CELLS FOR ABO SERUM TESTING

Testing a patient's serum or plasma with commercial group A_1 and group B red cells confirms the ABO typing performed on the patient's red cells. Known as ABO reverse grouping or ABO serum testing, this procedure detects ABO antibodies. Patients possess the antibody directed against the antigen of the ABO system that is lacking on their red cells. Patients with A antigen on their red cells (e.g., group A) possess the A antigen and lack the B antigen. These patients possess anti-B antibodies in their plasma. Serum or plasma samples from group A individuals agglutinate with reagent B red cells but not with reagent A_1 red cells. Patients with the B antigen on their red cells (e.g., group B) possess the B antigen and lack the A antigen. These patients possess anti-A antibodies in their plasma. Serum or plasma samples from group B individuals agglutinate with reagent A_1 red cells but not with reagent B red cells. Compared with red cell testing with commercial anti-A and anti-B reagents, the ABO antibody results provide an additional confirmation or check of the assigned ABO typing (Table 2-7).

TABLE 2-6	Examples of Low-Protein Reagent Controls in ABO and D Typing			
REACTION WITH ANTI-A	REACTION WITH ANTI-B	REACTION WITH ANTI-D	RED CELL ANTIGENS PRESENT	REAGENT CONTROL PRESENT?
+	0	+	A and D	Yes; no agglutination with anti-B
0	+	0	B	Yes; no agglutination with anti-A
0	+	+	B and D	Yes; no agglutination with anti-A
+	+	0	A and B	Yes; no agglutination with anti-D
+	+	+	Cannot interpret typing	No; reagent control must be tested to determine ABO and D typing results

+, Agglutination; 0, no agglutination.

TABLE 2-7	ABO Serum Testing (Reverse Grouping)		
ABO BLOOD GROUP ANTIGENS	REACTION WITH REAGENT A₁ CELLS	REACTION WITH REAGENT B CELLS	ABO ANTIBODY DEFINED
A	0	+	Anti-B
B	+	0	Anti-A
AB	0	0	No anti-A or anti-B present
O	+	+	Anti-A and anti-B

+, Agglutination; 0, no agglutination.

Reagent red cells for serum testing are obtained from selected human donors and are manufactured in several optional packages. The most commonly used package consists of a two-vial set of A_1 and B red cells. Depending on the manufacturer, the red cell source may be obtained from either a single donor or a pool of several donors.

During the manufacturing process, all reagent red cells are washed to remove blood group antibodies and are resuspended to a 2% to 5% concentration in a buffered preservative solution to minimize hemolysis and loss of antigenicity during the dating period. These red cell preparations are usually negative for the Rh antigens D, C, and E. Each reagent lot is tested to meet the FDA standards of specificity; however, no potency standard requirement exists for this reagent. Reagent red cells should not be used if the red cells darken, spontaneously agglutinate in the reagent vial, or exhibit significant hemolysis.[8]

SCREENING CELLS

Screening cells are used in antibody screen (antibody detection) tests. This procedure looks for antibodies with specificity to red cell antigens in patient and donor samples. Patients and donors may have preformed antibodies to red cell antigens as a result of exposure to foreign red cell antigens from previous transfusions or pregnancies. For transfusion purposes, detection of these preformed red cell antibodies in a patient or donor sample is an important step in the provision of red cell products.

The reagent red cells are obtained from group O donor sources and are commercially available as two-vial or three-vial sets. Group O donors are selected because the group O phenotype lacks A and B antigens, and so these red cells do not react with ABO antibodies present in patient or donor serum or plasma. Serum or plasma from any ABO type may be used in the antibody screen test without interference from the ABO antibodies. Each vial in these sets represents the red cells harvested from a single donor. In addition, a product with pooled screening cells is commercially available and contains group O red cells derived from two donors in equal proportions.

According to the AABB *Standards for Blood Banks and Transfusion Services,* tests for antibodies performed on **recipient** specimens (e.g., specimens of a patient who may be receiving a transfusion) require unpooled screening cells.[7] Recipient testing must maximize sensitivity to detect the presence of weakly reactive antibodies. Because a pooled red cell reagent decreases the ability to detect a weakly reactive antibody, this reagent is not recommended for recipient samples. Pooled screening cells are acceptable in screening donors for red cell antibodies.

Each lot of reagent screening cells arrives with an accompanying antigenic profile, or **antigram,** of each donor (Fig. 2-7). Screening cells licensed by the FDA require an antigenic profile capable of detecting most clinically significant red cell antibodies. Blood group antigens that must be expressed on the screening cells include D, C, E, c, e, M, N, S, s, P_1, Le^a, Le^b, K, k, Fy^a, Fy^b, Jk^a, and Jk^b.[5] Diminished reagent reactivity may be observed as the screening cells approach the end of their dating period. Because of the danger of antigen deterioration, these screening cells should not be used beyond their expiration date.[9] Any signs of significant hemolysis, discoloration, or agglutination might indicate contamination.

Recipient: patient receiving the transfusion.

Antigram: profile of antigen typings of each donor used in the manufacture of commercially supplied screening and panel cells.

Cell		Rh							MNSs				P_1	Lewis		Lutheran		Kell		Duffy		Kidd				
	D	C	E	c	e	f	C^w	M	N	S	s	P_1	Le^a	Le^b	Lu^a	Lu^b	K	k	Fy^a	Fy^b	Jk^a	Jk^b			
I R1R1 (56)	+	+	0	0	+	0	0	+	+	0	+	0	+	0	0	0	+	+	+	0	+	+			
II R2R2 (89)	+	0	+	+	0	0	0	0	+	+	0	+	0	+	0	+	0	+	0	+	+	0			

Fig. 2-7 Example of an antigram for commercial screening cells. The antigram is a profile of antigen typings of each donor used in the screening cells. +, The antigen is present on the screening cell; *0,* the antigen is absent on the screening cell.

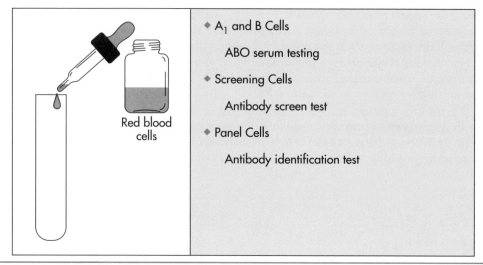

Fig. 2-8   Summary of reagent red cells. (Modified from Immucor, Norcross, GA.)

ANTIBODY IDENTIFICATION PANEL CELLS

Reagent red cell antibody identification panels are required to determine the specificity of a red cell antibody in a blood banking procedure called antibody identification (discussed in Chapter 7). Patient or donor serum is tested with the reagent panel cells to identify an antibody to red cell antigens. These reagent red cells possess the same sources as the screening cells (individual group O donors). Antibody identification panels are packaged in sets of 10 or more, depending on the individual manufacturer. The selected donors for the identification panels possess the majority of the most frequently inherited red cell antigens. An antigenic profile of each donor is provided with each lot number of panel cells. A laboratory often has several in-dated panels to help resolve antibody problems. It is important to use the correct antigram according to the panel lot number when selecting the panel used for antibody identification. Fig. 2-8 summarizes the various types of reagent red cells.

> An antibody identification panel is performed when the antibody screen test is positive.

SECTION 5
ANTIGLOBULIN TEST AND REAGENTS

PRINCIPLES OF ANTIGLOBULIN TEST

In 1945 Coombs, Mourant, and Race[10] showed that red cells may combine with antibodies without producing agglutination. These investigators prepared an antibody that reacted with human globulins (e.g., a family of human proteins) and used this reagent to agglutinate antibody-coated red cells. The reagent was called antihuman globulin (AHG); the procedure is referred to as the antiglobulin test. This test is applied to many blood banking testing protocols and provides important information. The antiglobulin test is important because it detects IgG antibodies and complement proteins that have attached to red cells either in-vitro or in vivo but do not show visible agglutination in testing.

The principle of the antiglobulin test is not complicated. The test uses a reagent that has been prepared by injecting animals (e.g., rabbits) with human antibody molecules (human IgG) and complement proteins. In these animals, the injected proteins are recognized as foreign antigens, stimulating the animal's immune system to produce antibodies to human antibody molecules and complement proteins. The reagent, polyspecific AHG, contains antibodies to IgG molecules (anti-IgG) and complement proteins (anti-C3d, anti-C3b). This AHG reagent reacts with human IgG antibody and complement proteins whether freely present in serum or bound to antigens on the red cells. It is essential that red cells first be washed with physiologic saline to remove any unbound molecules before the addition of the AHG reagent. The washing step of an antiglobulin test requires the filling of test tubes with saline to mix with the red cells already present in the tube. The saline-suspended red cells are centrifuged. The saline wash is decanted from the red cell button, and this process is repeated for two to three additional cycles. On completion of the third or fourth wash, the saline is removed, and the tube is blotted dry to remove most traces of the saline.

Red cell washing is an important technical aspect in the performance of an antiglobulin test. If the test red cells are inadequately washed, any unbound antibody or complement present in serum can potentially bind to the AHG reagent and inhibit its reaction with antibody or complement molecules attached to the red cells. This effect is known as **neutralization** of the AHG reagent. Neutralization of the AHG reagent is a source of error in antiglobulin testing because it can mask a positive antiglobulin test.[5] To detect potential neutralization, IgG-sensitized cells are added to tubes with negative reactions. After centrifugation, a positive reaction should be observed to confirm that washing was adequate.

After adequate red cell washing, the AHG reagent is added to the test. If the red cells in the test are **sensitized** with IgG or complement, the AHG reagent crosslinks and causes agglutination. The anti-IgG in the AHG reagent attaches to the Fc portion of the IgG molecule that is bound to the red cell; the anti-C3 in the AHG reagent attaches to C3 molecules bound to the red cell as the consequence of complement activation. The formation of agglutinated red cells after the addition of AHG shows that IgG or complement proteins were attached to the red cells (Fig. 2-9). Agglutination is interpreted as a positive antiglobulin test. No agglutination at the completion of the antiglobulin test is interpreted as a negative antiglobulin test and indicates that no IgG or complement proteins were attached to the red cells.

Two types of antiglobulin tests are performed in the immunohematology laboratory: **direct antiglobulin test** (DAT) and **indirect antiglobulin test** (IAT). The distinction between these tests is often difficult for individuals entering this field because both tests use the AHG reagents. The DAT is a test in immunohematology to detect antibody bound to red

Neutralization: blocking antibody sites, causing a negative reaction.

Neutralization causes false-negative AHG test results.

Sensitized: immunoglobulin or complement attached to the cells from the immune system (in-vivo) or from a test procedure (in-vitro).

Direct antiglobulin test: test used to detect antibody bound to red cells in-vivo.

Indirect antiglobulin test: test used to detect antibody bound to red cells in-vitro.

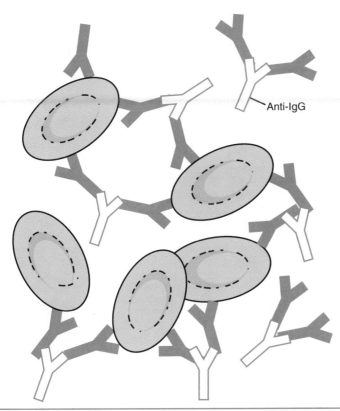

Anti-IgG

Fig. 2-9 Antiglobulin test. The antiglobulin test detects IgG molecules and complement protein molecules that have attached (sensitized) to red cells but have not resulted in a visible agglutination reaction. (Modified from Stroup MT, Treacy M: *Blood group antigens and antibodies*, Raritan, NJ, 1982, Ortho Diagnostic Systems, Inc.)

cells in-vivo or within the body. In contrast, the IAT is used in immunohematology testing to detect antibody bound to red cells in-vitro or within a test tube.

Direct Antiglobulin Test

Under normal circumstances, red cells are not sensitized with either IgG or complement in-vivo. The DAT is ordered to detect IgG or complement proteins bound to patient cells, which is a consequence of certain clinical events, including **autoimmune hemolytic anemia**, HDFN, a drug-related mechanism, or an antibody reaction to transfused red cells. A positive DAT is an important indicator of potential immune-mediated red cell destruction in the body. As a consequence of IgG or complement attachment to red cells, macrophages are signaled to clear them using the mononuclear phagocytic system, particularly in the spleen. This event can signal immune destruction of red cells and often leads to anemia.

In the DAT procedure, the patient's red cells are first washed three or four times with physiologic saline to remove unbound proteins. The AHG reagent is added after the washing process. Agglutination with AHG reagent indicates that IgG antibodies, complement molecules, or both are bound to the patient's red cells. Agglutination after the addition of the AHG reagent is interpreted as a positive DAT (Fig. 2-10). If polyspecific antiglobulin reagent is used, it can detect both IgG and complement molecules on the red cell. If the test result is positive, the test is repeated using **monospecific AHG reagents** that are specific for IgG and complement separately to determine which molecule was on the red cell. No agglutination after the addition of polyspecific AHG reagent is interpreted as a negative DAT. Retesting with monospecific AHG is unnecessary.

As noted earlier, a positive DAT recognizes attached antibody or complement as a result of a clinical process or event (Table 2-8). Incubation is not necessary because the antibody attached in-vivo. The significance of a positive DAT should be assessed in relation to the patient's medical history and clinical condition.

The sample of choice for a DAT is collected in an ethylenediaminetetraacetic acid (EDTA) tube. Because complement can attach nonspecifically to red cells when samples are stored, it is important to use an anticoagulated EDTA sample when performing this test. Because EDTA negates the in-vitro activation of the complement pathway, the test detects only complement proteins that have been bound to the red cells in-vivo.[5] In other words, complement-dependent antibodies will not be detected when plasma is used.

Autoimmune hemolytic anemia: immune destruction of autologous or self–red cells.

Monospecific AHG reagents: reagents prepared by separating the specificities of the polyspecific AHG reagents into individual sources of anti-IgG and anti-C3d/anti-C3b.

TABLE 2-8 Clinical Examples Causing a Positive Direct Antiglobulin Test

CLINICAL CONDITION	CAUSED BY	SOURCE OF IgG
Transfusion reaction	Donor cells coated with IgG	Recipient (patient) antibody
Hemolytic disease of the fetus and newborn	Fetal red cells coated with IgG	Maternal antibody crossing the placenta
Autoimmune hemolytic anemia	IgG or C3 on patient red cells	Patient autoantibody
Drug-related mechanism	IgG-drug complex attached to cells	Immune complex formed with drug

Fig. 2-10 Direct antiglobulin test. **A,** In the DAT, patient red cells are washed to remove unbound immunoglobulins. **B,** AHG reagent, either polyspecific or monospecific, is added. If either IgG or C3d molecules are present on the patient's red cells, agglutination is observed. The patient has a positive DAT result. (Modified from Immucor, Norcross, GA.)

Indirect Antiglobulin Test

The IAT is designed to detect in-vitro sensitization of red cells. This test is a two-stage procedure. Antibodies first must combine with red cell antigens in-vitro through an incubation step. In this first stage, a serum source is incubated at body temperature with a red cell source to allow the attachment of IgG antibodies to specific red cell antigens. The red cell suspension is washed with physiologic saline to remove unbound antibody or complement proteins. After red cell washing, the AHG reagent is added to the test and centrifuged. Any agglutination at this step is interpreted as a positive IAT. A positive IAT indicates a specific reaction between an antibody in the serum and an antigen present on the red cells (Fig. 2-11). No agglutination at this step is interpreted as a negative IAT.

The IAT is routinely used in immunohematology in testing both patient and donor samples. Several immunohematologic tests incorporate an indirect antiglobulin **reaction phase** in their procedures. These procedures include antibody screening, antibody identification, crossmatching, and antigen typing (Table 2-9). All of these procedures are important in the immunohematology laboratory and are discussed in subsequent chapters.

Reaction phase: observation of agglutination at certain temperatures, after incubation, or after addition of AHG.

Table 2-10 compares the DAT and IAT procedures.

SOURCES OF ERROR IN ANTIGLOBULIN TESTING

Sources of error in antiglobulin testing can lead to either false-negative or false-positive results. A **false-negative result** is a test result that incorrectly indicates a negative reaction. In the antiglobulin test, no agglutination is observed, yet the red cells in the test are sensitized with IgG or complement. An Ag-Ab reaction has occurred but is not shown in testing. Conversely, a false-positive result is a test result that incorrectly indicates a

False-negative result: test result that incorrectly indicates a negative reaction (the lack of agglutination); an antigen-antibody reaction has occurred but is not detected.

TABLE 2-9	Applications of Indirect Antiglobulin Test in the Immunohematology Laboratory
PROCEDURE	**PURPOSE**
Antibody screening	Detects antibodies with specificity to red cell antigens
Antibody identification	Identifies specificity of red cell antibodies
Crossmatch	Determines serologic compatibility between donor and patient before transfusion
Antigen typing	Identifies a specific red cell antigen in a patient or donor

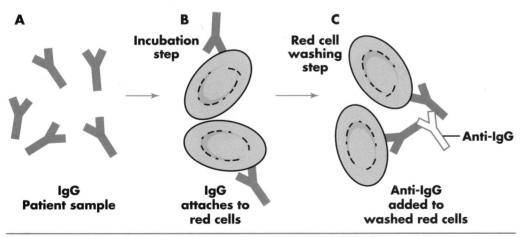

Fig. 2-11 Indirect antiglobulin test. In the IAT, a source of antibody and red cells are incubated at 37° C for a specified time to allow Ag-Ab reactions to occur. Following incubation, the red cells are washed to remove unbound molecules. AHG reagent, monospecific anti-IgG is added. If IgG are present on the red cells, agglutination is observed. The result is a positive IAT. (Modified from Stroup MT, Treacy M: *Blood group antigens and antibodies*, Raritan, NJ, 1982, Ortho Diagnostic Systems, Inc.)

TABLE 2-10	Comparison of Direct Antiglobulin Test and Indirect Antiglobulin Test Procedures
DIRECT ANTIGLOBULIN TEST	INDIRECT ANTIGLOBULIN TEST
Detects IgG- and complement-coated red cells	Detects IgG- and complement-coated red cells
IgG attachment to red cells has occurred within the patient's body	IgG attachment to red cells occurred during the incubation step
One-stage procedure	Two-stage procedure
Patient's red cells are tested with antiglobulin reagent without an incubation step	Test requires an incubation step before the addition of antiglobulin reagent
Test for certain clinical conditions: hemolytic disease of the fetus and newborn, hemolytic transfusion reaction, and autoimmune hemolytic anemia	Used as a reaction phase of several tests in immunohematology

TABLE 2-11	Common Sources of False-Positive Error in Antiglobulin Testing
FALSE-POSITIVE	POSSIBLE EXPLANATIONS
Red cells are agglutinated before washing step and addition of antihuman globulin reagent	Potent cold reactive antibody of patient origin
Use of dirty glassware	Particles or contaminants
Improper centrifugation—overcentrifugation	Red cell button packed so tightly on centrifugation that nonspecific clumping cannot be dispersed

TABLE 2-12	Common Sources of False-Negative Error in Antiglobulin Testing
FALSE-NEGATIVE	POSSIBLE EXPLANATIONS
Failure to wash cells adequately during the test procedure before the addition of AHG reagent	Unbound human serum globulins neutralize AHG reagent
Testing is interrupted or delayed; AHG reagent is not added immediately after washing	Bound IgG or complement molecules may detach from the coated red cells
Failure to identify weak positive reactions	Technical error in testing
Loss of reagent activity	Improper reagent storage, bacterial contamination, or contamination with human serum
Failure to add AHG reagent	Technical error in testing
Improper centrifugation: undercentrifugation	Conditions for promoting agglutination are not optimal
Inappropriate red cell concentrations—red cell suspensions fall outside the optimal 2%-5%	Concentration of red cells influences the reaction

AHG, Antihuman globulin.

positive reaction. In antiglobulin testing, agglutination is observed, but the red cells in the test are not sensitized with IgG or complement. No Ag-Ab reaction has occurred in testing. With careful attention to the test procedures, individuals who perform the AHG tests can avoid many of these false-positive and false-negative results. Common sources of error in antiglobulin testing are summarized in Tables 2-11 and 2-12.[5]

ANTIGLOBULIN REAGENTS

The antiglobulin test is important for the detection of IgG antibodies and complement proteins that have attached to the red cells but have not resulted in visible agglutination.

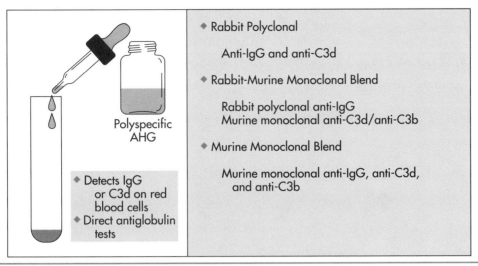

Fig. 2-12 Polyspecific antihuman globulin reagents. (Text from *Code of federal regulations*, 21CFR 660.55, Washington, DC, US Government Printing Office, revised annually. Illustration modified from Immucor, Norcross, GA.)

Two categories of antiglobulin reagents exist: polyspecific and monospecific. The AHG reagents can be either monoclonal antibody products or polyclonal antiserum products.

Polyspecific Antihuman Globulin Reagents

Polyspecific AHG reagents are used primarily in the DAT to determine whether either IgG or complement molecules have attached to the red cells in vivo. This reagent contains both anti-IgG and anti-C3d antibodies and detects both IgG and C3d molecules on red cells. The detection of either molecule implies that red cell Ag-Ab complex formation has clinically occurred. Several reagent preparations are commercially available for polyspecific products derived from either polyclonal or monoclonal antibody sources. Other complement antibodies may also be present, including anti-C3b. All these products meet the FDA requirements for licensure and are outlined in Fig. 2-12.

Monospecific Antihuman Globulin Reagents

Monospecific AHG reagents are used in the investigation of a positive DAT to determine the nature of the molecules attached to the red cells. Are the patient's red cells sensitized with IgG, complement, or both proteins? To answer this question, a **differential DAT** is performed with monospecific AHG reagents using individual sources of anti-IgG and anti-C3d/anti-C3b (Table 2-13). Monospecific AHG reagents are prepared by separating the specificities of the polyspecific AHG reagents.

Anti-IgG monospecific AHG products contain antibodies to human gamma chains. They are commercially available as either polyclonal or monoclonal antibody products. Often these products are labeled heavy-chain specific, meaning that the antiserum contains antibodies specific for the gamma heavy chains of the IgG molecule. Products without this label may contain antibodies that react with immunoglobulin light chains. Recall from the immunology discussion in Chapter 1 that immunoglobulin light chains (kappa and lambda) are common to all immunoglobulin classes (e.g., IgG, IgM, IgA). In addition to their use in the investigation of a positive DAT, anti-IgG reagents are used in many laboratories for antibody detection, antibody identification, and crossmatching procedures. Fig. 2-13 summarizes monospecific anti-IgG products.

Anti-C3b and anti-C3d monospecific reagents contain no reactivity to human immunoglobulin molecules. These reagents specifically detect complement proteins that have been attached to the red cell surface as a result of the activation of complement's classical pathway. Activation of the complement pathway can lead to red cell destruction in vivo through either **intravascular hemolysis** or **extravascular hemolysis**. For the detection of any complement proteins bound in vivo, a product requires specificity for the C3d fragment. This fragment of complement is usually the only protein that remains attached to

Differential DAT: immunohematologic test that uses monospecific anti-IgG and monospecific anti-C3d/anti-C3b reagents to determine the cause of a positive DAT with polyspecific antiglobulin reagents.

Intravascular hemolysis: destruction of red cells and release of hemoglobin within the vascular compartment through immune or nonimmune mechanisms; antibodies of the ABO system can cause this type of hemolysis.

Extravascular hemolysis: removal of red cells from circulation by the phagocytic cells of the reticuloendothelial system (liver and spleen).

TABLE 2-13   Differential Direct Antiglobulin Test Procedure

INTERPRETATION	MONOSPECIFIC ANTI-IgG	MONOSPECIFIC ANTI-C3d
Patient red cells sensitized with IgG only	+	0
Patient red cells sensitized with IgG and C3d	+	+
Patient red cells sensitized with C3d only	0	+

+, Agglutination; *0*, no agglutination.

Fig. 2-13   Monospecific anti-IgG antihuman globulin reagents. (Text from *Code of federal regulations*, 21CFR 660.55, Washington, DC, US Government Printing Office, revised annually. Illustration modified from Immucor, Norcross, GA.)

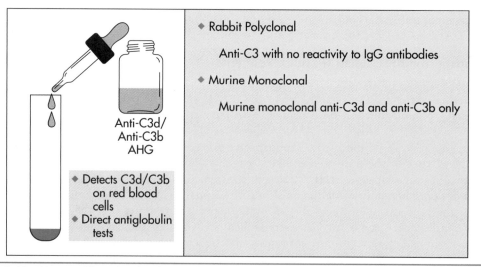

Fig. 2-14   Monospecific anti-C3d and anti-C3b antihuman globulin reagents. (Text from *Code of federal regulations*, 21CFR 660.55, Washington, DC, US Government Printing Office, revised annually. Illustration modified from Immucor, Norcross, GA.)

the patient's red cells. Anti-C3d is commercially available as either polyclonal or monoclonal antibody products (Fig. 2-14).

IgG-Sensitized Red Cells

The AABB *Standards for Blood Banks and Transfusion Services*[7] requires a control system for antiglobulin tests interpreted as negative. The control system consists of red cells that have been commercially prepared with IgG antibodies attached. The addition of

IgG-sensitized red cells to negative AHG tests is required for antibody detection and crossmatch procedures. This control is often referred to as check cells or Coombs control cells. Because antiglobulin testing has its own set of test limitations that might affect interpretation of results, IgG-sensitized red cells were designed as an additive system for negative antiglobulin tests to control the possibility of false-negative results. On addition to a negative AHG test, the IgG-sensitized red cells should react with the AHG reagent and show agglutination.

IgG-sensitized red cells cannot provide assurance that all causes of false-negative results are controlled. Following are three potential reasons for a false-negative result detected by the use of IgG-sensitized red cells in an antiglobulin test:

- Failure to add the antiglobulin reagent to the test
- Failure of the added antiglobulin reagent to react
- Failure to wash red cells adequately

> IgG-sensitized red cells are added to negative AHG tests. Agglutination should be present after the control cells are added.

SECTION 6
PRINCIPLES OF ANTIBODY POTENTIATORS AND LECTINS

As discussed in Chapter 1, the zeta potential, or the force of repulsion between red cells in a physiologic saline solution, exerts an influence on the agglutination reaction. Because of the larger size, pentameteric shape, and multivalent properties of IgM molecules, agglutination is facilitated between adjacent red cells that have IgM attached to them. IgM antibodies can easily react in a saline medium. In contrast, IgG antibody molecules are smaller and less able to span the distance between adjacent red cells generated by the zeta potential. IgG molecules may attach, but visible agglutination might not occur.

Antibody potentiators, or **enhancement media,** are commercially available reagents that enhance the detection of IgG antibodies by increasing their reactivity. Enhancement media can reduce the zeta potential of the red cell membrane by adjusting the in-vitro test environment to promote agglutination. Potentiators are also added to blood bank tests to enhance the detection of Ag-Ab complex formation. In this role, potentiators may enhance antibody uptake (first stage of agglutination), promote direct agglutination (second stage of agglutination), or serve both functions. The major types of potentiators used in the blood bank laboratory include antiglobulin reagents, low-ionic-strength saline (LISS), polyethylene glycol (PEG), and **proteolytic enzymes** (ficin and papain). These reagents are summarized in Table 2-14.

Antibody potentiators: reagents or methods that enhance or speed up the antibody-antigen reaction.

Enhancement media: reagents that enhance or speed up the antibody-antigen reaction.

Proteolytic enzymes: enzymes that denature certain proteins.

LOW-IONIC-STRENGTH SALINE (LISS)

The incubation of serum and red cells in a reduced ionic environment increases the rate of antibody binding to specific antigen receptor sites on red cells.[11] In physiologic saline, sodium and chloride ions cluster around the antigen and antibody molecules. Ag-Ab complex formation is influenced by the attraction of opposite charges, and the clustering of these free sodium and chloride ions hinders the complex formation. When the ionic

TABLE 2-14	Summary of Antibody Potentiators
POTENTIATOR	**MECHANISM OF ACTION**
Antiglobulin reagents	Cross-linking of IgG-sensitized red cells
LISS	Increases rate of antibody uptake
PEG	Concentrates the antibody in the test environment in LISS
Proteolytic enzymes (papain and ficin)	Removes negative charges from the red cell membrane, which reduces the zeta potential; denatures some red cell antigens

LISS, Low-ionic-strength saline; *PEG,* polyethylene glycol.

strength is reduced, the antigen and antibody molecules are capable of combining at a faster rate.[12] In 1974, Löw and Messeter[13] applied this principle in routine testing to detect unknown red cell antibodies by using LISS as the suspending medium for red cells (the source of known antigens in the test). Other investigators confirmed that LISS enhanced antibody reactions, especially in the indirect antiglobulin phases of testing.[14]

The low-ionic environment can be accomplished in two ways:

- Suspending red cells of the test in LISS reagent
- Using additive LISS reagent in conjunction with saline-suspended red cells

The LISS reagent contains sodium chloride, glycine, and salt-poor albumin (approximately 0.03 M) ionic strength compared with saline (approximately 0.17 M) and is formulated to prevent hemolysis of red cells, which is a concern when using LISS.[15] In addition, some low-ionic–saline solution reagents may contain macromolecular additives to potentiate the direct agglutination of antigen-positive red cells by some antibodies. The reagent supplies a low-ionic environment to enhance antibody uptake and improve detection at antiglobulin phases of testing. The final result is sensitization or the potentiation of the first stage in the agglutination reaction. The advantage of the increased antibody uptake is the reduction of incubation time and time to a final result.

POLYETHYLENE GLYCOL

Polyethylene glycol (PEG) additive in a low-ionic–saline medium effectively concentrates antibody in the test mixture, while creating a low-ionic environment that enhances the rate of antibody uptake. The enhancement medium is a water-soluble polymer, which has been reported to increase the sensitivity of the IAT.[16] The PEG reagent removes water molecules in the test environment to allow a greater probability of collision between antigen and antibody molecules.[17] Because PEG can directly affect the aggregation of red cells, the reagent can be used only in indirect antiglobulin testing. Tubes should not be centrifuged and read prior to washing. Only monospecific anti-IgG AHG reagent is suitable for use with PEG because of reports of nonspecific agglutination with polyspecific AHG reagents.

> LISS and PEG enhance reactivity of antibodies and reduce incubation time.

ENZYMES

Proteolytic enzymes commonly used in the immunohematology laboratory include papain, ficin, and bromelin, all of which are commercially available. The term proteolytic refers to the breakdown of protein molecules. These enzymes possess the property to modify red cell membranes by removing the negatively charged molecules from the red cell membrane and denaturing certain antigenic determinants. The loss of these negatively charged molecules reduces the zeta potential and enhances the agglutination of some antigens to their corresponding antibodies. If the antibody specificity is in the Rh, Kidd, and Lewis blood group systems, there is an enhanced reaction using enzymes. Certain other red cell antigens are denatured when exposed to these proteolytic enzymes. These red cell antigens include M, N, S, Xg^a, Fy^a, and Fy^b. Depending on the red cell antibody, the use of enzymes in testing may enhance, depress, or inhibit entirely the Ag-Ab complex formation. A good knowledge of the blood group systems aids in the interpretation of these enzyme tests.

> Proteolytic enzymes are not used routinely in testing. They are a tool that can be useful to solve complex antibody identification problems.

BOVINE SERUM ALBUMIN

Bovine serum albumin (BSA) is prepared from bovine serum or plasma and is commercially available in either a 22% or a 30% concentration. This reagent is less commonly used than other enhancement media. In contrast to LISS, albumin does not promote the antibody uptake stage of agglutination, but it influences the second stage by allowing antibody-sensitized cells to become closer together than is possible in a saline medium without additives. The addition of BSA to reaction tubes favors the direct agglutination of Rh antibodies and enhances the sensitivity of the IAT for a wide range of antibody specificities.

TABLE 2-15	Summary of Common Lectins in the Blood Bank
LECTIN	**ANTIGEN SPECIFICITY**
Dolichos biflorus	A_1
Ulex europaeus	H
Vicia graminea	N
Iberis amara	M

Various hypotheses have been proposed to explain the enhancement properties of BSA. Pollack et al[18] suggested that albumin reduces the zeta potential by dispersing some of the positively charged ions surrounding each negatively charged red cell. In this theory, albumin increases the dielectric constant of the medium, defined as a measure of the ability to dissipate a charge. Other investigators believe that albumin bound to the cell membrane affects the degree of water hydration of the red cell membrane itself.[19]

LECTINS

Lectins are useful alternatives to antisera for blood typing purposes in blood group serology. Some extracts of seeds known as lectins have specificity toward certain red cell antigens. These extracts contain proteins that behave in a manner identical to that of antibodies but are not immunoglobulin in nature. Lectins bind specifically to the carbohydrate determinants of certain red cell antigens with resultant agglutination. Although no antibodies exist in these reagents, lectins can be useful in identifying antigens present on patient or donor red cells. Table 2-15 reviews the major lectins used in blood group serology.

Lectins: plant extracts useful as blood banking reagents; they bind to carbohydrate portions of certain red cell antigens and agglutinate the red cells.

SECTION 7
OTHER METHODS OF DETECTING ANTIGEN-ANTIBODY REACTIONS

Blood bank reagents have been used in testing designed to detect agglutination in test tubes. Other commercially available methods for detecting Ag-Ab reactions use different techniques for detection of agglutination. This section presents a brief overview of these techniques.

GEL TECHNOLOGY METHOD

The FDA licensed gel technology by Micro Typing Systems, Inc. (Pompano Beach, Florida) as the ID-MTS Gel Card in 1994. Developed by Lapierre et al[20] in 1985, the technology uses dextran acrylamide gel particles to trap agglutinated red cells. Lapierre et al developed gel technology to standardize traditional tube testing methods. Tube-shaking techniques to resuspend the red cell button in tube testing vary among technologists. This technical variation affects the grading and interpretation of the test results. Gel technology provides stable and defined endpoints of hemagglutination, providing a method where objective and consistent interpretations of agglutination are possible.

In the gel test, the gel particles combined with diluent or reagents are predispensed into specially designed microtubes manufactured in plastic cards. The gel card is approximately the size of a credit card and contains six microtubes. Each microtube consists of an upper reaction chamber and a section that contains predispensed gel and reagents. The gel acts as the medium to separate agglutinated red cells from unagglutinated red cells. A foil strip is present on the top of the gel card to prevent spillage or drying of microtube contents. The six-microtube configuration of the gel card allows for possible sample batch testing (i.e., more than one patient sample can be tested in one gel card).

The gel test is a hemagglutination reaction. The red cells migrate through the gel matrix to separate agglutinated from unagglutinated red cells.

Because this technology is suitable for automation, blood bank instrumentation is available for the performance of gel testing.

Two major categories of gel cards are licensed for blood bank testing. Specific reagent antibody is incorporated into the gel.

- Phenotyping cards for ABO and D typing and other Rh antigens (C, c, E, e)
- AHG cards (anti-IgG and anti-IgG, -C3d) for IAT (antibody screen, antibody identification, and compatibility testing) and DAT

To perform a gel test, measured volumes of red cells and plasma/serum are added to the reaction chamber of the microtube. The reaction chamber allows red cell sensitization to occur during the incubation of an IAT. The centrifugation step allows time for contacts of red cells with antisera and gel particles. Centrifugation also separates positive and negative agglutination results. In positive reactions, agglutinated red cells are trapped in the gel at various levels, depending on the agglutination strength and size of the agglutinates. In negative reactions, unagglutinated red cells pass through the gel and form a button on the bottom of the microtube.[21]

Gel technology is applied in antibody screening as follows:
1. Add 50 μL of 0.8% suspension of reagent screening cells to the microtubes of the anti-IgG gel cards.
2. Add 25 μL of patient serum or plasma to the microtubes.
3. Incubate the gel card at 37° C for a predetermined time and centrifuge.
4. After centrifugation, the test results are read and graded. No washing step is required for antiglobulin testing. No IgG-sensitized red cells are required.

Larger agglutinates are trapped at the top of the gel microtubes and do not travel through the gel during the centrifugation process. Smaller agglutinates travel through the gel microtubes and may be trapped in either the top or the bottom half of the microtubes. Unagglutinated screening cells travel unimpeded through the length of the microtube and form a red cell button at the bottom after centrifugation (Fig. 2-15).

MICROPLATE TESTING METHODS

Microplate techniques apply the same principle of hemagglutination as the tube test.

Since the late 1960s, microplate methods have been used for routine processing in blood donor centers. A microtiter plate with 96 wells serves as the substituted test tubes to which the principles of blood banking are applied. Each well is considered a short test tube. The microplate technique can be adapted to red cell antigen testing or serum testing for antibody detection. The principles that apply to agglutination in test tubes also apply to testing in microplate methods. The microplate may have either a U-shaped or a V-shaped bottom in the microtiter plate well; the U-bottom well is more widely used. Small quantities of red cells and antisera are added to the microtiter wells, followed by centrifugation of the microtiter plates. The cell buttons are resuspended by manually tapping the plate or with the aid of a mechanical shaker. A concentrated button of red cells is indicative of Ag-Ab reactions, whereas the red cells in a negative result are dispersed throughout the well (Fig. 2-16). Automated photometric devices are available to read and interpret the reactions on the plates. Alternatively, the microtiter plates may be observed for a streaming pattern of red cells when the plate is placed on an angle.[5]

The microplate test method for red cell phenotype is performed as follows[5]:
1. 1 drop of anti-A and 1 drop of anti-B are placed in separate wells of a U-bottom microplate.
2. 1 drop of a 2% to 5% saline suspension of red cells is added to each well.
3. Wells are mixed by gently tapping them.
4. The plate is centrifuged at an appropriate time and speed
5. The cell button is resuspended by manually tapping the plate or using a mechanical shaker, or placed at an angle for the tilt and stream method.
6. Reactions are read, interpreted, and recorded.

Agglutination or hemolysis in any well is a concentrated button of red cells and is interpreted as a positive result. A smooth suspension of red cells after resuspension of the cell button or a streaming pattern of red cells when the plate is placed on an angle is interpreted as no agglutination and a negative test result (Fig. 2-17).

1. Add test reactants
   • Add 50 μL of the 0.8% red cell suspension of screening cells I and II to each microtube.
   • Add 25 μL of the test serum or plasma to each microtube that contains screening cells.

Anti-IgG

2. Incubation step
   • Incubate gel card at 37°C for 15 minutes.

3. Reaction step
   • Centrifuge gel card for 10 minutes.

4. Results
   • Observe and grade reactions in gel card.
   • Record test interpretation: positive antibody screen or negative antibody screen

0 0 4⁺ 0 0 0

A

| 0 | 1+ | 2+ | 3+ | 4+ | MF |

Range of Reactions

B

Fig. 2-15 Gel testing. **A,** Gel Test Antibody Screen (IAT). 0.8% suspensions of screening cells and patient serum or plasma are added to the microtubes of MTS Anti-IgG Card. The gel card is incubated for 15 minutes at 37° C. The gel card is centrifuged. After centrifugation, the gel card is observed for agglutination reactions. **B,** Range of reactions in gel testing. The agglutination reaction is graded from 4+ to 0. The assigned grade is dependent on the position of the red cells in the gel microtube. (**A,** Modified from Immucor, Norcross, GA. **B,** Courtesy Ortho-Clinical Diagnostics, Raritan, New Jersey; and Micro Typing Systems, Pompano Beach, Florida.)

Fig. 2-16 Microtiter plate method. Microtiter plate wells are used to add reagents and samples for hemagglutination tests. (Courtesy Thermo Fisher Scientific, Rochester, NY.)

REACTIONS OF MICROPLATE TESTING

Negative reaction wells   **Positive reaction well**

Positive Reaction:	A concentrated button of red blood cells
Negative Reaction:	Smooth suspension of red blood cells or a streaming pattern of red blood cells when the plate is placed on an angle

Fig. 2-17   Positive and negative reactions in microplate wells. A concentrated button of red cells is a positive reaction. Red cells are dispersed throughout the well in a negative reaction.

SOLID-PHASE RED CELL ADHERENCE METHODS

Another serologic method used in the blood bank is solid-phase red cell adherence.[22] Commercial solid-phase test procedures have been available for the detection of both red cell and platelet antibodies since the late 1980s (Capture; Immucor, Norcross, Georgia). This technology uses microplate test wells with immobilized reagent red cells. Solid-phase technology is currently licensed for antibody screening, antibody identification, and compatibility testing. As previously identified with gel technology, the major advantages of solid-phase technology include standardization and stable, defined endpoints, leading to more objective and consistent interpretations of agglutination reactions. This technology is also suitable for automation, and blood bank instrumentation is available.

The antigen or antibody is immobilized to the bottom and sides of the microplate wells. In a direct test, the antibody is fixed to the wells. Antigen-positive red cells from donor or patient sources adhere to the sides and bottom of the wells. Antigen-negative red cells from donor or patient sources settle to the bottom of the well and form a red cell button after centrifugation. In an indirect test, red cell membranes are bound to the wells. Unknown patient or donor serum is added and allowed to react. This step allows for the capture of IgG antibodies from the patient or donor serum to the red cell membranes. A washing step removes unbound IgG antibodies and is followed by the addition of anti-IgG–coated indicator red cells. In a positive indirect test, the indicator cells adhere to the sides and bottom of the well. In a negative indirect test, the indicator cells settle to the bottom of the wells and form a red cell button after centrifugation.[23]

The procedure for the red cell antibody detection test is as follows:
1. Polystyrene microplates are purchased with red cell membranes such as screening cells bound to the surface of the wells.
2. Patient or donor serum and low-ionic-strength saline are added to these wells.
3. The microplate is incubated 37° C for a predetermined time.
4. The microplate is washed to remove unbound antibodies.
5. Indicator cells (anti-IgG–coated red cells) are added to the wells.
6. The microplate is centrifuged.
7. The test results are read and interpreted.

A negative agglutination reaction appears as a red cell button on the bottom of the wells. A positive agglutination reaction is indicated by attachment of indicator cells to the sides and bottom of the wells. Weak agglutination reactions give intermediate results. The red cells are said to have adhered to the wells (Fig. 2-18).

Microplate techniques apply the same principle of hemagglutination as the tube test. In contrast, solid-phase technology reactions are opposite. A positive reaction is adherence to the wells; a negative reaction is a red cell button.

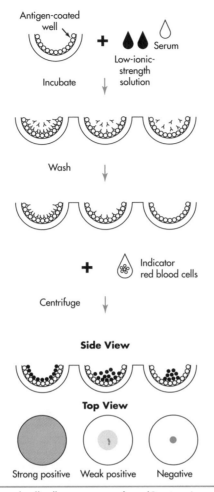

Fig. 2-18 Solid-phase red cell adherence procedure. (Courtesy Immucor, Norcross, Georgia.)

CHAPTER SUMMARY

- The reagents used in the immunohematology laboratory provide the tools to detect Ag-Ab reactions.
- Principles of routine testing are based on the combination of a source of antigen and a source of antibody in a test environment.
- Sources of antigen and antibody are derived from commercially available reagents and patient or donor samples.
- Agglutination or hemolysis is indicative of Ag-Ab recognition.
- The purposes of reagents used in the immunohematology laboratory are to:
    a. Determine the ABO/Rh-type of donors and patients
    b. Detect antibodies produced by patients or donors who have been exposed to red cells through transfusion or pregnancy
    c. Identify the specificity of antibodies detected in the antibody screen procedure
    d. Determine the presence or absence of additional antigens on the red cells in addition to the A, B, and D antigens
    e. Perform crossmatches to evaluate serologic compatibility of donor and patient before transfusion
- Potency in blood banking reagents refers to the strength of an Ag-Ab reaction. Specificity in blood banking reagents refers to recognition of antigen and antibody to make the Ag-Ab reaction.
- Polyclonal antibodies are made from several different clones of B cells that secrete antibodies of different specificities. Monoclonal antibodies are made from a single clone of B cells that secrete antibodies of the same specificity.

- Reagents for ABO typing are derived from monoclonal antibody sources and may be blended to create reagents that recognize the corresponding A or B antigen. These reagents contain IgM antibodies in a low-protein environment.
- Reagents for D typing are derived from monoclonal antibody sources and may be monoclonal antibody blends or monoclonal-polyclonal antibody blends. The reagents can contain either IgM or IgG antibodies in a low-protein environment.
- The low-protein control reagent checks for the presence of spontaneous agglutination of patient or donor red cells in testing. The control should always show no agglutination.
- Reagent red cells are used as sources of antigen in antibody screens, ABO reverse grouping, and antibody identification tests.
- The antiglobulin test detects IgG molecules and complement protein molecules that have attached (sensitized) to red cells but have not resulted in a visible agglutination reaction.
- The DAT detects antibody or complement molecules that have sensitized red cells as a result of a clinical event within the body.
- The IAT requires an incubation step for sensitization and is an in-vitro test. The IAT is commonly used in antibody screens, antibody identification, and testing of donor and recipient compatibility.
- The AHG test can possess sources of error that cause false-positive or false-negative AHG test results. Recognition and prevention of these sources of error aid the correct interpretation of the AHG test result.
- Polyspecific AHG reagents are used primarily in direct antiglobulin testing to determine whether IgG or complement molecules have attached to the red cells in vivo. This reagent contains both anti-IgG and anti-C3d antibodies and detects both IgG and C3d molecules on red cells.
- Monospecific AHG reagents are used in the investigation of a positive DAT to determine the nature of the molecules attached to the red cells. Monospecific AHG reagents are prepared by separating the specificities of the polyspecific AHG reagents into individual sources of anti-IgG and anti-C3d/anti-C3b.
- Antibody potentiators, or enhancement media, are commercially available reagents that enhance the detection of IgG antibodies by increasing their reactivity. Examples of enhancement media include AHG reagents, LISS, PEG, and enzymes.
- Enhancement media can reduce the zeta potential of the red cell membrane by adjusting the in-vitro test environment to promote agglutination.
- Enhancement media are added to improve the detection of Ag-Ab complex formation. In this role, potentiators may enhance antibody uptake (first stage of agglutination), promote direct agglutination (second stage of agglutination), or serve both functions.
- Lectins are plant extracts that bind to carbohydrate portions of certain red cell antigens and agglutinate the red cells. Although no antibodies exist in these reagents, lectins can be useful in identifying antigens present on patient or donor red cells.
- Gel technology uses gel particles combined with diluent or reagents to trap agglutination reactions within the gel matrix.
- Microplate techniques use a microtiter plate with 96 wells to serve as the substituted test tubes. The microplate technique can be adapted to red cell antigen testing or serum testing for antibody detection. The principles that apply to agglutination in test tubes also apply to testing in microplate methods.
- In solid-phase red cell adherence testing, the antigen or antibody is immobilized to the bottom and sides of the microplate wells. IgG antibodies or red cell antigens adhere to the microplate wells if an Ag-Ab reaction is observed.
- An awareness of the proper use and limitations of reagents enhances the ability of laboratory personnel to provide accurate interpretations of results generated in testing and ultimately affects overall transfusion safety.

CRITICAL THINKING EXERCISES

EXERCISE 2-1

The quality control procedure for commercial anti-A and anti-B reagents is performed using A_1 and B reagent red cells. The results of the daily quality control for ABO reagents for your facility are presented in the following chart. Do the quality control results meet acceptable performance criteria, or are they unacceptable for the commercial ABO typing reagents? Discuss your answer.

ABO Typing Reagent	Reactions with Reagent Red Cells	
	A_1 Cells	B Cells
Anti-A	4+	0
Anti-B	0	4+

EXERCISE 2-2

The results of anti-D reagent quality control for the past week are presented in the following chart. What are the implications of these results regarding reagent potency and specificity?

	Anti-D Quality Control	
	Reactions of Anti-D Reagent with D-Positive and D-Negative Red Cells	
Days	D-Positive	D-Negative
1	3+	0
2	3+	0
3	2+	0
4	2+	0
5	1+	0

EXERCISE 2-3

Using several product inserts as resources, what are the visible signs of possible reagent deterioration in both reagent red cells and antisera as outlined by the manufacturers?

EXERCISE 2-4

Using a product insert for a commercial source of antisera, identify the product limitations as described by the manufacturer.

EXERCISE 2-5

Read a reagent quality control procedure from a transfusion service and identify the criteria for acceptable performance for each reagent.

EXERCISE 2-6

The saline in an automated red cell washer did not fill the test tubes consistently when the instrument was evaluated during a routine quality control check. Would this situation affect the results of the AHG test? How would this problem be detected in testing?

EXERCISE 2-7

You have added IgG-sensitized red cells to the negative indirect antiglobulin test result of the antibody screen procedure. You observe agglutination in the tube. Is the antibody screen interpretation positive or negative? Explain your answer.

EXERCISE 2-8

A donor unit obtained from Central Blood Bank was labeled group O, D-positive. When the hospital transfusion service confirmed the donor unit's typing, the result was group O, D-negative. Investigation of the label issued at the blood bank was performed and the label was verified to be correct. How can you explain the discrepancy in the D typing of this donor unit?

STUDY QUESTIONS

1. What is the purpose of including a reagent control when interpreting group AB, D-positive red cells after testing with a low-protein anti-D reagent?
   a. to detect false-positive agglutination reactions
   b. to detect false-negative agglutination reactions
   c. to identify a mix up with patient's sample
   d. to confirm ABO typing results

2. Monospecific AHG reagents:
   a. increase the dielectric constant in-vitro
   b. contain either anti-IgG or anti-C3d antibody specificities
   c. are not useful in identifying the molecule causing a positive DAT
   d. contain human IgG or complement molecules

3. You have added IgG-sensitized red cells to a negative indirect antiglobulin test. You observe agglutination in the tube. What situation was *not* controlled for in testing by adding these control cells?
   a. the addition of patient serum
   b. the addition of AHG reagent
   c. adequate washing of cell suspension
   d. adequate potency of AHG reagent

4. Part of the daily quality control in the blood bank laboratory is the testing of reagent antisera with corresponding antigen-positive and antigen-negative red cells. What does this procedure ensure?
   a. antibody class
   b. antibody titer
   c. antibody specificity
   d. antibody sensitivity

5. Group O red cells are used as a source for commercial screening cells because:
   a. anti-A is detected using group O cells
   b. anti-D reacts with most group O cells
   c. weak subgroups of A react with group O cells
   d. ABO antibodies do not react with group O cells

6. Information regarding reagent limitations is located in the:
   a. SOPs
   b. blood bank computer system
   c. product inserts
   d. product catalogs

7. What regulatory agency provides licensure for blood banking reagents?
   a. AABB
   b. FDA
   c. American Red Cross
   d. College of American Pathologists

8. What antibodies are present in polyspecific AHG reagent?
   a. anti-IgG
   b. anti-IgM and anti-IgG
   c. anti-IgG and anti-C3d
   d. anti-C3d

9. In which source are the regulations regarding the manufacturing of blood banking reagents published?
   a. *Code of Federal Regulations*
   b. *AABB Standards for Blood Banks and Transfusion Services*
   c. *AABB Technical Manual*
   d. *AABB Accreditation Requirements Manual*

10. After the addition of anti-D reagent to a patient's red cell suspension, agglutination was observed. The result with anti-A reagent was negative. What is the interpretation of this patient's D typing?
    a. patient is D-negative
    b. patient is D-positive
    c. cannot interpret the test
    d. invalid result

11. What reagent would be selected to detect the presence of unexpected red cell antibodies in a patient's serum sample?
    a. A_1 and B cells
    b. panel cells
    c. IgG-sensitized cells
    d. screening cells

12. Select the method that uses the principle of sieving to separate larger agglutinates from smaller agglutinates in Ag-Ab reactions.
    a. gel technology
    b. solid-phase adherence
    c. microplate
    d. none of the above

13. To determine the specificity of a red cell antigen in a patient sample, what source of antibody is selected?
    a. commercial reagent red cells
    b. commercial antisera
    c. patient serum
    d. patient plasma

14. To determine the presence of a red cell antibody in a patient sample, what source of antigen is selected?
    a. commercial reagent red cells
    b. commercial antisera
    c. patient serum
    d. patient's red cells

15. What reagents are derived from plant extracts?
    a. panel cells
    b. commercial anti-B
    c. lectins
    d. antiglobulin reagents

REFERENCES

1. Food and Drug Administration: *Code of federal regulations*, 21 CFR 211-800, Washington, DC, US Government Printing Office, revised annually.
2. Sazama K: *Accreditation requirements manual*, ed 6, Bethesda, Md, 1995, AABB.
3. Lomas-Francis C: *The potential of monoclonal antibodies to Rh, MNS, and other blood group antigens: the compendium*, Arlington, Va, 1997, AABB.
4. Walker PS: *Using FDA-approved monoclonal reagents: the compendium*, Arlington, Va, 1997, AABB.
5. Roback JD: *Technical manual*, ed 17, Bethesda, Md, 2011, AABB.
6. Beck ML, Kirkegaard JR: Annotation-monoclonal ABO blood grouping reagents: a decade later, *Immunohematology* 11:67, 1995.
7. Carson TH, editor: *Standards for blood banks and transfusion services*, ed 27, Bethesda, Md, 2011, AABB.
8. *Reagent red cells (pooled cells) Affirmagen, Product Insert (rev)*, Raritan, NJ, 2000, Ortho-Clinical Diagnostics.
9. *Reagent red cells Selectogen, Product Insert (rev)*, Raritan, NJ, 2004, Ortho-Clinical Diagnostics.
10. Coombs RRA, Mourant AE, Race RR: A new test for the detection of weak and "incomplete" Rh agglutinins, *Br J Exp Pathol* 26:255, 1945.
11. Hughes-Jones NC, Polley MJ, Telford R: Optimal conditions for detecting blood group antibodies by the antiglobulin test, *Vox Sang* 9:385, 1964.
12. Elliot M, Bossom E, Dupuy ME, et al: Effect of ionic strength on the serologic behavior of red cell isoantibodies, *Vox Sang* 9:396, 1964.
13. Löw B, Messeter L: Antiglobulin test in low ionic strength salt solution for rapid antibody screening and crossmatching, *Vox Sang* 26:53, 1974.
14. Wicker B, Wallas CH: A comparison of a low ionic strength saline medium with routine methods for antibody detection, *Transfusion* 16:469, 1976.
15. Harmening D: *Modern blood banking and transfusion practices*, ed 5, Philadelphia, 2005, FA Davis.
16. Nance SJ, Garratty G: A new potentiator of red cell antigen-antibody reactions, *Am J Clin Pathol* 87:633, 1987.
17. de Man AJ, Overbeeke MA: Evaluation of the polyethylene glycol antiglobulin test for detection of red cell antibodies, *Vox Sang* 58:207, 1990.
18. Pollack W, Hager HJ, Reckel R, et al: A study of forces involved in the second stage of hemagglutination, *Transfusion* 5:158, 1965.
19. Steane EA: Red cell agglutination: a current perspective. In Bell CA, editor: *Seminar on antigen-antibody reactions revisited*, Arlington, Va, 1982, AABB.

20. Lapierre Y, Rigal D, Adam J, et al: The gel test: a new way to detect red cell antigen-antibody reactions, *Transfusion* 30:109, 1990.
21. *ID-Microtyping System interpretation guide*, Raritan, NJ, 2004, Ortho-Clinical Diagnostics.
22. Plapp FV, Rachel JM, Beck ML, et al: Blood antigens and antibodies: solid phase adherence assays, *Lab Med* 22:39, 1984.
23. *Ortho W.I.R.E.* www.ortho-wire.com. Accessed May 18, 2011.

Genetic Principles in Blood Banking

3

CHAPTER OUTLINE

LEARNING OBJECTIVES

On completion of this chapter, the reader should be able to:

1. Define the term blood group system with regard to serologic and genetic classifications.
2. Distinguish the term phenotype from genotype using the ABO system as an example.
3. Using a Punnett square, illustrate the potential offspring from group A and group B parents.
4. Contrast the terms allele and antithetical with regard to genes and antigens.
5. Predict the potential phenotypes of the offspring of a trait with an X-linked inheritance pattern.
6. Illustrate the genetic and serologic characteristics of the terms homozygous and heterozygous and dosage using the M and N blood group antigens.
7. Draw a diagram to illustrate the difference between *cis* and *trans* and their effect on gene interactions.
8. Apply the terms codominant, recessive, and dominant to the possible inheritance patterns in the ABO blood group system.
9. Calculate the probability of finding compatible red blood cell (RBC) units for a recipient with multiple antibodies.
10. Apply the Hardy-Weinberg law to calculate the percentage of homozygous and heterozygous expressions in a select population given the frequency of a certain phenotype.
11. Evaluate examples of paternity results to determine if direct or indirect exclusions are present.
12. Demonstrate the principles of Mendelian laws of independent assortment and independent segregation by describing how they apply to blood group antigen inheritance.
13. Evaluate the results of a family study to predict the potential phenotype of untested family members.
14. List the applications of molecular testing methods to the field of blood banking.
15. Compare and contrast molecular techniques used to identify HLA antigens: SSP, SSOP, and SBT.
16. Describe the theory of STR testing and its application to hematopoietic progenitor cell engraftment evaluations.
17. Outline the principle of molecular techniques used to identify red cell antigens and the applications to patient care.

The concept of an antigen as a molecule that can elicit an immune response was introduced in Chapter 1. In the study of immunohematology, the antigens of interest are part of the red cell membranes. These antigens are inherited characteristics or traits categorized into **blood group systems** based on their genetic and serologic properties. Similarly, human leukocyte antigens (HLAs) are defined and named based on serologic and genetic information.

Blood group systems: groups of antigens on the red cell membrane that share related serologic properties and genetic patterns of inheritance.

The study of blood group systems requires an understanding of certain genetic principles and terminology. The characteristics that make each blood group system unique are the structure and location of the antigens present on the red cells, the antibodies they elicit, and the genetic control of antigen expression. Because these properties can be shown by serologic and molecular methods, each blood group system is said to be serologically and genetically defined. Classification of some blood group systems has been modified because of enhanced knowledge regarding the molecular structure of the genes producing the antigens.[1]

In subsequent chapters describing the blood group systems, the reader is introduced to the specific genetic pathways that create each antigen. In some systems, such as the Rh blood group system, the gene directly encodes a protein on the red cell, which is recognized by the immune system as an Rh antigen. With other blood group systems, several interacting genes encode a particular antigen on the red cell. For example, expression of the ABO antigens requires the interaction of the *ABO, Hh,* and *Se* genes. Appreciating that each blood group system is the product of a gene or a group of genes assists in their classification and further enhances the understanding of their related serologic properties.

The following section reviews molecular genetics as it applies to the field of immunohematology. Molecular genetics has enhanced the understanding of the molecular basis of blood group antigens, provided more sensitive methods for viral antigen testing in donors, and contributed to more accurate methods for "relationship testing" (previously called paternity tests). Methods for the detection of viral nuclear material by nucleic amplification tests for viral markers in donors have reduced the exposure window for hepatitis C virus and human immunodeficiency virus (HIV). The antigens in the HLA system, described in Chapter 1, are also more accurately identified by molecular methods that are outlined in this chapter.

SECTION 1
BLOOD GROUP GENETICS

GENETIC TERMINOLOGY

Gene: segment of DNA that encodes a particular protein.

Chromosomes: structures within the nucleus that contain DNA.

Mitosis: cell division in somatic cells that results in the same number of chromosomes.

Meiosis: cell division in gametes that results in half the number of chromosomes present in somatic cells.

A **gene** is a unit of inheritance that encodes a particular protein and is the basic unit for inheritance of a trait. Genetic information is carried on double strands of DNA known as **chromosomes** (Fig. 3-1). Humans have 23 pairs of chromosomes: 22 pairs of autosomes and 1 pair of sex chromosomes.

Cell division allows the genetic material in cells to be replicated so that identical chromosomes can be transmitted to the daughter cells. This cell division occurs through a process called **mitosis** in somatic cells and through **meiosis** in gametes.

Before knowledge of genes and DNA was established, the inheritance patterns of certain detectable traits were observed, and theories of inheritance were established. These theories are applicable to the study of blood group genetics. In this section, genetic terms are described as they pertain to red cell antigen inheritance patterns and as products of specific genes.

Cell   Nucleus   Chromosome   DNA   Gene ⟶ Protein

Fig. 3-1   Chromosomes. Chromosomes are found in the cell nucleus and contain double-stranded DNA that have specific areas called genes that code for proteins.

Phenotype versus Genotype

Serologic testing determines the presence or absence of antigens on the red cells. The **phenotype,** or the physical expression of inherited traits, is determined by reacting red cells with known antisera and observing for the presence or absence of hemagglutination. Reagents used for this purpose were described in Chapter 2. For example, testing red cells with anti-A or anti-B reagents can determine whether a person has the A or B antigen. If neither anti-A nor anti-B shows agglutination, the red cells are classified as group O. This determination is called the phenotype.

The **genotype,** or the actual genes inherited from each parent, may be inferred from the phenotype. Family studies or molecular tests are required to determine the actual genotype. If an individual's phenotype is A, the genotype may be *A/A* or *A/O*. *A/A* indicates that both parents contributed the *A* gene. The *A/O* genotype indicates that one parent contributed the *A* gene, and the other contributed the *O* gene. Because the *O* gene has no detectable product, only the A antigen is expressed when the *A/O* genotype is inherited. If the *A/O* individual has a group O child, it becomes evident that the individual carried the *O* gene. Two people with group A red cells have the same phenotype but can have different genotypes.

Punnett Square

Examination of family history is an important component in the investigation of inheritance patterns. Fig. 3-2 is an example of genotypes and phenotypes for the ABO blood group system.

A **Punnett square** illustrates the probabilities of phenotypes from known or inferred genotypes. It visually portrays the genotypes of the potential offspring or the probable genotypes of the parents. Fig. 3-3 shows possible ABO blood group system gene combinations through the use of Punnett squares. From this figure, it would be easy to determine that two group A parents can have a group O child. It could also be illustrated that the parents of a group AB child can be group A, B, or AB but not group O.

Genes, Alleles, and Polymorphism

Genes, the basic units of inheritance on a chromosome, are located in specific places called **genetic loci.** Several different forms of a gene, called **alleles,** may exist for each locus (Fig. 3-4). For example, *A, B,* and *O* are alleles on the *ABO* gene locus. The term **antithetical,** meaning opposite, refers to the antigens produced by allelic genes. For example, the Kp^a antigen is antithetical to the Kp^b antigen. *Kp^a* and *Kp^b* are examples of alleles in the Kell blood group system.

The term **polymorphic** refers to having two or more alleles at a given locus, as with the ABO blood group system. Some blood group systems are more polymorphic than others; in other words, many more alleles exist at a given locus. The Rh blood group system is highly polymorphic compared with the ABO blood group system because of

---

Phenotype: observable expression of inherited traits.

The patient's red cell phenotype is determined by hemagglutination of red cell antigens using specific antisera.

Genotype: actual genetic makeup; determined by family studies or molecular typing.

The patient's genotype is not determined in routine blood bank testing. DNA-based assays or family studies are used for the determination of genotype.

Punnett square: square used to display the frequencies of different genotypes and phenotypes among the offspring of a cross.

Genes are written in italics, whereas red cell antigens are not.

Genetic loci: sites of a gene on a chromosome.

Alleles: alternate forms of a gene at a given locus.

Antithetical: opposite antigens encoded at the same locus.

Polymorphic: genetic system that expresses two or more alleles at one locus.

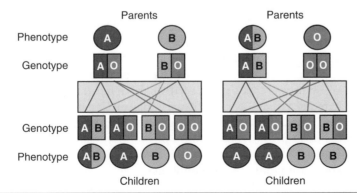

Fig. 3-2 Difference between phenotype and genotype. The difference between the genotype and phenotype is illustrated in this diagram of ABO system inheritance patterns.

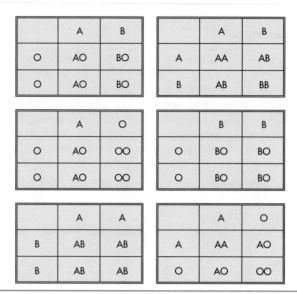

Fig. 3-3 Punnett squares showing ABO inheritance.

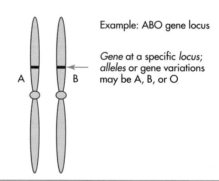

Fig. 3-4 Genes and alleles in relation to a chromosome.

the greater number of alleles. The frequency of a particular phenotype in a population depends on the degree of polymorphism within a blood group system. A highly polymorphic system makes it less likely to find two identical individuals. An example of a highly polymorphic system is one involving the genes that encode HLA. Because bone marrow and organ transplants require HLA matching, HLA polymorphism contributes to the challenge of finding suitable donors. If several polymorphic systems are used to determine a phenotype of an individual, finding two identical individuals becomes increasingly difficult.

Inheritance Patterns

Codominant: equal expression of two different inherited alleles.

In most cases, blood group antigens are inherited in an autosomal **codominant** pattern, or the equal expression of both inherited alleles found on autosomes. The product of each allele can be identified when inherited as a codominant trait. If one parent passed on an *A* gene and the other parent passed on a *B* gene, both the A and the B antigens would be expressed equally on the red cells. **Recessive** inheritance would require that the same allele from both parents be inherited to show the trait. An example is a group O phenotype that requires both parents to pass on an *O* gene (*O/O*). In blood group genetics, a recessive trait can be caused by red cells expressing a null phenotype such as Lu (a–b–), Rh_{null} or O phenotypes because of homozygosity for a silent or amorphic gene.[2]

Recessive: trait expressed only when inherited by both parents.

Dominant: gene product expressed over another gene.

A **dominant** expression would require only one form of the allele to express the trait, such as a group A phenotype that inherits an *A* gene from one parent and an *O* gene from the other parent (*A/O*). The alleles of the ABO blood group system display dominant, recessive, and codominant patterns of inheritance.

Silent Genes

In some blood group systems, genes do not produce a detectable antigen product. These silent genes are called **amorphs.** The phenotypes are often called null types because expressions of the blood group system antigens are not apparent. For example, an Rh_{null} individual lacks the presence of all Rh system antigens. The amorphic gene must be inherited from both parents (homozygous) to produce a null phenotype. If the gene is rare, this phenomenon is uncommon. Because the O allele has a high frequency in the population, however, the O phenotype is common. Examples of null phenotypes include Rh_{null}, O, and Lu(a–b–).[2]

Unusual phenotypes may also result from the action of **suppressor genes.** These genes act to inhibit the expression of another gene to produce a null expression. The occurrence of suppressor genes that affect blood group antigen expression is rare. An example of a suppression gene is *In(Jk)*, which affects the Kidd blood group system expression causing the Jk(a–b–) phenotype. In addition to the silent gene, *Lu*, the *In(Lu)* gene suppresses Lutheran blood group system antigens resulting in the Lu(a–b–) phenotype. Null phenotypes can be a result of either an amorphic or a suppressor gene. Table 3-1 includes examples of suppressor and amorphic genes.

Mendelian Principles

Mendel observed certain hereditary patterns in his early genetic experiments that subsequently were applied to the study of blood group system genetics. Mendel's law of **independent segregation** refers to the transmission of a trait in a predictable fashion from one generation to the next.[2] This concept was described previously with the Punnett square using the ABO blood group system genes. Independent segregation illustrates that each parent has a pair of genes for a particular trait, either of which can be transmitted to the next generation. The genes "segregate" and allow only one gene from each parent to be passed on to each child. Another important law, **independent assortment,** is demonstrated by the fact that blood group antigens, inherited on different chromosomes, are expressed separately and discretely. Fig. 3-5 illustrates that the ABO blood group system genes,

Amorphic: describes a gene that does not express a detectable product.

Suppressor genes: genes that suppress the expression of another gene.

Inheritance of the group O phenotype is an example of a recessive trait.

Independent segregation: passing of one gene from each parent to the offspring.

Independent assortment: random behavior of genes on separate chromosomes during meiosis that results in a mixture of genetic material in the offspring.

TABLE 3-1	Amorph and Suppressor Genes in Blood Groups		
BLOOD GROUP SYSTEM	AMORPH GENE	SUPPRESSOR GENE	RESULTING PHENOTYPE
ABO	O		O
H	*h*		Bombay
Kell	K^0		Kell_null
Lutheran	*Lu*	*In(Lu)*	Lu(a–b–)
Kidd	*Jk*	*In(Jk)*	Jk(a–b–)
Duffy	*Fy*		Fy(a–b–)

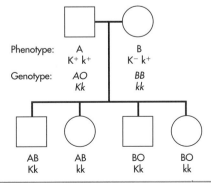

Fig. 3-5 Independent assortment. ABO system genes are sorted independently from Kell system genes because they are inherited on different chromosomes.

located on chromosome 1, and the Kell blood group system genes, located on chromosome 7, are inherited independent of each other.

Chromosomal Assignment

The genetic loci of most of the blood group system genes have been determined. Table 3-2 shows the chromosomal assignment for common blood group systems.[1] Most of the blood group–associated genes are on **autosomes.** Inheritance patterns are the same regardless of gender. The Xg blood group system is an exception. Genes coding for this system are found on the X chromosome. In this system, if the Xg^a allele is carried on the father's X chromosome, he would pass it on to all of his daughters but none of his sons. Conversely, if the father lacked the Xg^a gene and the mother carried the gene, both the sons and the daughters would express the Xg^a antigen.

Heterozygosity and Homozygosity

An individual whose genotype is made up of identical genes, such as *AA, BB,* or *OO,* is called **homozygous.** An individual who has inherited different alleles from each parent, such as *AO, AB,* or *BO,* is called **heterozygous** (Fig. 3-6).

Autosomes: chromosomes other than the sex chromosomes.

Homozygous: two alleles for a given trait are identical.

Heterozygous: two alleles for a given trait are different.

TABLE 3-2	Chromosomal Assignment of Genes for Common Blood Group Systems
BLOOD GROUP SYSTEM	**CHROMOSOME**
Rh	1
Duffy	1
MNS	4
Chido/Rodgers	6
Kell	7
ABO	9
Kidd	18
Lewis	19
Landsteiner-Wiener	19
Lutheran	19
Hh	19
P	22

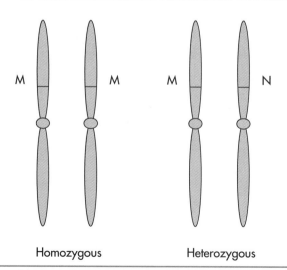

Fig. 3-6 Homozygosity and heterozygosity. A homozygous expression means that both parents contributed the same gene, giving a "double dose" of antigen expression. In some blood group systems, the antigen may appear to have stronger expression.

In serologic testing, the concept of homozygous and heterozygous inheritance is important with some blood group antigens. As discussed in the previous chapters, agglutination reactions vary in strength. This variation can be due to the strength of the antibody or the density of the antigens on the red cells. When antigen density varies between red cells of different individuals, it is often due to the inheritance of the antigen expression. An individual who inherits different blood group system alleles from each parent (*MN*) has a "single dose" of that antigen on the red cells (one M and one N). The agglutination reaction may demonstrate a weaker antigenic expression, or lower antigen density, on the red cell. When the same allele is inherited from both parents (*MM* or *NN*), a stronger red cell antigen is apparent because a "double dose" of the M or N antigen is present on the red cells. The variation in antigen expression because of the number of alleles present is called the **dosage effect** (Fig. 3-7). The dosage effect is not observed with all blood group antigens or with all antibodies of a given specificity.

Dosage effect: stronger agglutination when a red cell antigen is expressed from homozygous genes.

Genetic Interaction

Sometimes genes can interact with each other, depending on whether they are inherited on the same chromosome (*cis*) or on the opposite chromosome (*trans*). This interaction may weaken the expression of one of the antigens encoded by the genes. For example, the *Ce* and *D* genes of the Rh blood group system are inherited on different genetic loci. The *Ce* gene encodes the Ce antigen, and the *D* gene encodes the D antigen. When *Ce* is inherited in *trans* to *D*, it weakens the D antigen expression on the red cell (Fig. 3-8).[2]

cis: two or more genes on the same chromosome of a homologous pair.

trans: genes inherited on opposite chromosomes of a homologous pair.

Linkage and Haplotypes

In some blood group systems, antigens are encoded by two or more genes close together on the same chromosome and are inherited from each parent as a unit. Genes that are so close together on a chromosome that they are inherited as a unit are

Cell	| Rh							| MNSs				| P1	| Lewis		| Lutheran		| Kell		| Duffy		| Kidd		| Antibody reaction
	D	C	E	c	e	f	Cw	M	N	S	s	P1	Lea	Leb	Lua	Lub	K	k	Fya	Fyb	Jka	Jkb	
1 R1R1	+	+	0	0	+	0	0	+	0	+	0	+	0	+	0	+	+	+	+	+	+	0	3+
2 R2R2	+	0	+	+	0	0	0	+	+	+	+	+	+	0	0	+	0	+	+	0	+	+	1+

Fig. 3-7 Dosage effect. Homozygous expressions of some red cell antigens react more strongly than heterozygous expressions. This antibody screen result shows that the antibody reacts more strongly (3+) with the red cell #1 homozygous (M+N−) expression than with the red cell #2 heterozygous (M+N+) expression of the antigen.

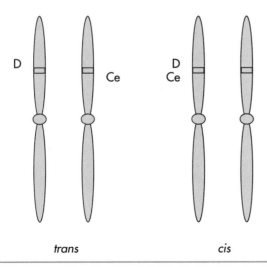

trans   *cis*

Fig. 3-8 *Cis* and *trans* position genes. When the *Ce* gene is inherited on opposite chromosomes or in *trans* to the *D* gene, the D antigen expression is weaker than when the *Ce* gene is inherited in *cis*, or on the same chromosome.

Linked: when two genes are inherited together because they are very close on a chromosome.

Haplotype: linked set of genes inherited together because of their close proximity on a chromosome.

Linkage disequilibrium: occurrence of a set of genes inherited together more often than would be expected by chance.

Crossing over: exchange of genetic material during meiosis between paired chromosomes.

linked. Independent assortment does not occur when genes are linked. These gene units are called **haplotypes.** For example, in the MNS blood group system, *M* and *N* are alleles on one gene whereas *S* and *s* are alleles on another gene. Because the genes are close, they are inherited as haplotypes: *MS, Ms, NS,* or *Ns* (Fig. 3-9). Haplotypes occur in the population at a different frequency than would be expected if the genes were not linked. **Linkage disequilibrium** refers to the phenomenon of antigens occurring at a different frequency in the population, depending on whether they were inherited by linked or unlinked genes. In other words, if the *M* and *S* gene were not linked, the expected frequency of the M and S antigen in the population would be 17% according to calculated frequency probabilities.[2] Because of linkage disequilibrium, the observed frequency of the MS haplotype is actually 24%.

Linkage in the HLA system occurs because these genetic loci are very close. The major histocompatibility (MHC) genes that encode HLA antigens are inherited as haplotypes. Each sibling could potentially share at least one haplotype with the other and has a 25% chance of having the same HLA typing. Fig. 3-10 illustrates this concept. For this reason, siblings are likely matches when organ or bone marrow transplants are required.

Crossing Over

Another exception to the law of independent assortment occurs if two genes on the same chromosome recombine. **Crossing over** is the exchange of genetic material during meiosis after the chromosome pairs have replicated (Fig. 3-11). The resulting genes are exchanged during this process but are not lost. The recombination results in two new and different chromosomes. Crossing over can be observed with genes on the same chromosome but does not usually occur when the genes are close together. Because the genes expressing

Phenotype: MNSs
Genotype: MS, Ns

Fig. 3-9   Haplotypes. Haplotypes are genes that are very close on a chromosome and often inherited together.

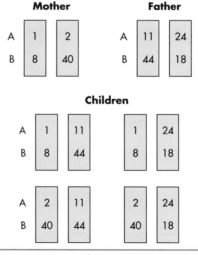

Fig. 3-10   Linkage in the HLA system. Inheritance of the *A* and *B* genes in the HLA system occurs as a set or a haplotype.

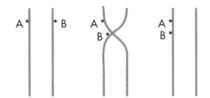

Fig. 3-11 Unequal crossing over meiosis. Crossing over causes the predicted inheritance patterns to be changed.

blood group systems are either close (linked) or on different chromosomes, crossing over rarely affects the inheritance of the blood group system. Crossover frequencies are used to map the relative locations of genes on a chromosome because the closer the genes, the rarer the possibility for the genes to be separated.

SECTION 2
POPULATION GENETICS

Population genetics is the statistical application of genetic principles to determine genotype and phenotype occurrence, which is dependent on the gene frequency.[2] Two types of calculations are applicable in the study of blood group population genetics. The first calculation involves combined phenotype frequencies, and the second involves gene or allele frequency estimates.

COMBINED PHENOTYPE CALCULATIONS

Determining the frequency of a particular phenotype in the population enables finding a donor unit of RBCs with certain antigen characteristics. For example, patients with multiple antibodies may require RBCs that are negative for several different antigens. The calculation of combined phenotype frequencies provides an estimate of the number of units that may need to be tested to find the unit with the desired antigens.

The frequency of multiple traits inherited independently is calculated by multiplying the frequency of each trait. If a patient produced red cell antibodies from exposure to previous transfusions or pregnancies, red cells that were negative for the corresponding antigens would be required for transfusion. For example, if a patient produced antibodies such as anti-C, anti-E, and anti-S, RBC units that are negative for the antigens C, E, and S would be required for transfusion. The percentage of donors negative for the individual antigens is expressed as a decimal point and then multiplied.

68% C positive	32% C negative	= 0.32 C negative
29% E positive	71% E negative	= 0.71 E negative
52% S positive	48% S negative	= 0.48 S negative

$$0.32 \times 0.71 \times 0.48 = 0.109, \text{ rounded to } 0.11 \text{ or } 11\%$$

Thus 11% of the population has a probability of being negative for all three antigens. This means that approximately 1 in 10 units of RBCs are likely to be negative for the combined antigens.

The percentages used are established antigen frequencies and can be found in the *AABB Technical Manual,* package inserts for the corresponding antisera, and *The Blood Group Antigen Facts Book.*[1] Antigen frequencies vary with race. The predominant race found in the donor population for the area should be used when calculating antigen frequencies. The frequency of an antigen in the population is the occurrence of the positive phenotype. Subtracting the frequency from 100 yields the percentage that is negative.

For example, if a patient has an anti-Fy^a, an anti-Jk^b, and an anti-K, how many units should be tested to find 2 units of the appropriate phenotype?

68% Fy^a positive	32% Fy^a negative
74% Jk^b positive	26% Jk^b negative
9% K positive	91% K negative

$$0.32 \times 0.26 \times 0.91 = 0.076, \text{ rounded to } 0.08 \text{ or } 8\%$$

If 2 units are needed, solve for X:

$$\frac{8}{100} = \frac{2}{X}$$

The calculation shows the probability of finding a unit of RBCs negative for all three antigens to be 8 of 100 units. Solving for X shows that antigen typing 25 units may be required to find 2 units that are negative for all three antigens.

GENE FREQUENCIES

The concept of genetic equilibrium was developed independently in 1908 by the English mathematician Hardy and the German physician Weinberg.[3] Their theories led to the formulation of the Hardy-Weinberg law. The statistical formulas derived from these principles are used to estimate the frequency of genetic diseases or observed traits. The formula is based on the principle that the sum of the gene frequencies, when expressed as a decimal, is equal to 1. This formula is used for predictions of populations at equilibrium, meaning that there is no migration, mutations, or natural selection. In addition, random mating must occur. By observing phenotypes or traits in a large number of individuals, the percentage of trait occurrences is established. The Hardy-Weinberg formula can be used to calculate a determination of the gene frequencies that produced that trait. The probability of heterozygous and homozygous expression for each of the genes in a system can be predicted. With the ability to characterize genes and determine the zygosity through molecular methods, this formula is less frequently used.

For example:

p is the frequency of allele A

q is the frequency of allele a

$$\text{Genotype proportions are: } p + q = 1.0$$

$$p^2(AA) + 2\,pq\,(Aa) + q^2(aa) = 1.0$$

If the frequency of p is 0.3, what is the value of q?

$$1 - 0.3 = 0.7$$

What proportion of the population is homozygous for A, or AA, heterozygous, or Aa, and homozygous for a, or aa?

$$AA = p^2 \text{ or } 0.09 \qquad Aa \text{ is } 2pq \text{ or } 0.42 \qquad aa = q^2 \text{ or } 0.49$$

RELATIONSHIP TESTING

The high degree of polymorphism of the HLA and blood group systems has made them valuable tools in cases of disputed paternity. Although paternity, or relationship, testing is typically performed by molecular methods, recognizing inheritance patterns of blood group and HLA using family studies helps reinforce the genetic concepts important in understanding blood groups.

If maternity is assumed, paternity can be excluded by either indirect or direct exclusion. In a **direct exclusion**, the child has inherited a genetic marker that is not found in the mother or **alleged father** (the *B gene* in the following example). This gene is also called

Direct exclusion: exclusion of paternity when a child has a trait that neither parent shows.

Alleged father: man accused of being the biological father; the putative father.

the **obligatory gene,** the gene that should be passed on by the father to establish probability of paternity.

Obligatory gene: gene that should be inherited from the father to prove paternity.

	Mother	Alleged Father	Child
Phenotype	Group O	Group A	Group B
Genotype	O/O	A/A or A/O	B/O

In an **indirect exclusion,** the child lacks a genetic marker that the father should have transmitted to all of his offspring. Refer to the Jk^b allele in the following example. Because an indirect exclusion can be caused by a silent gene, it is not used as the only marker to exclude paternity.

Indirect exclusion: failure to find an expected marker in a child when the alleged father is apparently homozygous for the gene.

	Mother	Alleged Father	Child
Phenotype	Jk(a+b−)	Jk(a−b+)	Jk(a+b−)
Genotype	Jk^a/Jk^a	Jk^b/Jk^b	Jk^a/Jk^a

If an alleged father cannot be excluded, the probability of paternity can be calculated based on the gene frequency of the obligatory gene in the population with the same race or ethnic group as the alleged father. The result is expressed as a likelihood ratio (paternity index) or as a percentage.[2]

SECTION 3
MOLECULAR GENETICS

APPLICATION OF MOLECULAR GENETICS TO BLOOD BANKING

Procedures based on the detection or analysis of DNA and RNA have made important contributions to biological science. Applications of molecular technology in the field of blood banking and transplantation include HLA typing, red cell typing, viral marker testing, and determination of engraftment in **hematopoietic progenitor cell (HPC)** transplantation (Table 3-3).[4] Nucleic acid testing (NAT) is a general term used for molecular-based methods of screening for infectious agents. This methodology further reduces the "window period" in viral testing when antibodies may be below detectable levels. NAT is discussed further in Chapter 13. DNA-based assays have also largely replaced red cell and HLA typing for identity (relationship) testing, also referred to as DNA fingerprinting.[2] The next section outlines the concept of the polymerase chain reaction (PCR) and its application in transplantation and transfusion medicine.

Hematopoietic progenitor cells (HPC): type of stem cells committed to a blood cell lineage that are collected from marrow, peripheral blood, and cord blood and used to treat certain malignant diseases and congenital immune deficiencies.

TABLE 3-3	Applications of Molecular Testing in the Blood Bank
Transplantation	HLA antigen-level and allele-level typing for HPC and organ transplants Engraftment studies for HPC transplants
Transfusion	Red cell typing in multiply transfused patients Determine blood type when the DAT is positive Complex Rh genotypes, weak D expression Screen for antigen-negative donor units when antisera are unavailable Donor antigen screening for prevention of alloimmunization
HDFN	Determine parental RhD zygosity Type fetal blood
Donor testing	Detect virus in donors that may be below detectable levels by antibody detection methods
Relationship testing	Establish paternity and legal relationships for immigration

From Alexander L: Personalized therapy reaches transfusion medicine, *AABB News* 13:10, 2011.
DAT, Direct antiglobulin test; *HDFN,* hemolytic disease of the fetus and newborn; *HLA,* human leukocyte antigen; *HPC,* hematopoietic progenitor cell.

POLYMERASE CHAIN REACTION

The genes encoding many of the red cell and HLA antigens have been sequenced and cloned, providing "maps" for the specific nucleotide differences that define each allele. Most HLA and red cell antigen differences are the result of single nucleotide substitutions in the coding sequence of each unique allele. DNA-based assays identify single-nucleotide polymorphisms (SNPs) by amplifying the part of the DNA where the SNPs are located.[5] This amplification is performed by PCR, which allows specific DNA sequences to be multiplied rapidly and precisely (Fig. 3-12). PCR is an in vitro technique used to amplify specific DNA sequences of interest through cycles of denaturation, annealing of primers that select the area of the DNA to be amplified, and replication that result in a millionfold copies of a specific area of DNA. Components of the PCR reaction are listed in Table 3-4.

Polymerase Chain Reaction–Based Human Leukocyte Antigen Typing Procedures

HLA typing procedures are based on the amplification by PCR of one or more alleles. The test methods vary in the techniques used to detect and identify the amplified

Fig. 3-12   Polymerase chain reaction.

TABLE 3-4	Polymerase Chain Reaction Components
COMPONENT	**DESCRIPTION**
Target DNA	DNA that contains the region of the DNA fragment to be amplified
Taq polymerase	Thermostabile enzyme that catalyzes the replication of template DNA into copies
Primers	Short pieces of single-stranded DNA that are complementary to the opposite strands that flank the target DNA. Primers mark the sequence to be amplified and provide the initiation site on each DNA
Nucleotides	dNTPs, which are the building blocks for the newly synthesized DNA
MgCl$_2$ and buffer	Allows proper pH and divalent cations for the enzyme to function

dNTPs, Deoxynucleotide triphosphates.

products.[6] This section describes the principles and application of several methods used in HLA typing.

Sequence-Specific Primers

In the sequence-specific primers (SSP) test method, primers that are specific for a particular sequence select the area of the DNA to be evaluated during the PCR reaction.[7] As described previously, the specificity of the genetic material being amplified is determined by the primer. Each primer pair can amplify one or several alleles. Primers can be either low or high resolution, resulting in either antigen-level or allele-level results. Low-resolution results are similar to identification by serologic testing, whereas high-resolution primers define more specific alleles. The primers are purchased in PCR trays in various configurations for most common HLA specificities. The DNA to be tested is added to the tray wells and amplified by a thermal cycler according to the manufacturer's recommended protocol.[8]

After PCR, the specificity of the amplified DNA, or **amplicons**, is assessed using gel electrophoresis. The amplified DNA from each well is transferred to an agarose gel prepared with ethidium bromide to allow for DNA detection under ultraviolet light. Electrophoresis of the gel is then performed. Low-molecular-weight amplicons migrate faster than high-molecular-weight amplicons. A blank well indicates that the primer did not detect the portion of DNA in question. The identity of the allele that defines the antigen is determined by comparing the migration pattern of the gel with the primer specificities and patterns provided by the manufacturer (Fig. 3-13).

Sequence-Specific Oligonucleotide Probes

In the sequence-specific oligonucleotide probes (SSOP) technique, the target DNA is amplified using group-specific primer in separate wells (e.g., A, B, C, DR, DQ, DP).[9] After amplification by PCR, the DNA is denatured and **hybridized** to a mixture of complementary **DNA probes** conjugated to fluorescently coded microspheres (Fig. 3-14). There can be 30 to 70 probes per locus to characterize the various alleles. The hybridized solution is evaluated with a flow analyzer such as the Luminex. The fluorescent intensity is measured, and the reaction pattern is analyzed by the instrument software and compared with patterns associated with published HLA gene sequences. An assignment of the HLA

Amplicon: short sequences of amplified DNA flanked on either end by the primer.

Hybridize: to attach a complementary sequence of DNA using the properties of complementary base pair sequencing.

DNA probe: short sequence of DNA complementary to the area being identified. It is attached to a marker (usually fluorescent) that can be read by an instrument such as a flow cytometer.

Fig. 3-13 Diagram of the SSP process.

Fig. 3-14 Diagram of the SSOP process.

typing is then determined. The SSOP typing test provides serologic and allele-level evaluations.

Sequence-Based Typing

Donor and recipient typing for HPC transplants require high-resolution typing at the allele level.[2] This resolution is most accurately performed by sequence-based typing (SBT). In SBT, the amplified DNA is purified after the PCR reaction, and a fluorescent locus-specific sequencing mix is added.[10] Following a sequencing step on the thermal cycler, the DNA is washed and denatured. The actual nucleotide sequence and predicted amino acid sequence, corresponding to the allele, can be read and analyzed by a capillary array instrument. The allele identification is not limited to available primers, but rather the nucleotide sequences define the allele.[11] Instrument software helps to facilitate the analysis and the assignment of alleles.

Short Tandem Repeats

Most of our DNA is identical to DNA of others. However, there are inherited regions of DNA that can vary from person to person. Variations in DNA sequence between individuals are termed polymorphisms.[2] Sequences with the highest degree of polymorphism are very useful for relationship testing, forensics, and determining engraftment after HPC transplants. Engraftment evaluations, also called **chimerism** studies, determine the percentage of hematopoietic and lymphoid cells from the donor that have engrafted into the recipient at several intervals after transplant. This test can determine how successful the transplant is and if further treatment is necessary. Because the HLA alleles of the donor and recipient have been closely matched, testing HLA alleles would be of little value to differentiate the donor and recipient cells in a sample.

Short tandem repeats (STR) are short sequences of DNA, normally 2 to 5 base pairs in length, that are repeated 4 to more than 50 times. The number of times the repeats occur varies between individuals and is genetically determined. STR identification can therefore be used to establish genetic relationships between individuals. If six to 12 STR loci are used, the ability to discriminate between individuals has a high degree of accuracy.

STR testing is performed by amplifying DNA from the donor, the recipient and the posttransplant samples. Locus-specific primers for the STR are added to the DNA that has been isolated from donor, pretransplant recipient, and posttransplant recipient samples. Following amplification by PCR, the amplicons are denatured and labeled with fluorescent dyes that can be analyzed on a sequencing instrument such as the capillary array used for SBT. The STRs in the pretransplant samples from the donor and recipient are identified and compared with the STRs in the posttransplant sample. A calculation of the percent of donor-to-recipient STRs is made. In 100% engraftment the only STRs detected are those from the donor. In chimerism studies where less than 100% engraftment is determined, early relapses or graft failures can be detected and treated with this knowledge.

MOLECULAR TESTING APPLICATIONS IN RED CELL TYPING

Molecular determination of red cell antigens has become more available in recent years to supplement traditional hemagglutination methods. There are several situations where molecular testing yields more accurate results and can be a more cost-effective method for donor red cell antigen typing. Table 3-3 lists molecular applications for red cell typing.

Polymerase Chain Reaction–Based Red Cell Typing Procedures

Bead-Chip Technology

After the genes encoding the major blood group antigens had been sequenced and cloned, the correlation of the differences in DNA sequences with red cell antigen expression could be applied to the development and standardization of laboratory tests.[6] In many of the blood group systems, single-nucleotide substitutions, described earlier, code for the unique blood group allele.

Chimerism: mixture of donor and recipient cell populations after hematopoietic stem cell transplants.

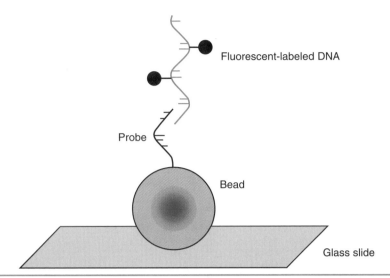

Probe

Bead

Glass slide

Fluorescent-labeled DNA

Fig. 3-15 BeadChip Technology concept. (Courtesy BioArray Solutions, An Immucor Company, Warren, New Jersey.)

The antigen-defining SNPs are identified through PCR methods combined with bead-chip technology.[12] The principle of human erythrocyte antigen (HEA) bead chip technology uses oligonucleotide primers attached to silica beads of various colors. The beads are attached to a substrate (e.g., a glass slide). A "map" identifying the color and the specific oligonucleotide (primer) is made. When the chip is used, the PCR is amplified, and digested DNA in question is exposed to the surface of the chip, allowing the primers to bind to the matches in the single-stranded DNA. Unbound DNA is washed away, and the bound DNA is labeled with fluorescent-labeled deoxynucleotide triphosphates (dNTPs). Computer analysis determines which beads fluoresced and which primers attached (Fig. 3-15).

CHAPTER SUMMARY

- Blood group systems are serologically and genetically defined because they can be categorized by molecular and serologic properties.
- Various forms of genes at the same gene locus are called alleles and encode the blood group antigens.
- The testing of red cell antigens determines the phenotype. Inferences regarding the genotype or genetic makeup are often made; however, molecular methods or family studies are necessary to determine the genotype.
- When identical alleles for a given locus are present on both chromosomes, a person is homozygous for the allele; nonidentical alleles are heterozygous. Inheriting homozygous blood group system alleles can code for a greater antigen density, causing agglutination reactions to be stronger.
- Two or more closely linked genes can be inherited as a haplotype.
- Genes with two or more possible alleles are termed polymorphic; the HLA system is the most polymorphic.
- Techniques of molecular genetics, such as PCR, have made possible significant improvements in HLA tissue typing and viral marker testing on donated blood products.
- PCR is the basis of most molecular tests used in blood banking; variations in the identification of the DNA products of this technique are what distinguish SSOP, SSP, SBT, STR, and bead-chip technology.

CRITICAL THINKING EXERCISES

EXERCISE 3-1

Given the following pedigree for a family study involving the ABO system, determine the phenotype and the probable genotype of the father:

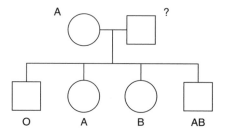

EXERCISE 3-2

While working in the blood bank, the laboratory staff receives a call from a father who wants to know if his group O son could possibly belong to him. He knows that he is group B, and the mother is group A. Provide an explanation in terms understandable to a person without a background in basic genetics.

EXERCISE 3-3

Is a person whose phenotype is M+, N– homozygous or heterozygous for the *M* gene? Would you expect reactions with this person's red cells to be stronger or weaker than red cells that phenotyped as M+, N+?

EXERCISE 3-4

The following pedigree represents a family study of the Xg blood group system. What are the phenotypes of the sons?

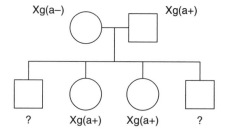

EXERCISE 3-5

A patient's antibodies are identified to be anti-K, anti-Jk^a, and anti-E. How many RBC units are needed to find 2 antigen-negative units? The antigens occur in the population with the following frequency: E, 30%; K, 9%; Jk^a, 77%.

EXERCISE 3-6

You performed a population study on your class and found that 84% are D-positive. Using the Hardy-Weinberg calculation, determine the percentage of your classmates who are heterozygous for D antigen.

EXERCISE 3-7

A family study was performed for a potential bone marrow transplant. The father was unavailable for testing, but the rest of the family members were present. Predict the father's phenotype and explain how nonidentical twins can have the same HLA type.
Mother: A2, A11, B7, B44, DR4, DR17
Child 1: A2, A28, B51, B44, DR17, DR8
Child 2: A2, A28, B51, B44, DR17, DR8
Child 3: A11, A30, B44, B8, DR4, DR15
Child 4: A11, A28, B7, B51, DR17, DR8

STUDY QUESTIONS

1. Which of the following describes the expression of most blood group inheritance?
   a. dominant
   b. recessive
   c. sex-linked
   d. codominant

2. With which of the following red cell phenotypes would anti-Jk^a react most strongly?
   a. Jk (a–b+)
   b. Jk (a+b–)
   c. Jk (a+b+)
   d. Jk (a–b–)

3. In relationship testing, a "direct exclusion" is established when a genetic marker is:
   a. absent in the child but present in the mother and alleged father
   b. absent in the child, present in the mother, and absent in the alleged father
   c. present in the child, absent in the mother, and present in the alleged father
   d. present in the child but absent in both the mother and the alleged father

4. Which of the following items is a useful genetic marker for relationship testing?
   a. all races have the same gene frequencies
   b. the genetic system is polymorphic
   c. there are no amorphic genes
   d. recombination is common

5. The term used when two of the same alleles of a gene are inherited from each parent is:
   a. homozygous
   b. allele
   c. heterozygous
   d. syntenic

6. Alternate forms of a gene at given genetic loci are called:
   a. alleles
   b. amplicons
   c. nucleotides
   d. amorphs

7. The technique that uses a small amount of DNA and amplifies it for identification is called:
   a. RFLP
   b. a DNA probe
   c. PCR
   d. gene mapping

8. A gene that can inhibit the expression of another gene is called:
   a. an amorph
   b. a *cis* gene
   c. a null gene
   d. a regulator gene

9. The phosphate, sugar, and base that constitute DNA and RNA are called:
   a. amplicons
   b. polymerases
   c. nucleotides
   d. anticodons

10. Synthetic single-stranded DNA that determines the sequence of DNA to be amplified in the PCR reaction is referred to as:
    a. amplicons
    b. nucleotides
    c. DNA primer
    d. *Taq* polymerases

11. Genes located close together on the same chromosome are more likely to:
    a. be inherited as a haplotype
    b. cross over
    c. show independent assortment
    d. suppress each other

12. In molecular techniques for HLA typing, which high-resolution method analyzes the nucleotide sequence to define the allele?
    a. SSP
    b. SSO
    c. STR
    d. SBT

13. What is the best source of an HLA-matched kidney?
    a. mother
    b. cousin
    c. father
    d. sibling

14. A gene inherited in a *cis* position to another gene is:
    a. on an opposite chromosome
    b. on a different chromosome number
    c. on the same chromosome
    d. antithetical

15. In PCR testing, the initial step involves adding the DNA in question to a mixture of taq polymerase, excess nucleotides, $MgCl_2$, and primers. This mixture is placed in which of the following instruments to allow the amplification to take place?
    a. flow cytometer
    b. capillary array sequencer
    c. thermal cycler
    d. electrophoresis chamber

16. A group O patient with anti-D and anti-K alloantibodies requires a unit of red cells. What percentage of the white population would be compatible with her serum (Type O: 0.45, D neg 0.15, K neg 0.91)?
    a. 50%
    b. 20%
    c. 6%
    d. 3%

17. Molecular tests on samples from hematopoietic progenitor cell transplant recipients are used to determine if engraftment is successful. The method used for this is called:
    a. sequence-specific primers (SSP)
    b. sequence-based typing (SBT)
    c. short tandem repeats (STR)
    d. sequence-specific oligonucleotide probes (SSOP)

18. In a relationship test, the mother and the alleged father were both typed Jk(a–b+), and the was child typed Jk(a+b+). This is an example of:
    a. direct exclusion
    b. indirect exclusion
    c. no exclusion of paternity
    d. none of the above

19. The term antithetical is most closely defined as a(an):
    a. similar gene
    b. opposite allele
    c. opposite antigen
    d. heterozygous gene

REFERENCES

1. Reid ME, Lomas-Francis C: *The blood group antigen facts book*, New York, 2003, Elsevier Academic Press.
2. Roback JD, editor: *Technical manual*, ed 17, Bethesda, Md, 2011, AABB.
3. Watson JD, Baker TA, Bell SP: *Molecular biology of the gene*, ed 5, San Francisco, 2004, Pearson.
4. Alexander L: Personalized therapy reaches transfusion medicine, *AABB News* 13:10, 2011.10
5. Anstee DJ: Goodbye to agglutination and all that? *Transfusion* 45(5):652-653, 2005.
6. Reid ME: Applications of DNA based assays on blood group antigen and antibody identification, *Transfusion* 43:1748, 2003.
7. Rodey GE: *HLA beyond tears*, ed 2, Durango, CO, 2000, DeNovo Inc.
8. *Olerup package insert*, SSP. Stockholm, Sweden, Olerup SSP AB, Franzengatan 5, 112 51.
9. *LABType SSO Typing Tests package insert*, Canoga Park, CA, One Lambda, Inc.
10. Invitrogen SeCore Locus Sequencing Kit instructions for use, rev 009, Brown Deer, WI, 2011, Invitrogen Corporation.
11. Hillyer CD, Silberstein LE: *Blood banking and transfusion medicine, basic principles and practice*, ed 2, Philadelphia, 2007, Churchill-Livingstone.
12. BioArray Solutions. http://www.immucor.com/bioarray/html/press.html. Accessed January, 2012.

ABO and H Blood Group Systems and Secretor Status

4

CHAPTER OUTLINE

LEARNING OBJECTIVES

On completion of this chapter, the reader should be able to:

1. Define a blood group system with regard to blood group antigens and their inheritance.
2. Explain Landsteiner's rule.
3. List the cells, body fluids, and secretions where ABO antigens can be located.
4. Describe the relationships among the *ABO, H,* and *Se* genes.
5. Differentiate between type 1 and type 2 oligosaccharide structures, and state where each is located.
6. Describe the formation of the H antigen from the gene product and its relationship to ABO antigen expression.
7. List the glycosyltransferases and the immunodominant sugars for the *A, B, O,* and *H* alleles.
8. Compare and contrast the A₁ and A₂ phenotypes with regard to antigen structure and serologic testing.
9. Compare and contrast serologic testing among A₃, Aₓ, and Aₑₗ subgroups.
10. Predict the possible ABO genotypes with an ABO phenotype.

11. Describe the ABO blood group system antibodies with regard to immunoglobulin class, clinical significance, and in vitro serologic reactions.
12. Discuss the selection of whole blood, red blood cell, and plasma products for transfusions.
13. Define the terms universal donor and universal recipient as they apply to red blood cell and plasma products.
14. Apply concepts of ABO compatibility in the selection of blood products for recipients.
15. List the technical errors that may result in an ABO discrepancy.
16. Define the acquired B antigen and the B(A) phenotypes; interpret the ABO discrepancies that would result from these phenotypes and methods used in resolving these discrepancies.
17. List reasons for missing or weakly expressed ABO antigens, and identify the test methods used to resolve these discrepancies.
18. Describe ABO discrepancies caused by extra reactions in serum testing and how they can be resolved.

19. Illustrate the Bombay phenotype with regard to genetic pathway, serologic reactions, and transfusion implications.
20. Define the terms secretor and nonsecretor.
21. Identify and resolve ABO typing discrepancies from ABO typing results.
22. Apply concepts to solve case studies with ABO discrepant information.

> Blood group antigens form part of the red cell membranes. Antigens differ depending on inheritance of blood group genes as described in Chapter 3.

This chapter begins a section of the textbook dedicated to the basic understanding of blood group systems and their significance in the practice of transfusion medicine. A blood group system is composed of antigens that are produced by alleles at a single genetic locus or at loci so closely linked that genetic crossing over rarely occurs.[1] Blood group antigens are molecules located primarily on the red cell membrane. These molecules can be classified biochemically as proteins and as carbohydrates linked to either a lipid (glycolipid) or a protein (glycoprotein) as shown in Fig. 4-1. With adequate immunologic exposure, a blood group antigen may elicit the production of its corresponding antibody in individuals who lack the antigen. During transfusions, the recipient is exposed to many blood group antigens. Patients receiving transfusions may produce alloantibodies in response to the exposure to blood group antigens not present on their own red cells.

Because the terminology for red cell antigens is inconsistent, the International Society of Blood Transfusion (ISBT) created a Working Party on Terminology for Red Cell Antigens in 1980 to standardize blood group systems and antigen names. The committee's goal was not to create replacement terminology, but rather to provide additional terminology suitable for use with computer software. The ISBT Working Party has assigned genetically based numeric designations for red cell antigens and presently has defined 30 blood group systems (Table 4-1).[2,3] According to ISBT criteria, genetic studies and serologic data are required before an antigen is assigned to a blood group system. The ABO blood group system has been assigned the ISBT number 001 and includes four antigens, whereas the H blood group system is ISBT number 018 with one antigen. This textbook addresses blood group systems with commonly used names and includes ISBT symbols and numbers.

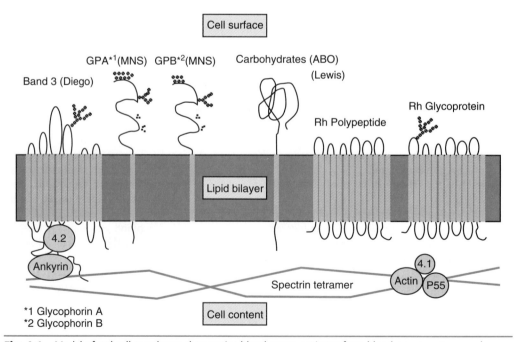

Fig. 4-1   Model of red cell membrane that carries blood group antigens from blood group systems and collections. The red cell antigens are molecules that form part of the red cell membrane's lipid bilayer or extend from the surface of the red cell. (Redrawn from Reid ME, Lomas-Francis C: *The blood group antigen facts book,* ed 2, San Diego, 2004, Elsevier Academic Press.)

TABLE 4-1	ISBT Blood Group System Assignments	
BLOOD SYSTEM NAME	**ISBT GENE NAME**	**ISBT NUMBER**
ABO	ABO	001
MNS	MNS	002
P1PK	P1	003
Rh	RH	004
Lutheran	LU	005
Kell	KEL	006
Lewis	LE	007
Duffy	FY	008
Kidd	JK	009
Diego	DI	010
Cartwright (Yt)	YT	011
Xg	XG	012
Scianna	SC	013
Dombrock	DO	014
Colton	CO	015
Landsteiner-Wiener	LW	016
Chido/Rodgers	CH/RG	017
Hh	H	018
Kx	XK	019
Gerbich	GE	020
Cromer	CROM	021
Knops	KN	022
Indian	IN	023
Ok	OK	024
Raph	RAPH	025
JMH	JMH	026
I	IGNT	027
Globoside	GLOB	028
Gil	GIL	029
Rh-associated glycoprotein	RHAG	030

ISBT, International Society of Blood Transfusion.

SECTION 1

HISTORICAL OVERVIEW OF ABO BLOOD GROUP SYSTEM

The discovery of the ABO blood group system by Landsteiner[4] in 1900 marked the beginning of modern blood banking and transfusion medicine. In a series of experiments designed to show serologic incompatibilities between humans, Landsteiner recognized different patterns of agglutination when human blood samples were mixed in random pairings. He described the blood groups as A, B, and O. Several years later, Landsteiner's associates, von Decastello and Sturli,[5] added group AB to the original observations. In his investigations, Landsteiner noted the presence of agglutinating antibodies in the serum of individuals who lacked the corresponding ABO antigen. He observed that group A red cells agglutinated with the serum from group B individuals. This observation has been termed **Landsteiner's rule** (or Landsteiner's law). Landsteiner's rule established that

Landsteiner's rule: rule stating that normal, healthy individuals possess ABO antibodies to the ABO blood group antigens absent from their red cells.

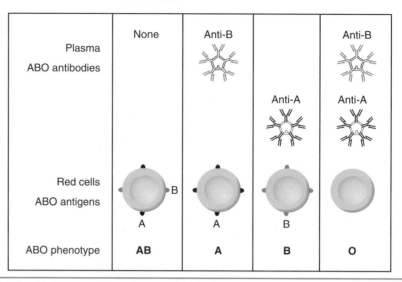

Fig. 4-2   Relationship between ABO antigens and antibodies. ABO antigens are located on the red cells. Group AB possesses both A and B antigens; group A possesses A antigens; group B possesses B antigens; group O lacks both A and B antigens. ABO antibodies are located in plasma. Group AB lacks ABO antibodies; group A possesses anti-B; group B possesses anti-A; group O possesses anti-A and anti-B. (Modified from Immunobase, Bio-Rad Laboratories, Inc., Hercules, CA.)

normal, healthy individuals possess ABO antibodies to the ABO blood group antigens lacking on their red cells. Individuals with group A red cells possess the A antigen and lack the B antigen. Therefore, these individuals possess anti-B antibodies. Individuals with group B red cells possess the B antigen and lack the A antigen. Therefore, these individuals possess anti-A antibodies. Antigens and antibodies associated with each ABO phenotype are illustrated in Fig. 4-2. Four major phenotypes are derived from the two major antigens (A and B) of the system. These phenotypes are group A, group B, group AB, and group O.

The first blood group system to be described, the ABO blood group system, remains the most important blood group system for transfusion purposes. Accurate donor and recipient ABO types are fundamental to transfusion safety because of the presence of ABO antibodies in individuals with no previous exposure to human red cells. The transfusion of ABO-incompatible blood to a recipient can result in intravascular hemolysis and other serious consequences of an **acute hemolytic transfusion reaction.**

Acute hemolytic transfusion reaction: complication of transfusion associated with intravascular hemolysis, characterized by rapid onset with symptoms of fever, chills, hemoglobinemia, and hypotension; major complications include irreversible shock, renal failure, and disseminated intravascular coagulation.

SECTION 2
ABO AND H BLOOD GROUP SYSTEM ANTIGENS

GENERAL CHARACTERISTICS OF ABO ANTIGENS

ABO antigens are widely distributed and are located on red cells, lymphocytes (adsorbed from plasma), platelets (adsorbed from plasma), most epithelial and endothelial cells, and organs such as the kidneys.[6] Soluble forms of the ABO blood group system antigens can also be synthesized and secreted by tissue cells. As a result, ABO blood group system antigens are found in association with cellular membranes and as soluble forms. Soluble antigens are detected in secretions and all body fluids except cerebrospinal fluid.[6] ABO blood group system antigens, which are intrinsic to the red cell membrane, exist as either glycolipid or glycoprotein molecules, whereas the soluble forms are primarily glycoproteins.

ABO antigens are detectable at 5 to 6 weeks in utero. A newborn possesses fewer antigen copies per red cell compared with an adult. For example, adult red cells carry 610,000 to 830,000 B antigens; whereas newborn red cells carry 200,000 to 320,000 B antigens.[7] Newborns' red cells also lack the fully developed antigen structures of adults' red cells. In **cord blood** samples, ABO antigens have fewer numbers and partially developed antigen structures and may demonstrate weaker ABO phenotyping reactions. Antigen development occurs slowly until the full expression of adult levels is reached at about 2 to 4 years of age.

The worldwide frequency of ABO phenotypes within the white population has been well documented. Group O and group A individuals constitute 45% and 40% of whites. These two blood groups are the most common ABO phenotypes, followed by group B with an 11% frequency and group AB with a 4% frequency.[8] ABO phenotype frequencies differ in selected populations and ethnic groups. For example, the group B phenotype has a higher frequency in blacks and Asians compared with whites (Table 4-2).

INHERITANCE AND DEVELOPMENT OF A, B, AND H ANTIGENS

A discussion of the inheritance and formation of ABO antigens requires an understanding of the H antigen, which is inherited independent of the ABO blood group system antigens. The production of H antigen is genetically controlled by the *H* gene, which is located on a different chromosome from the ABO genetic locus. In addition to the *ABO* and *H* genes, the expression of soluble ABO antigens is influenced by inheritance of the *Se* gene (see the section on Secretor Status later in this chapter). The *Se* gene genetically influences the formation of ABO antigens in saliva, tears, and other body fluids. Consequently, occurrence and location of the ABO antigens are influenced by three genetically independent loci: *ABO*, *H*, and *Se*.

ABO antigens are assembled on a common carbohydrate structure that also serves as the base for the formation of the H, Lewis, I/i, and P_1 antigens. Consequently, this common carbohydrate structure is capable of antigen expression for more than one blood group system (Fig. 4-3). This common structure is analogous to an antigen building block. Because of the interrelationship between the common antigen building block and multiple blood group systems, it is important to recognize that the action of genes of one blood group system can affect the expression of antigens in another system.

Cord blood: whole blood obtained from the umbilical vein or artery of the fetus.

When phenotyping cord blood samples, blood grouping reagents, anti-A and anti-B, may show weaker agglutination reactions.

TABLE 4-2	Frequency Distributions of ABO Phenotypes (U.S. Population)		
ABO PHENOTYPE	**WHITE (%)**	**BLACK (%)**	**ASIAN (%)**
A	40	27	28
B	11	20	27
AB	4	4	5
O	45	49	40

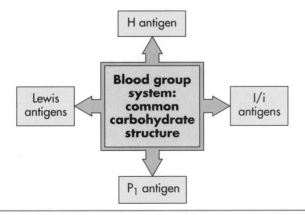

Fig. 4-3 Antigens in several blood group systems are formed from the same carbohydrate precursor structure.

Type 1: Body Fluids and Secretions

Type 2: Red Blood Cells*
Body Fluids and Secretions

Fig. 4-4   Type 1 and type 2 oligosaccharide chain structures. *Gal,* Galactose; *GlcNAc, N*-acetylglucosamine; *, most type 2 chains are located on the red cells. (Modified from Brecher ME, editor: *Technical manual*, ed 15, Bethesda, MD, 2005, AABB.)

Common Structure for A, B, and H Antigens

Oligosaccharide chain: chemical compound formed by a small number of simple carbohydrate molecules.

The common structure (antigen building block) for A, B, and H antigens is an **oligosaccharide chain** attached to either a protein or a lipid carrier molecule. The oligosaccharide chain comprises four sugar molecules linked in simple linear forms or in more complex structures with a high degree of branching. The two terminal sugars, D-galactose and N-acetylglucosamine, may be linked together in two different configurations. When the number 1 carbon of D-galactose is linked with the number 3 carbon of N-acetylglucosamine, the linkage is described as β1→3. Type 1 oligosaccharide chains are formed. When the number 1 carbon of D-galactose is linked with the number 4 carbon of N-acetylglucosamine, the linkage is described as β1→4. Type 2 oligosaccharide chains are formed (Fig. 4-4). Type 2 structures are associated primarily with glycolipids and glycoproteins on the red cell membrane, and type 1 structures are associated primarily with body fluids. Some type 2 glycoprotein structures are located in body fluids and secretions.[9]

Development of H Antigen

Transferase: class of enzymes that catalyzes the transfer of a chemical group from one molecule to another.

The H antigen is the only antigen in the H blood group system. This blood group system has been assigned to a locus on chromosome 19 and is closely linked with the *Se* locus. The *H* locus has two significant alleles: *H* and *h*. The *H* allele is a dominant allele with high frequency (>99.99%), whereas the *h* allele is classified as an amorph with rare frequency. Genes encode for the production of proteins, and the gene product of the *H* allele is a protein classified biochemically as a **transferase** enzyme. Transferase enzymes promote the transfer of a biochemical group from one molecule to another. A **glycosyltransferase** enzyme catalyzes the transfer of glycosyl groups (simple carbohydrate units) in biochemical reactions.

Glycosyltransferase: enzyme that catalyzes the transfer of glycosyl groups (simple carbohydrate units) in biochemical reactions.

In the formation of H antigen, a glycosyltransferase enzyme transfers a sugar molecule, L-fucose, to either type 1 or type 2 common oligosaccharide chains. The biochemical name for this enzyme is L-fucosyltransferase *(FUT-1)*. The L-fucose added to the terminal galactose of the type 1 and type 2 chain is called the **immunodominant sugar** for H antigens because the sugar confers H specificity (Fig. 4-5).[10] Formation of the H antigen is the end product of an enzymatic reaction. This formation is crucial to the expression of A and B antigens because the gene products of the *ABO* alleles require that the H antigen be the acceptor molecule. The *FUT-1* gene adds galactose to both oligosaccharide chains on red cells and in secretions.

Immunodominant sugar: sugar molecule responsible for specificity.

Bombay phenotype: rare phenotype of an individual who genetically has inherited the h allele in a homozygous manner; the individual's red cells lack H and ABO antigens.

This section previously described the *h* allele as an amorph with no detectable gene product. The red cells from an *h* homozygote *(hh)* are classified as the **Bombay phenotype**. These rare individuals lack both H antigen and ABO antigen expression on their red cells. The Bombay phenotype is discussed in more detail at the end of this chapter.

> The precursor of A and B antigens is the H antigen.

Development of A and B Antigens

Genetic control of A and B antigens has been mapped to chromosome 9. Three major alleles exist within the *ABO* locus: *A*, *B*, and *O*. The *A* and *B* alleles, similar to the *H*

Fig. 4-5 Biochemical structures of the H, A, and B antigens. *Gal*, D-Galactose; *GlcNAc, N*-acetylglucosamine; *Fuc*, L-fucose; *GalNAc, N*-acetylgalactosamine. (Modified from Brecher ME, editor: *Technical manual*, ed 15, Bethesda, MD, 2005, AABB.)

allele, are glycosyltransferases. The *A* allele produces *N*-acetylgalactosaminyltransferase, which transfers the sugar *N*-acetylgalactosamine to an oligosaccharide chain; the chain was previously converted to H antigen. The *B* allele produces D-galactosyltransferase, which transfers the sugar D-galactose to an oligosaccharide chain; the chain was previously converted to H antigen (see Fig. 4-5).[10] *N*-acetylgalactosamine is the immunodominant sugar for A specificity, and D-galactose is the immunodominant sugar for B specificity.

The *O* allele is considered nonfunctional because the resulting gene product is an enzymatically inactive protein. As a result, group O red cells carry no A or B antigens but are rich in unconverted H antigens. Adult group O red cells have about 1.7 million H-antigen copies per red cell and possess the greatest concentration of H antigens per red cell.[6] Other ABO phenotypes have fewer copies of H antigens because the H antigen is the acceptor molecule for the A and B enzymes. Group A_1B phenotype possesses the lowest number of unconverted H sites. Fig. 4-6 illustrates the variation of H-antigen concentration in ABO phenotypes.

Yamamoto et al[11] defined the molecular basis of the ABO phenotypes. These investigators discovered that a few mutations exist in the glycosyltransferase gene at the ABO locus. On the molecular level, the A and B glycosyltransferases differ slightly in their nucleic acid compositions. Additionally, the nucleic acid composition of the O allele has revealed that it does not produce an enzymatically active protein capable of acting on the H-antigen precursors. Readers are encouraged to review the article by Poole and Daniels in the Suggested Readings for greater detail on the molecular basis of the ABO phenotypes.

The specificity of A and B antigen is defined by immunodominant sugars: *N*-acetylgalactosamine (A antigen) and D-galactose (B antigen).

A and B antigens are not primary gene products.

$$O > A_2 > B > A_2B > A_1 > A_1B$$

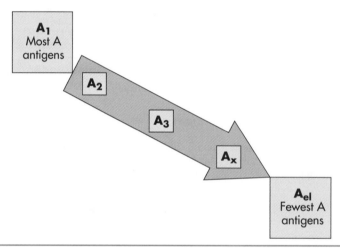

Most
H antigens   Fewest
                                              H antigens

Fig. 4-6   Variation of H-antigen concentrations in ABO phenotypes. Group O red cells possess the most H antigens; group A_1B red cells possess the fewest H antigens.

A_1
Most A
antigens

A_2

A_3

A_x

A_{el}
Fewest A
antigens

Fig. 4-7   Gradient of the subgroups of A: number of A antigen sites per red cell. Red cells classified as subgroups of A possess fewer A antigens than the A_1 phenotype.

ABO SUBGROUPS

Comparison of A_1 and A_2 Phenotypes

The ABO phenotypes can be divided into categories termed subgroups. Subgroups differ in the amount of antigen expressed on the red cell membrane, representing a quantitative difference in antigen expression (Fig. 4-7). Some evidence also exists to support the theory of qualitative differences in antigen expression. Some subgroups possess more highly branched, complex antigenic structures, whereas others have simplified linear forms of antigen.[12]

The group A phenotype is classified into two major subgroups: A_1 and A_2. These glycosyltransferase gene products, which are genetically controlled by the A^1 and A^2 genes differ slightly in their ability to convert H antigen to A antigen. The A_1 phenotype, encoded by the A^1 gene, exists in about 80% of group A individuals. In the A_1 phenotype, A antigens are highly concentrated on branched and linear oligosaccharide chains. The A^1 gene effectively acts on the H antigens in the production of A antigens. The A_2 phenotype, encoded by the A^2 gene, constitutes about 20% of group A individuals. In the A_2 phenotype, A-antigen copies are fewer than in the A_1 phenotype. This phenotype is assembled on the simplified linear forms of the oligosaccharide chains. An alloantibody, anti-A_1, can be detected in 1% to 8% of A_2 individuals and in 22% to 35% of A_2B individuals.

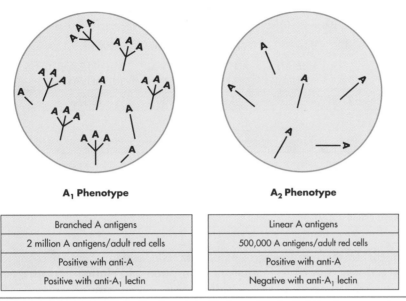

Fig. 4-8 Comparison of A_1 and A_2 red cells. (From Issitt PD, Anstee DJ: *Applied blood group serology*, ed 4, Durham, NC, 1998, Montgomery Scientific Publications.)

In routine ABO phenotyping, both A_1 and A_2 red cells agglutinate with commercially available anti-A reagents. These red cells can be distinguished in serologic testing only with a reagent called *Dolichos biflorus* lectin. This lectin is extracted from the seeds of the plant *Dolichos biflorus* and possesses anti-A_1 specificity. When properly diluted, the *Dolichos biflorus* lectin (anti-A_1 lectin) agglutinates A_1, but not A_2, red cells. The anti-A_1 lectin is not used in routine ABO testing of donors and recipients because it is unnecessary to distinguish between the A_1 and A_2 phenotypes for transfusion purposes. This reagent is useful in resolving ABO typing problems and identifying infrequent subgroups of A. Fig. 4-8 compares the A_1 and A_2 phenotypes.

Additional Subgroups of A and B

Subgroups of A

Although more infrequent than A_1 and A_2, other A subgroups have been described that involve reduced expression of A antigens. The decreased number of A antigen sites per red cell result in weak or no agglutination when tested with commercial anti-A reagents. The subgroups are genetically controlled by the inheritance of rare alleles at the *ABO* locus and collectively occur at less than 1% frequency. Because these subgroups occur so infrequently, they are mainly of academic interest. The A subgroups have been classified as A_{int}, A_3, A_x, A_m, A_{end}, A_{el}, and A_{bantu}, based on the reactivity of red cells with human anti-A and anti-A,B. Historically, human polyclonal-based anti-A,B contained an antibody with specificity toward both the A and the B antigens that could not be separated into anti-A and anti-B components. This reagent possessed an enhanced ability to detect weaker subgroups compared with anti-A. Current anti-A,B monoclonal antibody reagents blend anti-A and anti-B clones for formulations to detect the weaker subgroups.

Weak or no agglutination with commercial anti-A monoclonal antibody reagents is a key factor in recognizing a subgroup in this category. Murine monoclonal blends of commercial anti-A have been formulated to enhance the detection of these weaker subgroups in ABO phenotyping. These monoclonal antibody anti-A reagents are blended to ensure that some subgroups of A are readily detected. Some subgroups may characteristically demonstrate **mixed-field agglutination** patterns (e.g., A_3 subgroup) or possess anti-A_1 in the serum (e.g., A_3, A_x, and A_{el} subgroups).[13] Some subgroups of A continue to react weakly or not react with murine monoclonal blends of anti-A. In these circumstances, saliva studies for the detection of soluble forms of A and H antigens and testing with anti-H lectin *(Ulex europaeus)* may provide additional information. The amount of H

Dolichos biflorus: plant lectin with specificity for the A_1 antigen.

A_1 and A_2 phenotypes demonstrate 3+ to 4+ reactions with commercial anti-A reagents.

Anti-A_1 lectin agglutinates *only* A_1 red cells. This lectin is used to distinguish the A_1 and A_2 phenotypes in resolving ABO typing problems when A_2 phenotypes develop anti-A_1.

Mixed-field agglutination: agglutination pattern in which a population of the red cells has agglutinated and the remainder of the red cells are unagglutinated.

Ulex europaeus: plant lectin with specificity for the H antigen.

TABLE 4-3	Serologic Characteristics of A_3, A_x, and A_{el} Subgroups					
			RED CELL AGGLUTINATION WITH			
SUBGROUP	ANTI-A	HUMAN ANTI-A,B	ANTI-H LECTIN*	ANTI-A₁ LECTIN†	SOLUBLE ANTIGENS IN SALIVA‡	ANTI-A₁ IN SERUM
A_3	++mf	++mf	+++	0	A and H	0 to ++§
A_x	weak/0	+ to ++	++++	0	H	0 to ++§
A_{el}	0	0	++++	0	H	0 to ++§

mf, Mixed field.
**Ulex europaeus.*
†*Dolichos biflorus.*
‡If secretor.
§Variable occurrence of anti-A₁.

Adsorption: immunohematologic technique that uses red cells (known antigens) to remove red cell antibodies from a solution (plasma or antisera); group A red cells can remove anti-A from solution.

Elution: process that dissociates antigen-antibody complexes on red cells; freed IgG antibody is tested for specificity.

antigen present on the weak subgroups of A is usually equivalent to group O red cells (3+ to 4+ reactions). Special techniques of **adsorption** and **elution** may also be necessary to demonstrate the presence of the A antigen (e.g., A_{el} subgroup). However, these techniques are not performed routinely.

The serologic classification of rare A subgroups is determined by the following:
• Weak or no red cell agglutination with anti-A and anti-A,B commercial reagents
• No agglutination with anti-A₁
• Presence or absence of anti-A₁ in the serum
• Strong agglutination reactions with anti-H
• Presence of A and H in saliva
• Adsorption and elution studies

Table 4-3 provides information regarding the serologic characteristics of A_3, A_x, and A_{el} subgroups.[10] Weak subgroups of A are difficult to classify using serologic techniques. Usually the phenotype is described as A subgroup or A subgroup B. For definitive classification, molecular techniques are available to characterize the genotype, if necessary. For an in-depth presentation of the other subgroups, the reader is referred to the Suggested Readings.

Subgroups of B

B subgroups are rarer than the A subgroups. The criteria for the recognition and differentiation of these subgroups are similar to criteria of the A subgroups. Typically, these subgroups demonstrate weak or no agglutination of red cells with anti-B reagents.

Importance of Subgroup Identification in Donor Testing

Although subgroups of A and B are considered to be of academic interest, the failure to detect a weak subgroup could have serious consequences. If a weak subgroup is missed in a recipient (the individual receiving the transfusion), the recipient would be classified as group O. Classification as a group O rather than a weak subgroup would probably not harm the recipient because group O red cells would be selected for transfusion and can be transfused to any ABO phenotype. However, an error in donor phenotyping and the subsequent labeling of the donor unit as group O (rather than group A) might result in the decreased survival of the transfused cells in a group O recipient. Group O recipients would possess ABO antibodies capable of reacting with the weak subgroup antigens in vivo, resulting in the decreased survival of these transfused red cells in the recipient's circulation.

SECTION 3

GENETIC FEATURES OF ABO BLOOD GROUP SYSTEM

Inheritance of genes from the *ABO* locus on chromosome 9 follows the laws of Mendelian genetics. An individual inherits two *ABO* genes (one from each parent). The three major alleles of the ABO blood group system are *A*, *B*, and *O*. The *A* gene subsequently can be divided into the A^1 and A^2 alleles. The *A* and *B* genes express a codominant mode of inheritance, whereas the O allele is recessive. The A^1 allele is dominant over the A^2 allele, and both alleles are dominant over the O allele. The major ABO phenotypes and possible corresponding genotypes for the phenotypes are outlined in Table 4-4. Correct use of terminology regarding the ABO blood group system should be mentioned. When reference is made to the alleles A^1 and A^2, the numbers are always indicated as superscripts. In references to the A_1 and A_2 phenotypes, the numbers are always indicated in a subscript format.

Because the O allele is recessive, it is not always possible to determine the ABO genotype from the corresponding phenotype without family studies or molecular analysis. Red cells can be phenotyped only for the presence or absence of antigens and cannot be genotyped. Unless a family study has been performed with conclusive results, a genotype is only a probable interpretation of a phenotype. Deduction of the genotype from a family study is illustrated in Fig. 4-9. The Generation I female's phenotype is group B with possible genotypes of *BB* or *BO*, and the male's phenotype is group A with possible genotypes of *AA* or *AO*. The parental genotypes may be deduced only after phenotyping the offspring. The four offspring's phenotypes are presented in Generation II. To produce a group O offspring, both parents must have passed on the O allele. Therefore their genotypes must be *AO* and *BO*.

TABLE 4-4	ABO Phenotypes and Possible Genotypes
PHENOTYPE	**POSSIBLE GENOTYPES**
Group A_1	A^1A^1
	A^1A^2
	A^1O
Group A_2	A^2A^2
	A^2O
Group B	BB
	BO
Group A_1B	A^1B
Group A_2B	A^2B
Group O	OO

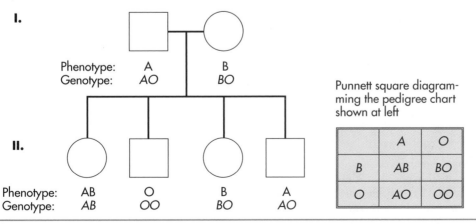

Fig. 4-9 Practical application: ABO inheritance patterns. Group A and group B phenotypes may produce offspring with group AB, O, B, and A phenotypes if the parents' genotypes are AO and BO.

SECTION 4

ABO BLOOD GROUP SYSTEM ANTIBODIES

As Landsteiner recognized in his early experiments, individuals possess the ABO antibody in their serum directed against the ABO antigen absent from their red cells. Landsteiner's rule remains an important consideration in the selection of blood products given that ABO antibodies exist in healthy individuals. These ABO antibodies, present in individuals with no known exposure to blood or blood products, were originally thought to be "naturally occurring." The current hypothesis is that biochemical structures similar to A and B antigens are present in the environment in bacteria, plants, and pollen. As a result of this environmental exposure to these similar forms of A and B antigens, individuals respond immunologically to these antigens and produce ABO antibodies detectable in plasma and serum.[14] Consequently, the term naturally occurring is a misnomer because an immunologic stimulus is present for antibody development. The term **non–red blood cell stimulated** is more appropriate for describing the ABO antibodies.

Newborns do not produce their own ABO antibodies until they are 3 to 6 months of age. ABO antibodies detected prior to this time are maternal in origin. Maximal ABO **titers** have been reported in children 5 to 10 years old. As a person ages, the ABO titers tend to decrease and may cause problems in ABO phenotyping. In addition to newborns and older patients, other situations exist where ABO antibody titers may be weak or not demonstrable in testing (Table 4-5).[15] Recognition of these circumstances can assist in resolving ABO phenotyping problems discussed later in this chapter.

GENERAL CHARACTERISTICS OF HUMAN ANTI-A AND ANTI-B

Immunoglobulin Class

The anti-A produced in group B individuals and the anti-B produced in group A individuals contain primarily antibodies of the IgM class along with small amounts of IgG. In contrast, anti-A and anti-B antibodies found in the serum of group O individuals are composed primarily of IgG class.

Hemolytic Properties and Clinical Significance

IgG and IgM forms of anti-A and anti-B are capable of the activation and binding of complement and eventual hemolysis of red cells in vivo or in vitro. Because of their ability to activate the complement cascade with resultant red cell hemolysis, the ABO antibodies are considered of **clinical significance** in transfusion medicine. An antigen-antibody reaction between a recipient's ABO antibody and the ABO phenotype of the transfused red cells can cause activation of complement and destruction of the transfused donor red cells, precipitating the clinical signs and symptoms of an acute hemolytic transfusion reaction. For example, a group A recipient has circulating anti-B antibodies in serum. If this individual is transfused with group B or AB donor red cells, the circulating anti-B would recognize the B antigen on the donor red cells and combine with the antigens. The

Non–red blood cell stimulated: immunologic stimulus for antibody production is unrelated to a red cell antigen.

Titers: extent to which an antibody may be diluted before it loses its ability to agglutinate with antigen.

Clinical significance: antibodies capable of causing decreased survival of transfused cells as in a transfusion reaction; have been associated with hemolytic disease of the fetus and newborn.

Congenital hypogammaglobulinemia: genetic disease characterized by reduced levels of gamma globulin in the blood.

Acquired hypogammaglobulinemia: lower than normal levels of gamma globulin in the blood associated with malignant diseases (chronic leukemias and myeloma) and immunosuppressive therapy.

Congenital agammaglobulinemia: genetic disease characterized by the absence of gamma globulin and antibodies in the blood.

Acquired agammaglobulinemia: absence of gamma globulin and antibodies associated with malignant diseases such as leukemia, myeloma, or lymphoma.

TABLE 4-5	Reduction in ABO Antibody Titers
Age-Related	
Newborn	
Elderly	
Pathologic Etiology	
Chronic lymphocytic leukemia	
Congenital hypogammaglobulinemia or **acquired hypogammaglobulinemia**	
Congenital agammaglobulinemia or **acquired agammaglobulinemia**	
Immunosuppressive therapy	
Bone marrow transplant	
Multiple myeloma	

complement system is readily activated, causing a decreased survival of transfused red cells.

In Vitro Serologic Reactions

ABO antibodies directly agglutinate a suspension of red cells in a physiologic saline environment and do not require any additional potentiators. They are optimally reactive in immediate-spin phases at room temperature (15° C to 25° C). The agglutination reactions do not require an incubation period and react without delay on centrifugation.

Anti-A and anti-B react in immediate-spin phases (direct agglutination reactions).

HUMAN ANTI-A,B FROM GROUP O INDIVIDUALS

Human anti-A,B is detected in the serum of group O individuals and possesses unique activities beyond mixtures of anti-A and anti-B antibodies. Activity of human anti-A,B is regarded as a specificity that is cross-reactive with both A and B antigens. A cross-reactive antibody is capable of recognizing a particular molecular structure (antigenic determinant) common to several molecules. This distinguishing characteristic enables the antibody to agglutinate with red cells of group A, B, and AB phenotype because this antibody recognizes a structure shared by both A and B antigens. Human anti-A,B also manifests the property of agglutinating red cells of infrequent subgroups of A, particularly A_x. Before the advent of monoclonal reagents, human anti-A,B was widely used to detect these infrequent subgroups in routine ABO typing. Monoclonal antibody reagents have since replaced the use of human anti-A,B in ABO phenotyping.

ANTI-A₁

In accordance with Landsteiner's rule for expected ABO antibodies, sera from group O and B individuals contain anti-A antibodies. The anti-A produced by group O and B individuals can be separated by adsorption and elution techniques into two components: anti-A and anti-A_1. Anti-A_1 is specific for the A_1 antigen and does not agglutinate A_2 red cells. The optimal reactivity of this antibody is at room temperature or lower. Anti-A_1 is not considered clinically significant for transfusion purposes. Anti-A_1 becomes a concern when it causes problems with ABO phenotyping results and **incompatible crossmatches** on immediate spin. Anti-A_2 does not exist because the A_2 phenotype possesses the same A antigens as A_1 phenotype but in reduced quantities. Individuals with A_1 phenotype do not respond immunologically when exposed to A_2 red cells.

Incompatible crossmatches: occur when agglutination or hemolysis is observed in the crossmatch of donor red cells and patient serum, indicating a serologic incompatibility. The donor unit would not be transfused.

Donor blood samples are routinely typed at the time of donation. The ABO-labeled red blood cell (RBC) donor units are confirmatory typed on receipt at the hospital transfusion service.

SECTION 5
ABO BLOOD GROUP SYSTEM AND TRANSFUSION

ROUTINE ABO PHENOTYPING

A fundamental procedure of immunohematologic testing is the determination of the ABO phenotype. The procedure is straightforward and is divided into two components: testing of the red cells for the presence of ABO antigens (or forward grouping) and testing of serum or plasma for the expected ABO antibodies (or reverse grouping). According to the *Standards for Blood Banks and Transfusion Services*, donor and recipient red cells must be tested using anti-A and anti-B reagents. Donor and recipient serum or plasma must be tested for the expected ABO antibodies using reagent A_1 and B red cells.[15] Neither human anti-A,B nor the monoclonal blend anti-A,B is required in ABO typing. Testing of cord blood and samples from infants younger than 4 months requires only red cell testing in ABO phenotyping because ABO antibody levels are not detectable.

The ABO phenotype is determined when the red cells are directly tested for the presence or absence of either A or B antigens. Serum testing provides a control for red cell testing because ABO antibodies would reflect Landsteiner's rule. Table 4-6 shows the expected reactions observed in ABO phenotyping. An **ABO discrepancy** occurs when red cell testing does not agree with the expected serum testing. Any discrepancy in ABO testing should be resolved before transfusion of recipients or labeling of donor units.

The procedure for ABO phenotyping is presented in the *Laboratory Manual* that accompanies this textbook.

Reverse grouping (serum or plasma testing) is not required for confirmatory testing of labeled, previously typed donor RBCs and in infants younger than 4 months of age.

ABO discrepancy: occurs when ABO phenotyping of red cells does not agree with expected serum testing results for the particular ABO phenotype.

Review the sections in Chapter 2 on ABO typing reagents.

TABLE 4-6   ABO Phenotype Reactions

| | RED CELL REACTIONS WITH | | SERUM OR PLASMA REACTIONS WITH | |
PHENOTYPE	ANTI-A	ANTI-B	A₁ CELLS	B CELLS
Group A	+	0	0	+
Group B	0	+	+	0
Group O	0	0	+	+
Group AB	+	+	0	0

+, Agglutination; *0*, no agglutination.

Agglutination reactions for ABO typing are usually 3+ to 4+ in strength.

TABLE 4-7   Practical Application: ABO Compatibility for Whole Blood, Red Blood Cells, and Plasma Transfusions

| RECIPIENT | DONOR | | |
ABO PHENOTYPE	WHOLE BLOOD	RED BLOOD CELLS	PLASMA
Group A	Group A	Groups A, O	Groups A, AB
Group B	Group B	Groups B, O	Groups B, AB
Group AB	Group AB	Groups AB, A, B, O	Group AB
Group O	Group O	Group O	Groups O, A, B, AB

SELECTION OF ABO-COMPATIBLE RED BLOOD CELLS AND PLASMA PRODUCTS FOR TRANSFUSION

In routine transfusion practices, donor products (RBCs and plasma) with identical ABO phenotypes are usually available to the recipient. This transfusion selection is referred to as providing ABO-identical (ABO group–specific) blood for the intended recipient. In situations where blood of identical ABO phenotype is unavailable, ABO-compatible (ABO group–compatible) blood may be issued to the recipient.

For RBC transfusions, ABO compatibility between the recipient and the donor is defined as the serologic compatibility between the ABO antibodies present in the recipient's serum and the ABO antigens expressed on the donor's red cells. For example, a group A recipient who concurrently demonstrates anti-B in serum would be compatible with either group A or group O donor red cells because serum anti-B would not react with either the group A or the group O red cells in vivo. However, if this individual receives a transfusion with either group B or group AB donor red cells, recipient anti-B antibodies would recognize the B antigens present on the red cells. Antigen-antibody complexes form, may activate the complement cascade, and result in the signs and symptoms of an acute hemolytic transfusion reaction. ABO compatibility applies to RBC transfusions but not to transfusions of whole blood. When whole blood is transfused, ABO-identical donor units must be provided because both plasma and red cells are present in the product. The concepts of ABO compatibility for whole blood and RBC transfusions are outlined in Table 4-7.

Persons with group O red cells are called **universal donors** because the RBC product lacks both A and B antigens and could be transfused to any ABO phenotype. Group O donor RBCs can be used in times of urgency for emergency release of donor units. Conversely, group AB recipients are considered **universal recipients** because these individuals lack circulating ABO antibodies and can receive RBCs of any ABO phenotype.

When plasma products are transfused, the selection of an ABO-identical phenotype is the ideal situation. When identical ABO phenotypes are unavailable, the rationale for compatible plasma transfusions is the reverse of RBC transfusions. In this case, the

Universal donors: group O donors for RBC transfusions; these RBCs may be transfused to any ABO phenotype because the cells lack both A and B antigens.

Universal recipients: group AB recipients may receive transfusions of RBCs from any ABO phenotype; these recipients lack circulating ABO antibodies in plasma.

donor's plasma must be compatible with the recipient's red cells. This concept translates to the serologic compatibility between the ABO antibodies in the donor unit with the ABO antigens present on the recipient's red cells. Group A recipients needing plasma would be compatible with group A and AB plasma products. Because group A plasma contains anti-B, and group AB has no ABO antibodies, these plasma products do not recognize the A antigen on recipient red cells. No adverse antigen-antibody reaction would ensue. For the transfusion of plasma, group AB is considered the universal donor and group O is the universal recipient (see Table 4-7).

> Universal donor for RBC transfusions is group O; universal donor for plasma transfusions is group AB.

> Universal recipient for RBC transfusions is group AB; universal recipient for plasma transfusions is group O.

SECTION 6
RECOGNITION AND RESOLUTION OF ABO DISCREPANCIES

The recognition and resolution of ABO discrepancies are challenging aspects of problem solving in the blood bank. As defined in a previous section, an ABO discrepancy is an ABO phenotype in which the results of the red cell testing do not agree with the results of expected serum testing. Discrepancies may be indicated when the following observations are noted in the results of ABO phenotyping:

* Agglutination strengths of the typing reactions are weaker than expected. Typically, the reactions in ABO red cell testing with anti-A and anti-B reagents are 3+ to 4+ agglutination reactions; the results of ABO serum testing with reagent A_1 and B cells are 2+ to 4+.
* Expected reactions in ABO red cell testing and serum testing are missing (e.g., group O individual is missing one or both reactions in serum testing with reagent A_1 and B cells).
* Extra reactions are noted in either the ABO red cell or serum tests.

   The source of these discrepancies can be either technical or sample-related problems. The first step in the resolution of an ABO discrepancy is to identify the source of the problem. Is the discrepancy a technical error in testing, or is the discrepancy related to the sample itself?

TECHNICAL CONSIDERATIONS IN ABO PHENOTYPING

Several types of technical errors can transpire in ABO typing and lead to erroneous results. An awareness and recognition of these technical errors can assist in the resolution of an ABO discrepancy. These technical errors can be classified into several categories, including identification and documentation errors, reagent and equipment problems, and standard operating procedure errors. By following the guidelines outlined in Table 4-8, technical

TABLE 4-8	Practical Application: Guidelines for Investigating ABO Technical Errors
Identification or Documentation Errors	
Correct sample identification on all tubes	
Results are properly recorded	
Interpretations are accurate and properly recorded	
Reagent or Equipment Errors	
Daily quality control on ABO typing reagents is satisfactory	
Inspect reagents for contamination and hemolysis	
Centrifugation time and calibration are confirmed	
Standard Operating Procedure Errors	
Procedure follows manufacturer's directions	
Correct reagents were used and added to testing	
Red blood cell suspensions are at the correct concentration	
Cell buttons are completely suspended before grading the reaction	

sources of error can be pinpointed more readily. A new sample can be obtained to eliminate possible contamination or identification problems. In addition, red cell suspensions prepared from patient samples can be washed three times before repeated testing. When a technical error is discovered and corrected, the ABO discrepancy can be quickly resolved with repeated testing. If the discrepancy still exists after repeated testing, the possibility of a problem related to the sample itself (e.g., related to the patient or donor) should be considered.

SAMPLE-RELATED ABO DISCREPANCIES

Sample-related problems can be divided into two groups: ABO discrepancies that affect the ABO red cell testing and discrepancies that affect the ABO serum or plasma testing. Is the problem associated with the patient or donor red cells, or is it associated with patient or donor antibodies? A logical approach to solving these sample-related problems is to select the side of the ABO test (red cell testing or serum or plasma testing) believed to be discrepant and to focus on the problem from this angle. The observed strengths of agglutination reactions in the testing of both the red cells and the serum or plasma are keys in determining whether to focus problem solving on a red cell or a serum/plasma problem. For success with this approach, a working knowledge of the multitude of potential problems relating to ABO red cell and serum testing is mandatory (Table 4-9). The most commonly encountered ABO discrepancies in the immunohematology laboratory are discrepancies relating to weak or missing ABO antibodies in serum/plasma testing. ABO discrepancies associated with red cell testing are reviewed first followed by discussion of discrepancies associated with serum/plasma testing.

ABO Discrepancies Associated with Red Cell Testing

ABO discrepancies that affect the testing of red cells (forward grouping) can be classified into three categories: extra antigens present, missing or weak antigens, and mixed-field reactions.

Extra Antigens Present

ABO red cell typing results may demonstrate unexpected positive agglutination reactions with commercial anti-A or anti-B reagents. Extra reactions are present in red cell testing or forward grouping. For the purposes of this textbook, the scope of the discussion on

TABLE 4-9 Overviews of ABO Discrepancies	
PROBLEMS WITH RED CELL TESTING	**PROBLEMS WITH SERUM/PLASMA TESTING**
Extra antigens	Extra antibodies
Group A with acquired B antigen	A subgroups with anti-A_1
B(A) phenotype	Cold alloantibodies
Polyagglutination	Cold autoantibodies
Rouleaux	Rouleaux
Hematopoietic progenitor cell transplants	IVIG
Missing or weak antigens	Missing or weak antibodies
ABO subgroup	Newborn
Pathologic etiology	Elderly
Transplantation	Pathologic etiology
	Immunosuppressive therapy for transplantation
Mixed-field reactions	
Transfusion of group O to group A, B, or AB	
Hematopoietic progenitor stem cell transplants	
A_3 phenotype	

IVIG, Intravenous immunoglobulin.

extra antigens in red cell testing is limited to the illustration of the **group A with acquired B antigen** and the **B(A) phenotype.**

Examples 1 and 2 follow to demonstrate extra antigens present with the acquired B and B(A) phenotype.

EXAMPLE 1

Group A with Acquired B Antigen			
ABO Testing Results			
Patient Red Cells with		Patient Serum with Reagent Red Cells	
Anti-A	Anti-B	A_1	B
4+	1+	0	4+

EVALUATION OF ABO TESTING RESULTS
1. The agglutination of the patient's red cells with anti-A is strong (4+).
2. The agglutination of the patient's red cells with anti-B is weaker (1+) than usually expected (3+ to 4+).
3. These red cells react as the phenotype group AB.
4. The results of serum testing reactions are typical of a group A individual.

CONCLUSION
These reactions are typical of individuals possessing the acquired B antigen. In group A acquired B antigen, a group A individual possesses an extra antigen in red cell testing (notice the weaker agglutination with anti-B reagents). Anti-B is observed in the serum testing. Serum testing reactions are typical for a group A individual.

BACKGROUND INFORMATION
Usually only group A_1 individuals with diseases of the lower gastrointestinal tract, cancers of the colon and rectum, intestinal obstruction, or gram-negative septicemia express the acquired B antigen. The most common mechanism for this phenotype is usually associated with a bacterial **deacetylating** enzyme that alters the A immunodominant sugar, N-acetylgalactosamine, by removing the acetyl group. The resulting sugar, galactosamine, resembles the B immunodominant sugar, D-galactose, and cross-reacts with many anti-B reagents.[16]

In the early 1990s, an increase in the detection of acquired B antigen with certain monoclonal anti-B blood grouping reagents licensed by the U.S. Food and Drug Administration was observed.[17] The observation was linked to the use of ES-4 monoclonal anti-B clone at pH levels of 6.5 to 7.0. If the formulation of the clone was acidified to pH 6.0, the acquired B antigen was not observed.

Red cells agglutinated strongly by anti-A and weakly by anti-B in combination with a serum containing anti-B suggest the acquired B antigen. These patients should receive units of group A red cells for transfusion purposes.

RESOLUTION OF ABO DISCREPANCY
1. Determine the patient's diagnosis and transfusion history. The first step in the resolution of any ABO discrepancy is to obtain more information about the patient. This information may provide additional clues about the root cause of the ABO discrepancy.
2. Test the patient's serum against **autologous** red cells. Anti-B in the patient's serum does not agglutinate autologous red cells with the acquired B antigen.
3. Test red cells with additional monoclonal anti-B reagents from other manufacturers that are documented not to react with the acquired B antigen or a source of human polyclonal anti-B.

Group A with acquired B antigen: group A_1 individual with disease of the lower gastrointestinal tract, cancer of the colon and rectum, intestinal obstruction, or gram-negative septicemia who acquires reactivity with anti-B reagents in ABO red cell testing and appears as group AB.

B(A) phenotype: group B individual who acquires reactivity with anti-A reagents in ABO red cell testing; in these individuals, the B gene transfers trace amounts of the immunodominant sugar for the A antigen and the immunodominant sugar for the B antigen.

Deacetylating: removal of the acetyl group (CH_3CO-).

Autologous: pertaining to self.

EXAMPLE 2

|---|---|---|---|
| Anti-A | Anti-B | A₁ | B |
B(A) Phenotype			
ABO Testing Results			
Patient Red Cells with		Patient Serum with Reagent Red Cells	
Anti-A	Anti-B	A_1	B
1+	4+	4+	0

EVALUATION OF ABO TESTING RESULTS
1. The agglutination of the patient's red cells with anti-A is weak (1+).
2. The agglutination of the patient's red cells with anti-B is strong (4+).
3. The results of serum testing are typical of a group B individual.

CONCLUSION
These reactions are characteristic of a possible B(A) phenotype. In the B(A) phenotype, a group B with an apparent extra antigen reaction is observed with anti-A in red cell testing.

BACKGROUND INFORMATION
The B(A) phenotype has been observed as a result of the increased sensitivity of potent monoclonal antibody reagents for ABO phenotyping.[18] These reagents can detect trace amounts of either A or B antigens that are nonspecifically transferred by the glycosyltransferase enzymes. In the B(A) phenotype, the *B* gene transfers trace amounts of the immunodominant sugar for the A antigen (*N*-acetylgalactosamine) and the immunodominant sugar for the B antigen (D-galactose) to the H-antigen acceptor molecules. The trace amounts of A antigens are detected with certain clones from the monoclonal antibody reagents. A similar mechanism can cause an A(B) phenotype analogous to the acquired B antigen.

RESOLUTION OF ABO DISCREPANCY
1. Determine the patient's diagnosis and transfusion history.
2. Test red cells with additional monoclonal antibody anti-A reagents from other manufacturers or a source of human polyclonal anti-A.

Other potential explanations for extra antigens in ABO red cell testing include the following:

a. **Polyagglutination** of red cells by most human sera as a result of the exposure of a hidden antigen on the red cell membrane because of a bacterial infection or genetic mutation. ABO discrepancies caused by polyagglutination are rarely detected because of the routine use of monoclonal antibody reagents, which have replaced human-derived ABO antisera.

b. Nonspecific aggregation of serum-suspended red cells because of abnormal concentrations of serum proteins or **Wharton's jelly** in cord blood samples (false-positive agglutination)

Polyagglutination: property of cells that causes them to be agglutinated by naturally occurring antibodies found in most human sera; agglutination occurs regardless of blood type.

Wharton's jelly: gelatinous tissue contaminant in cord blood samples that may interfere in immunohematologic tests.

Missing or Weakly Expressed Antigens

In the category of ABO discrepancies concerning missing or weakly expressed antigens, patient or donor red cells demonstrate weaker than usual reactions with reagent anti-A and anti-B or may fail to demonstrate any reactivity. Phenomena associated with this category include the following:

- ABO subgroups
- Weakened A and B antigen expression in patients with leukemia or Hodgkin's disease

Example 3 illustrates missing or weakly expressed antigens by presenting an ABO discrepancy typically observed with a subgroup of A.

EXAMPLE 3

Subgroup of A			
ABO Testing Results			
Patient Red Cells with		Patient Serum with Reagent Red Cells	
Anti-A	Anti-B	A₁	B
0	0	0	3+

EVALUATION OF ABO TESTING RESULTS

1. No agglutination of the patient's red cells with both anti-A and anti-B reagents is observed. The individual appears to be a group O phenotype.
2. The results of serum testing are typical of a group A individual. Agglutination of anti-B with reagent B red cells is strong (3+).

CONCLUSION

These reactions are characteristic of a missing antigen in the red cell testing. The serum testing results are those expected in a group A individual. Anti-A, found in group O individuals, is absent in the serum testing.

BACKGROUND INFORMATION

As previously discussed in this chapter, weak or missing reactions with anti-A and anti-B reagents correlate with subgroups of A and B. Subgroups of A represent less than 1% of the group A population, and the subgroups of B are even rarer. Inheritance of an alternative allele at the *ABO* locus results in a quantitative reduction of antigen sites per red cell and in weakened or missing reactions with anti-A and anti-B reagents.

RESOLUTION OF ABO DISCREPANCY

1. Determine the patient's diagnosis and transfusion history.
2. Repeat the red cell testing with extended incubation times and include human polyclonal anti-A,B or monoclonal blend anti-A,B. The extended incubation time may enhance the antigen-antibody reaction.

Additional Testing Results	
	Anti-A,B
Patient red cells	1+
Conclusion: Probable subgroup of A	

Additional Testing Results	
	Anti-A,B
Patient red cells	0
Next Step: Perform adsorption and elution studies with anti-A; these studies assist in determining the presence of A antigens on the patient's red cells	

Mixed-Field Reactions

Mixed-field reactions can occur in red cell testing with either anti-A or anti-B reagents. As noted earlier, a mixed-field reaction contains agglutinates with a mass of unagglutinated red cells. Usually a mixed-field reaction is due to the presence of two distinct cell populations. For example, testing red cells from a patient recently transfused with non–ABO-identical RBCs (group O donor RBCs to a group AB recipient) can yield mixed-field observations. In addition to the transfusion of group O RBCs to group A, B, or AB individuals, recipients of **hematopoietic progenitor transplants**, individuals with the A₃

Hematopoietic progenitor cell transplant: replacement of hematopoietic stem cells derived from allogeneic bone marrow, peripheral stem cells, or cord blood to treat certain leukemias, immunodeficiencies, and hemoglobinopathies.

Tn-polyagglutinable red cells:
type of polyagglutination that
occurs from a mutation in
the hematopoietic tissue,
characterized by mixed-field
reactions in agglutination testing.

The transfusion of red cell
donor units or stem cell
transplants can cause
mixed-field reactions. They are
called artificially induced
chimerisms.

phenotype, and patients with **Tn-polyagglutinable red cells** can demonstrate mixed-field reactions. Example 4 illustrates an ABO discrepancy showing mixed-field reactions.

EXAMPLE 4

Group B Patient Transfused with Group O RBCs			
ABO Testing Results			
Patient Red Cells with		**Patient Serum with Reagent Red Cells**	
Anti-A	**Anti-B**	**A₁**	**B**
0	2+mf	4+	0

mf, Mixed field.

EVALUATION OF ABO TESTING RESULTS
1. The strength of the agglutination reaction with anti-B is weaker than expected for group B individuals.
2. The anti-B mixed-field grading of reactivity is a 2+ reaction with a sufficient number of unagglutinated cells.
3. The results of serum testing are typical of a group B individual.

CONCLUSION
These results demonstrate a group B individual possibly transfused with group O RBCs.

BACKGROUND INFORMATION
In certain situations, ABO-identical RBC products might not be available for transfusion, and group O RBC products are transfused. If many group O donor RBC units are transfused in respect to the recipient's total body mass, mixed-field reactions may appear in the ABO red cell testing.

RESOLUTION OF ABO DISCREPANCY
1. Determine the patient's diagnosis and recent transfusion history.
2. Determine whether the patient is a recent hematopoietic progenitor cell recipient.
3. Investigate pretransfusion ABO phenotype history, if possible.

ABO Discrepancies Associated with Serum or Plasma Testing
ABO discrepancies that affect serum or plasma testing (reverse grouping) include the presence of additional antibodies other than anti-A and anti-B or the absence of expected ABO antibody reactions. The most commonly encountered ABO discrepancies involve the absence of expected ABO antibody reactions.

Cold alloantibodies: red cell
antibodies specific for other
human red cell antigens that
typically react at or below room
temperature.

Cold autoantibodies: red cell
antibodies specific for autologous
antigens that typically react at or
below room temperature.

Additional Antibodies in Serum or Plasma Testing
This section of ABO discrepancies addresses the detection of anti-A₁, **cold alloantibodies, cold autoantibodies,** and rouleaux in ABO typing. Example 5 is an illustration of group A₂ with anti-A₁. Example 6 illustrates a cold autoantibody and cold alloantibody. Example 7 illustrates rouleaux. In all of these situations, the ABO discrepancy manifests as additional antibodies in serum or plasma testing.

EXAMPLE 5

Group A₂ with Anti-A₁			
ABO Testing Results			
Patient Red Cells with		**Patient Serum with Reagent Red Cells**	
Anti-A	**Anti-B**	**A₁**	**B**
4+	0	2+	4+

EVALUATION OF ABO TESTING RESULTS

1. The agglutination pattern with anti-A and anti-B reagents is typical of a group A individual.
2. The results of serum testing with reagent A_1 and B red cells indicate a group O individual.

CONCLUSION

These results demonstrate an extra reaction in the serum testing with the reagent A_1 red cells (2+). Possible explanations for the extra reaction include an anti-A_1, a cold alloantibody, a cold autoantibody, or rouleaux. This example illustrates an ABO discrepancy resulting from group A_2 with anti-A_1.

RESOLUTION OF ABO DISCREPANCY

1. Determine the patient's diagnosis and transfusion history.
2. Test the patient's red cells with anti-A_1 lectin to ascertain whether a subgroup of A is present.

Additional Testing Results	
Patient Red Cells Tested with Anti-A_1 Lectin	Conclusion
0	Subgroup of A; suspect anti-A_1 antibody

3. Test the patient's serum with three examples of A_1 and A_2 reagent red cells to confirm the presence of anti-A_1 antibody.

Additional Testing Results					
Patient Serum Tested with					
A_1 Cells	A_1 Cells	A_1 Cells	A_2 Cells	A_2 Cells	A_2 Cells
2+	2+	2+	0	0	0

CONCLUSION

Agglutination is observed with A_1 red cells providing the evidence for anti-A_1. The serum does not agglutinate with A_2 red cells. Anti-A_1 may be present in 1% to 8% of the group A_2 phenotype.

EXAMPLE 6

Cold Autoantibody and Cold Alloantibody in Serum/Plasma Testing			
ABO Testing Results			
Patient Red Cells with		Patient Serum with Reagent Red Cells	
Anti-A	Anti-B	A_1	B
4+	4+	0	1+

EVALUATION OF ABO TESTING RESULTS

1. Strong agglutination reactions are observed in red cell testing and are consistent with a group AB individual.
2. The results of serum testing with reagent B red cells demonstrate a weaker extra reaction (1+). This serum testing appears to be consistent with a group A individual.

CONCLUSION

These results indicate a possible extra reaction in the serum testing with the reagent B red cells. Example 6 illustrates the presence of a cold alloantibody or a cold autoantibody.

BACKGROUND INFORMATION

Donors and patients may possess antibodies to other blood group system red cell antigens in addition to those of the ABO blood group system. These *alloantibodies* may appear as additional serum antibodies in ABO typing as one of the following specificities: anti-P_1, anti-M, anti-N, anti-Le^a, and anti-Le^b. Because they react at or below room temperature, these antibodies are sometimes referred to as *cold*. Reagent A_1 and B red cells used in ABO serum testing may possess these antigens in addition to the A and B antigens. Screening cells, which are group O reagent red cells, are used to detect an alloantibody because they lack A and B antigens. Any serum reactivity caused by an existing ABO antibody would be eliminated in the reaction with group O cells. It is logical to conclude that screening cells are valuable in distinguishing between ABO antibodies and alloantibodies.

Patients and donors may also possess serum antibodies directed toward their own red cell antigens. These antibodies are classified as autoantibodies. If autoantibodies are reactive at or below room temperature, they are also called *cold*. Cold autoantibodies usually possess the specificity of anti-I or anti-IH and react against all adult red cells, including screening cells, A_1 and B cells, and autologous cells. An **autocontrol** (autologous control) is tested to differentiate a cold autoantibody from a cold alloantibody. If the autocontrol is positive, the reactions observed with the A_1 and B cells and screening cells are probably the result of autoantibodies. See Chapter 7 for additional information on cold autoantibody test methods and techniques useful in negating their reactivity in ABO typing tests.

Autocontrol: testing a person's serum with his or her own red cells to determine whether an autoantibody is present.

RESOLUTION OF ABO DISCREPANCY

1. Determine the patient's diagnosis and transfusion history.
2. Test the patient's serum with screening cells and an autocontrol at room temperature. This strategy helps distinguish whether cold alloantibody or cold autoantibody is present.

Interpretation of Testing Results			
	Screening Cells	**Autologous Red Cells**	**Conclusion**
Patient serum	Pos*	Neg	Cold alloantibody
Patient serum	Pos	Pos	Cold autoantibody

*Positive reaction if the corresponding antigen is present on the screening cell.

3. If an alloantibody is detected, antibody identification techniques can be performed (see Chapter 7).
4. If an autoantibody is detected, special techniques to identify the antibody (a mini-cold panel) and remove antibody reactivity (prewarming techniques) can be used (see Chapter 7).

EXAMPLE 7

Rouleaux			
ABO Testing Results			
Patient Red Cells with		**Patient Serum with Reagent Red Cells**	
Anti-A	**Anti-B**	**A_1**	**B**
4+	4+	2+	2+

EVALUATION OF ABO TESTING RESULTS

1. Strong agglutination reactions are observed in red cell testing and are consistent with the expected results of a group AB individual.
2. Serum testing results are consistent with those of a group O individual.

CONCLUSION

Consider the possibility of extra reactions in serum testing with the reagent red cells because of an alloantibody, an autoantibody, or rouleaux. The phenomenon of rouleaux is demonstrated in this example.

BACKGROUND INFORMATION

Rouleaux can produce false-positive agglutination in testing. The red cells resemble stacked coins under microscopic examination. Increased concentrations of serum proteins can affect this spontaneous agglutination of red cells. Diseases associated with rouleaux include **multiple myeloma** and **Waldenström's macroglobulinemia.** In addition to creating problems with the serum testing in ABO phenotyping, rouleaux can create extra reactions in the ABO red cell typing if unwashed red cell suspensions are used.

RESOLUTION OF ABO DISCREPANCY

1. Determine the patient's diagnosis and transfusion history.
2. Wash red cell suspension and repeat the phenotyping.
3. Perform the **saline replacement technique** to help distinguish true agglutination from rouleaux (Fig. 4-10).

Missing or Weak ABO Antibodies in Serum or Plasma Testing

ABO antibodies may be missing or weakened in certain patient-related situations and may result in an ABO discrepancy. Example 8 illustrates this type of ABO discrepancy in serum/plasma testing.

Multiple myeloma: malignant neoplasm of the bone marrow characterized by abnormal proteins in the plasma and urine.

Waldenström's macroglobulinemia: overproduction of IgM by the clones of a plasma B cell in response to an antigenic signal; increased viscosity of blood is observed.

Saline replacement technique: test to distinguish rouleaux and true agglutination.

Missing or weak ABO antibodies in serum/plasma testing are the most commonly encountered ABO discrepancies.

Fig. 4-10   Saline replacement technique. Rouleaux causing false-positive reactions can be distinguished from agglutination through the use of this simple technique. (Modified from Mallory D: *Immunohematology methods and procedures,* Rockville, MD, 1993, American Red Cross.)

EXAMPLE 8

Missing or Weak ABO Antibodies in Serum or Plasma Testing			
ABO Testing Results			
Patient Red Cells with		Patient Serum with Reagent Red Cells	
Anti-A	Anti-B	A$_1$	B
0	0	0	0

EVALUATION OF ABO TESTING RESULTS

1. The agglutination pattern with anti-A and anti-B reagents is typical of a group O individual.
2. The results of serum testing with reagent A$_1$ and B red cells indicate a group AB individual.

CONCLUSION

Consider approaching this problem from the angle of missing serum reactions with reagent A$_1$ or B cells.

BACKGROUND INFORMATION

An investigation of the patient's history, including age, diagnosis, and immunoglobulin levels, provides clues to explaining the missing reactions in the serum testing. The patient's age is an important factor because the concentrations of ABO antibodies are reduced in newborns and elderly adults. Knowledge of the patient's diagnosis is essential; reduced immunoglobulin levels are also associated with several pathologic states (see Table 4-5). In conjunction with the patient's diagnosis, the immunoglobulin levels and serum protein electrophoretic patterns are helpful data in the resolution and identification of the root cause for this ABO discrepancy.

RESOLUTION OF ABO DISCREPANCY

1. Determine the patient's diagnosis, age, and immunoglobulin levels, if available.
2. Incubate serum testing for 15 minutes at room temperature, and then centrifuge and examine for agglutination. This simple incubation step often solves the problem. If the results are still negative, place the serum testing at 4° C for 5 minutes with an autologous control. The autologous control validates the test by ensuring that positive reactions are not attributable to a cold autoantibody.

Interpretation of Additional Testing Results				
4° C	A$_1$ Red Cells	B Red Cells	Autologous Red Cells	Conclusion
Patient serum	Pos	Pos	Neg	Group O
Patient serum	Pos	Pos	Pos	Cold autoantibody

SECTION 7

SPECIAL TOPICS RELATED TO ABO AND H BLOOD GROUP SYSTEMS

CLASSIC BOMBAY PHENOTYPE

The classic Bombay phenotype is an unusual genetic occurrence associated with the ABO and H blood group systems. A 1952 report describing a family living in Bombay, India, is the source of the descriptive term for the phenotype.[1] This family's red cells were unusual because they lacked H antigens and subsequently any ABO antigen expression. Both red cells and secretions were deficient in H and ABO antigen expression. The red cell reactions were characteristic of the group O phenotype in routine ABO testing. Serum testing demonstrated reactions similar to group O individuals. Another related antibody, anti-H, was detected in the family's serum in addition to the ABO antibodies of anti-A, anti-B, and anti-A,B. The anti-H in the Bombay phenotype is of clinical significance because this antibody is capable of high thermal activity at 37° C and complement activation with resulting hemolysis.

More than 130 Bombay phenotypes have been reported with a relatively greater incidence in India.[19] Genetic family studies have identified the genotype required for this phenomenon. An individual who is homozygous for the *h* allele *(hh)* expresses the Bombay phenotype (the *H* and *h* genes of the *H* locus were previously described in this chapter). The *hh* genotype does not produce the L-fucosyltransferase necessary to transfer the immunodominant sugar, L-fucose, to the acceptor oligosaccharide chain to form the H antigen. As a result, the H antigen is not assembled on the red cells. Because H antigen is the building block for the development of the A and B antigens, A and B glycosyltransferases cannot act on their substrate to produce the corresponding antigen structures, even though the ABO alleles are inherited. The resulting phenotype lacks expression of both H and ABO antigens. Transfusion for these individuals presents an especially difficult problem because they are compatible only with the Bombay phenotype. If transfusion is necessary, stored autologous units, siblings, and rare donor files are potential options.

> Bombay individuals have group O phenotype in routine ABO typing. These individuals are not compatible with group O donor units because their serum possesses anti-H.

SECRETOR STATUS

The interrelationship of the secretor locus with the expression of ABO antigens in body fluids has been mentioned several times throughout this chapter. There are two allelic genes at this locus: *Se* and *se*. The gene product of the *Se* allele, *FUT2*, is an L-fucosyltransferase that preferentially adds L-fucose to type 1 oligosaccharide chain structures in secretory glands. The *FUT2* gene may also act on type 2 chains in the secretory glands. The *H* gene, *FUT1*, preferentially adds fucose to type 2 chains.

The *FUT2* gene is directly responsible for regulating the expression of soluble A, B, and H antigens on the glycoprotein structures located in body secretions such as saliva. An individual who inherits the *Se* allele in either a homozygous *(SeSe)* or a heterozygous *(Sese)* manner is classified as a **secretor**. About 80% of the random population inherits the *Se* allele and is classified as secretors. These individuals express soluble forms of H antigens in secretions that can be converted to A or B antigens by the A and B glycosyltransferases. These soluble antigens are found in saliva, urine, tears, bile, amniotic fluid, breast milk, exudate, and digestive fluids. An individual with the genotype *sese* is classified as a **nonsecretor**. About 20% of the random population can be considered nonsecretors. The allele, *se*, is an amorph. A homozygote does not convert glycoprotein antigen precursors to soluble H substance and has neither soluble H antigens nor soluble A or B antigens present in body fluids. Fig. 4-11 illustrates the genetic interaction of the *ABO*, *H*, and *Se* loci.

> **Secretor:** individual who inherits *Se* allele and expresses soluble forms of H antigens in secretions.

> **Nonsecretor:** individual who inherits the genotype *sese* and does not express soluble H substance in secretions.

> Secretor studies may be helpful in identifying a subgroup of A or B antigens.

Example 1

Genes inherited			Antigen expression	
			RBC	Saliva
AB	HH	SeSe ⟶	A, B, H	A, B, H
AB	HH	sese ⟶	A, B, H	None

Example 2

Genes inherited			Antigen expression	
			RBC	Saliva
OO	HH	Sese ⟶	H	H
OO	HH	sese ⟶	H	None

Fig. 4-11 Practical application: interaction of ABO, H, and secretor genes in the expression of soluble antigens in saliva. *RBC,* Red blood cell.

CHAPTER SUMMARY

The major concepts of ABO antigens and ABO antibodies presented in this chapter are summarized in the following table.

Important Facts: ABO and H Blood Group System Antigens

Widespread antigen distribution	Blood cells, tissues, body fluids, secretions
Biochemical composition	Glycolipid/glycoprotein
Common structures	Type 1 and type 2 oligosaccharide chains
Gene products	Glycosyltransferases
Immunodominant sugars	H antigen: L-fucose A antigen: N-acetylgalactosamine B antigen: D-galactose
Antigen expression	Cord blood cells: weak
Genetic loci	ABO blood group system: chromosome 9 H system: chromosome 19
Major alleles	A^1, A^2, B, O H, h
Bombay phenotype	Genotype hh; no H or ABO antigens
Secretor status	Se allele; soluble H and ABO antigens
Landsteiner's rule	Serum possesses the ABO antibody directed toward the A or B antigen that is absent from red cells
Antibody production	No antibodies detectable in first few months of life; decreases in elderly adults
Antibody immunoglobulin class	IgM and IgG
In vitro reactions	At or below room temperature
Complement binding	Yes; some hemolytic
Clinical significance	Yes

CRITICAL THINKING EXERCISES

EXERCISE 4-1 Case Study

RT, a 37-year-old woman, is a first-time donor at your blood center. She is a healthy donor with an unremarkable medical history and is not taking any medications. Initial ABO phenotyping results indicate an ABO discrepancy.

ABO Testing Results			
Donor Red Cells with		**Donor Serum with Reagent Red Cells**	
Anti-A	**Anti-B**	**A_1**	**B**
0	4+	3+	1+

1. Evaluate the ABO phenotyping results. Is the discrepancy associated with the red cell testing or the serum testing? State the reasons for this selection.
2. How would you classify the category of ABO discrepancy shown in this problem?
3. What are the potential causes of an ABO discrepancy in this category?

Additional Testing

No technical errors were found. The donor's red cells were washed, and the ABO phenotyping was repeated. Red cell testing results were identical to the first set. In addition to A_1 and B reagent red cells, commercial screening cells and an autologous control were tested with the donor's serum. The results of the testing are depicted in the following table.

Additional Testing Results			
Donor's Serum Testing with			
A₁ Red Cells	B Red Cells	Screening Cells	Autologous Red Cells
3+	1+	1+	0

4. What conclusions can be drawn from the results of additional serum testing?
5. What additional steps are required to resolve this ABO discrepancy?

EXERCISE 4-2

What are the possible ABO phenotypes of offspring with parents possessing the genotypes A^1A^2 and BO?

EXERCISE 4-3

Group O individuals are considered universal donors for the transfusion of RBCs and universal recipients for plasma transfusions. Provide an explanation for this statement.

EXERCISE 4-4

Create a diagram to illustrate the genetic pathways for ABO antigen production and the Bombay phenotype.

EXERCISE 4-5

For a Bombay phenotype encountered in the immunohematology laboratory:
1. Predict the agglutination reactions of the patient's red cells with the following reagents: anti-A, anti-B, anti-A,B, and *Ulex europaeus*.
2. Predict the agglutination reactions of the patient's serum sample with the following reagent red cells: A₁, B, and O.

EXERCISE 4-6

Why does an individual with the genotyping of *AB*, *HH*, and *sese* possess A, B, and H antigens on red cells but not have any soluble forms of these antigens in the saliva?

STUDY QUESTIONS

1. Given the following ABO typing results, what conclusion can be drawn from these results?

ABO Testing Results			
Patient Red Cells with		Patient Serum with Reagent Red Cells	
Anti-A	Anti-B	A₁	B
4+	4+	1+	0

    a. expected results for a group O individual
    b. expected results for a group AB individual
    c. discrepant results; patient has A antigen on red cells with anti-A in serum
    d. discrepant results; patient has B antigen on red cells with no anti-B in serum

2. What are the gene products of the *A* and *B* genes?
    a. glycolipids
    b. glycoproteins
    c. oligosaccharides
    d. transferase enzymes

For questions 3 through 5, use the following ABO typing results:

ABO Testing Results			
Patient Red Cells with		Patient Serum with Reagent Red Cells	
Anti-A	Anti-B	A₁	B
0	0	4+	4+

3. What is the ABO interpretation?
   a. group O
   b. group A
   c. group B
   d. group AB

4. What ABO phenotypes would be compatible if the patient required a transfusion of RBCs?
   a. group AB, O, A, or B
   b. group O or B
   c. group AB or O
   d. only group O

5. What ABO phenotypes would be compatible if the patient required a transfusion of fresh frozen plasma?
   a. group AB, O, A, or B
   b. group O or B
   c. group AB or O
   d. only group O

6. Using known sources of reagent antisera (known antibodies) to detect ABO antigens on a patient's red cells is known as:
   a. Rh typing
   b. reverse grouping
   c. direct antiglobulin test
   d. forward grouping

7. Which result is discrepant if the red cell typing shown in the following chart is correct?

ABO Testing Results			
Patient Red Cells with		Patient Serum with Reagent Red Cells	
Anti-A	Anti-B	A₁	B
0	4+	0	0

   a. negative reaction with group B cells
   b. positive reaction with anti-B
   c. negative reaction with group A₁ cells
   d. no discrepancies in these results

8. What ABO antibody is expected in this patient's serum based on the following information?

Patient Red Cells with	
Anti-A	Anti-B
0	4+

   a. anti-B
   b. anti-A
   c. anti-A and anti-B
   d. none

9. According to Landsteiner's rule, if a patient has no ABO antibodies after serum testing, what ABO antigens are present on the patient's red cells?
   a. A
   b. B
   c. both A and B
   d. none

10. Select the ABO phenotypes, in order from most frequent to least frequent, that occur in whites:
    a. A, B, O, AB
    b. O, A, B, AB
    c. B, A, AB, O
    d. AB, O, B, A

11. Which of the following statements is true about ABO antibody production?
    a. ABO antibodies are present in newborns.
    b. ABO titers remain at constant levels throughout life.
    c. ABO antibodies are stimulated by bacteria and other environmental factors.
    d. All of these statements are true.

12. What immunoglobulin class is primarily associated with ABO antibodies?
    a. IgA
    b. IgG
    c. IgE
    d. IgM

13. What immunodominant sugar confers B blood group specificity?
    a. D-galactose
    b. L-fucose
    c. N-acetylgalactosamine
    d. L-glucose

14. An individual has the genotype of *AO, hh*. What antigens would be present on the red cells of this individual?
    a. A only
    b. A and H
    c. A and O
    d. none of the above

15. What gene controls the presence of soluble H substance in saliva?
    a. *H*
    b. *A*
    c. *Se*
    d. *B*

16. Which lectin agglutinates A$_1$ red cells?
    a. *Dolichos biflorus*
    b. *Ulex europaeus*
    c. *Dolichos europaeus*
    d. *Ulex biflorus*

17. What immunodominant sugar determines the specificity of H antigens?
    a. D-galactose
    b. L-fucose
    c. N-acetylgalactosamine
    d. L-glucose

18. Which of the following situations may produce ABO discrepancies in the serum testing?
    a. newborn
    b. patient with hypogammaglobulinemia
    c. cold alloantibody
    d. all of the above

19. What soluble antigen forms are detectable in saliva based on the following genotype: *AB, HH, SeSe?*
    a. none (nonsecretor)
    b. only H
    c. A, B, and H
    d. A and B

20. Which ABO discrepancy is the best explanation for the results shown in the following chart?

ABO Testing Results			
Patient Red Cells with		Patient Serum with Reagent Red Cells	
Anti-A	Anti-B	A$_1$	B
4+	0	2+	4+

    a. an elderly patient
    b. subgroup of A
    c. deterioration of reagents
    d. hypogammaglobulinemia

REFERENCES

1. Issitt PD, Anstee DJ: *Applied blood group serology*, ed 4, Durham, NC, 1998, Montgomery Scientific Publications.
2. Daniels GL, Cartron JP, Fletcher A, et al: International Society of Blood Transfusion Committee on terminology for red cell surface antigens: Vancouver report, *Vox Sang* 84:244, 2003.
3. Daniels GL, Anstee DJ, Cartron JP, et al: International Society of Blood Transfusion Working Party on Terminology for Red Cell Surface Antigens, *Vox Sang* 80:193, 2001.
4. Landsteiner K: Zur Kenntnis der antifermentativen, lytischen und agglutinierenden Wirkungen des Blutserums und der Lymphe, *Zbl Bakt* 27:357, 1900.
5. von Decastello A, Sturli A: Über die Isoagglutinine im Serum gesunder und kranker Menschen, *Munchen Med Wochenschr* 95:1090, 1902.
6. Reid ME, Lomas-Francis C: *The blood group antigen facts book*, ed 2, San Diego, 2004, Elsevier Academic Press.
7. Economidou J, Hughes-Jones N, Gardner B: Quantitative measurements concerning A and B antigen sites, *Vox Sang* 12:321, 1967.
8. Mourant AE, Kopeâc AC, Domaniewska-Sobczak K: *The distribution of the human blood groups and other biochemical polymorphisms*, ed 2, London, 1976, Oxford University Press.
9. Roback JD, editor: *Technical manual*, ed 17, Bethesda, Md, 2011, AABB.
10. Pittiglio DH: Genetics and biochemistry of A, B, H and Lewis antigens. In Wallace ME, Gibbs FL, editors: *Blood group systems: ABH and Lewis*, Arlington, VA, 1986, AABB.
11. Yamamoto F, Clausen H, White T, et al: Molecular genetic basis of the histo-blood group ABO blood group system, *Nature* 345:229, 1990.
12. Fukuda MN, Hakamori S: Structures of branched blood group A-active glycosphingolipids in human erythrocytes and polymorphism of A- and H-glycolipids in A_1 and A_2 subgroups, *J Biol Chem* 257:446, 1982.
13. Lopez M, Benali J, Bony V, et al: Activity of IgG and IgM ABO antibodies against some weak A (A_3, A_x, A_{end}) and weak B (B_3, B_x) red cells, *Vox Sang* 37:281, 1979.
14. Nance ST: Serology of the ABH and Lewis blood group systems. In Wallace ME, Gibbs FL, editors: *Blood group systems: ABH and Lewis*, Arlington, VA, 1986, AABB.
15. Carson TH, editor: *Standards for blood banks and transfusion services*, ed 27, Bethesda, Md, 2011, AABB.
16. Gerbal A, Maslet C, Salmon C: Immunological aspects of the acquired B antigen, *Vox Sang* 28:398, 1975.
17. Beck ML, Kowalski MA, Kirkegaard JR, et al: Unexpected activity with monoclonal anti-B reagents, *Immunohematology* 8:22, 1992.
18. Beck ML, Yates AD, Hardman J, et al: Identification of a subset of group B donors reactive with monoclonal anti-A reagent, *Am J Clin Pathol* 92:625, 1989.
19. Bhatia HM: Serologic reactions of ABO and Oh (Bombay) phenotypes due to variations in H antigens. In Mohn JF, Plunkett RW, Cunningham RK, et al, editors: *Human blood groups: Proceedings of the Fifth International Convocation on Immunology*, Basel, Switzerland, 1977, Karger.

SUGGESTED READINGS

Poole J, Daniels G: Blood group antibodies and their significance in transfusion medicine, *Transfus Med Rev* 21:58-71, 2007.

Rh Blood Group System

CHAPTER OUTLINE

LEARNING OBJECTIVES

On completion of this chapter, the reader should be able to:

1. Explain how the D antigen was named Rh.
2. Compare and contrast the current genetic theory of the inheritance of Rh blood group system antigens with theories proposed by Fisher-Race and Wiener.
3. Discuss the biochemistry of the Rh blood group system, including the gene products and antigen structures.
4. Translate between the Fisher-Race and Wiener terminology.
5. Express phenotyping results for the Rh blood group system antigens in the terminology currently accepted by the International Society of Blood Transfusion.
6. Predict the most probable Rh genotype given the Rh antigen typing results (phenotype).
7. Define weak D, and list the genetic circumstances that can cause this phenotype.
8. Describe the appropriate application and test procedure for the weak D antigen.

9. Interpret results of the weak D test when the control is positive, and explain why this would occur.
10. Define compound antigens, and give two examples of this phenotype.
11. Distinguish the G antigen from other antigens in the Rh blood group system, and explain the significance of anti-G.
12. Explain the significance of Rh_{null}, Rh_{mod}, and deletion phenotypes.
13. Describe the characteristics of the Rh blood group system antibodies and their clinical significance with regard to transfusion and hemolytic disease of the fetus and newborn (HDFN).
14. Compare and contrast the antibody and antigen characteristics of the LW blood group system to the Rh blood group system.

The Rh blood group system is highly complex, polymorphic, and the second most important blood group system after the ABO blood group system. Since the initial discovery of the D antigen in 1939, 50 related antigens have been assigned to the Rh blood group system by the International Society of Blood Transfusion (ISBT). This chapter focuses on the five principal antigens—D, C, E, c, and e—and their corresponding antibodies, which account for most clinical transfusion issues. Readers are encouraged to review the

Suggested Readings for more details regarding theoretical consideration, rare phenotypes, and less commonly encountered antibodies.

SECTION 1

HISTORICAL OVERVIEW OF THE DISCOVERY OF THE D ANTIGEN

The terms "Rh-positive" and "Rh-negative" refer to the presence or absence of the D red cell antigen; more correct terms are "D-positive" and "D-negative." In contrast to the ABO blood group system, the absence of the D or other Rh blood group system antigens on the red cell does not typically correspond with the presence of the antibody in the plasma. In other words, individuals who are typed as "A, D–negative" would be expected to have anti-B in their serum but not anti-D. The production of anti-D and other Rh blood group system antibodies requires immune red cell stimulation from red cells positive for the antigen. This exposure may occur during transfusion or pregnancy.

> If a person is D-negative, the production of anti-D may occur after exposure to D-positive blood following transfusion or pregnancy.

The discovery of the Rh blood group system, as with many other blood group systems, followed the investigation of an adverse transfusion reaction or hemolytic disease of the fetus and newborn (HDFN). In 1940, the cause of HDFN was linked to the Rh blood group system by Levine and Stetson.[1] Rh was the name given to the system because of the similarity of this antibody to one made from stimulating guinea pigs and rabbits with rhesus monkey cells.[2] This Rh antibody, described by Landsteiner and Wiener, agglutinated 85% of human red cells tested and was nonreactive with 15%. From this discovery, the population was characterized as Rh-positive or Rh-negative. A later experiment demonstrated that the Rh antibody made from the guinea pigs and rabbits was similar, but not identical, to the anti-Rh produced by humans. The rhesus antibody specificity was actually directed toward another red cell antigen. This antigen was named LW in honor of Landsteiner and Wiener. The name of the Rh blood group system had been established by then and was not changed.

SECTION 2

GENETICS, BIOCHEMISTRY, AND TERMINOLOGY

Current theory explaining genetic control of Rh antigen expression has been enhanced with the ability to characterize the amino acid sequences produced by genes that code for proteins on the red cell membrane. Originally postulated by Tippett,[3] the Rh blood group system antigens are encoded by two closely linked genes—*RHD* and *RHCE*—on chromosome 1. *RHD* determines the D antigen expression on the surface of red cells. D-negative individuals have no genetic material at this site.[4] An antithetical "d" antigen does not exist, although the small "d" notation is sometimes used to indicate a D-negative gene. Adjacent to the *RHD* locus, the gene *RHCE* determines the C, c, E, and e antigen specificities. The alleles at this locus are *RHCE*, *RHCe*, *RHcE*, and *RHce* and encode CE, Ce, cE, and ce, respectively (Fig. 5-1).[5] The *RHCE* gene codes for similar polypeptides, distinguished by two amino acid sequences as illustrated in Fig. 5-2.[6] The assortment of other antigens in the Rh blood group system occurs as a result of variations of these polypeptides embedded in the cell membrane bilayer in unique configurations. The *RHD* gene, which codes for the D antigen, can vary by many more amino acids creating much more variability among individuals. These differences between individuals help explain why exposure to D antigen can result in a likely immune response.[7] Commonly encountered Rh antigens are listed in Table 5-1.

The products of both the *RHD* and the *RHCE* genes are proteins of 416 amino acids that traverse the membrane 12 times and display short loops of amino acids on the exterior (see Fig. 5-2).[7] The Rh blood group system polypeptides, in contrast to most blood group–associated proteins, carry no carbohydrate residues. Rh antigens have been detected only on red cell membranes, and the proteins are not recognized by antibodies after the proteins separate from the membrane.[8] The functions of the Rh antigens on the red cells might be cation transport and membrane integrity.[9] The lack of Rh blood group system

Fig. 5-1 Comparison of Rh genetic theories. Comparison of three Rh genetic theories that have influenced the nomenclature of the Rh blood group system. Modern molecular techniques have established that the Rh blood group system antigens are determined by two genetic loci.

Antigen	Amino acid	Number
C	Serine	103 Cc
c	Proline	103 Cc
E	Proline	226 Ee
e	Alanine	226 Ee

Fig. 5-2 Model of the Rh polypeptide. Model of the differences in the amino acid sequence for the antigens produced by the *RHCE* gene. The basic structure is similar. Differences in the amino acid at the residue number indicated determine the serologic typing to be C or c, E or e.

TABLE 5-1	Common Antigens in the Rh Blood Group System: Equivalent Notations		
NUMERIC	**FISHER-RACE**	**OTHER NAMES**	**ISBT NO.**
Rh1	D	Rh+	004001
Rh2	C		004002
Rh3	E		004003
Rh4	c		004004
Rh5	e		004005
Rh6	ce	*cis*-ce or f	004006
Rh7	Ce	*cis*-Ce	004007
Rh8	C^w		004008
Rh9	C^x		004009
Rh10	ce^s	V	004010
Rh12	G		004012

ISBT, International Society of Blood Transfusion.

antigens, called Rh$_{null}$, causes a membrane abnormality that shortens red cell survival. Rh$_{null}$ is discussed in further detail later in this chapter.

Two systems of nomenclature were developed before more recent advances in molecular genetics. These systems reflect serologic observations and inheritance theories based on family studies. Because these systems are used interchangeably in the transfusion setting, it is necessary to understand these theories well enough to "translate" from one to another. Two additional systems were developed because of a need for a universal language compatible with computers. Table 5-1 lists the equivalent notations for the more common Rh antigens.

FISHER-RACE: CDE TERMINOLOGY

Fisher and Race[10] postulated that the Rh blood group system antigens were inherited as a gene complex or haplotype that codes for three closely linked sets of alleles. D gene is inherited at one locus, C or c genes are inherited at the second locus, and E or e genes are inherited at the third locus. Each parent contributes one haplotype or set of Rh genes. Fig. 5-1 illustrates this concept. Each gene expresses an antigen that is given the same letter as the gene except that when referring to the gene the letter is italicized. For example, the gene that produces the C antigen is *C*. Each red cell antigen can be recognized by testing with a specific antibody. The original theory assumed the *d* allele was present when the *D* allele was absent. The "d" is still sometimes written to denote the absence of the D antigen. According to the Fisher-Race theory, the order of the genes on the chromosome is *DCE*; however, it is often written alphabetically as *CDE*.

> The notation "d" is sometimes used to denote the absence of the D antigen; however, there is no gene or gene product for "d."

WIENER: RH-HR TERMINOLOGY

In contrast to the Fisher-Race theory, Wiener[11] postulated that alleles at *one* gene locus were responsible for expression of the Rh blood group system antigens on red cells. Each parent contributes one Rh gene. The inherited form of the gene may be identical (homozygous) to or different (heterozygous) from each parent. According to Wiener, eight alleles exist at the Rh gene locus: R^0, R^1, R^2, R^z, r, r', r'', and r^y. The gene encodes a structure on the red cell called an **agglutinogen**, which can be identified by its parts or factors. These factors are identified with the same antisera that agglutinate the D, C, c, E, and e antigens mentioned earlier in the Fisher-Race nomenclature. The difference between the Wiener and Fisher-Race theories is the inheritance of the Rh blood group system on a *single* gene locus rather than *three* separate genes. The antigen complex or agglutinogen is made up of factors that are identifiable as separate antigens (Table 5-2). For example, in Wiener terminology, the R^1 gene codes for the Rh$_1$ agglutinogen, which is made up of factors Rh$_0$, rh', and hr'' that correspond to D, C, and e antigens, respectively. The *r* gene codes for the rh agglutinogen, made up of factors hr' and hr'' that correspond to c and e

> **Agglutinogen:** term referring to a group of antigens or factors that are agglutinated by antisera.

TABLE 5-2	Wiener Theory: Genes and Antigens
GENE (WIENER)	**ANTIGENS (FISHER-RACE)**
R^0	cDe
R^1	CDe
R^2	cDE
R^z	CDE
r	ce
r'	Ce
r''	cE
r^y	CE

Note. Factors in the Wiener terminology are more easily translated to the Fisher-Race terminology, which defines the antigens more clearly.

TABLE 5-3	Converting Fisher-Race Terminology to Wiener Terminology		
FISHER-RACE ANTIGEN	**WIENER TERMINOLOGY**		**EXAMPLES**
D	R (D+)	r (D–)	$DCe = R_1$
C	1	'	$Ce = r'$, $DCe = R_1$
E	2	"	$cE = r''$, $DcE = R_2$
CE	z	y	$DCE = R_z$, $CE = r_y$
ce	0		$ce = r$

Upper-case R indicates that the D antigen is present; lower-case r indicates that the D antigen is absent; 1 and ' indicate C; 2 and " indicate E; 0 indicates ce; z indicates CE (with R); y indicates CE (with r).

antigens, respectively. The longhand factor notations of Rh_0, rh', hr', rh", and hr" that correspond to D, C, c, E, and e antigens, respectively, are outdated and rarely used.

Wiener terminology can be easily translated to Fisher-Race terminology when the following points are kept in mind: R is the same as D; r indicates no D antigen; the number 1 and the character ' denote C; and the number 2 and the character " denote E (Table 5-3). For example, in Wiener nomenclature, having the c, D, and E factors or antigens would be written as R_2. Although most workers prefer the Fisher-Race terminology to Wiener terminology, it is often easier to describe a phenotype as R_2R_2 than as D+, C–, c+, E+, e–. Subscripts refer to antigens, whereas italics and superscripts indicate genes.

R_1 is an antigen expression for DCe, which uses the subscript 1. R^1 is the allele for the antigen expression, which uses italics and the superscript 1.

ROSENFIELD: NUMERIC TERMINOLOGY

Both the Wiener and the Fisher-Race terminologies are based on genetic concepts. The Rosenfield system was developed to communicate phenotypic information more suited for computerized data entry; it does not address genetic information.[12] In this system, each antigen is given a number that corresponds to the order of its assignment in the Rh blood group system. The phenotype of a cell is expressed by the Rh followed by a colon and the numbers corresponding to the tested antigens. If a red cell sample is negative for the antigen tested, a minus sign is written before the number. For example, red cells that tested D+, C+, E–, c+, e+ would be written as Rh:1,2,–3,4,5. Table 5-1 compares Fisher-Race, Wiener, and Numeric terminology.

INTERNATIONAL SOCIETY OF BLOOD TRANSFUSION: STANDARDIZED NUMERIC TERMINOLOGY

The ISBT, in an effort to standardize blood group system nomenclature, assigned a six-digit number to each blood group specificity.[13] The first three numbers represent the system, and the remaining three represent the antigen specificity. The assigned number of the Rh blood group system is 004, and the remaining three numbers correspond to the Rosenfield system. For example, the ISBT number for the C antigen is 004002. An ISBT "symbol" or alphanumeric designation similar to the Rosenfield terminology is used to refer to a specific antigen. The term Rh is written in uppercase letters, and the antigen number immediately follows the system designation. The ISBT symbol for C is RH2. A partial list of Rh antigens that includes the ISBT numeric designation is given in Table 5-1.

DETERMINING THE GENOTYPE FROM THE PHENOTYPE

The term phenotype refers to the test results obtained with specific antisera, and the term genotype refers to the genetic makeup of an individual. The genotype cannot be absolutely determined without family studies or molecular testing but can be inferred from the phenotype based on the frequency of genes in a population. Five antisera, used to determine the Rh blood group system phenotypes, include anti-D, anti-C, anti-c, anti-E, and

TABLE 5-4	Order of Frequency of the Common Rh Blood Group System Haplotypes		
WHITE		**BLACK**	**Rare (both races)**
CDe (R^1)	Highest	cDe (R^0)	Ce (r')
ce (r)		ce (r)	cE (r'')
cDE (R^2)		CDe (R^1)	CE (r^y)
cDe (R^0)	Lowest	cDE (R^2)	CDE (R^z)

Note: The information in this table is useful when predicting the most probable genotype following the phenotype or antigen typing determination. Knowing that a cDe/cDe or R^0/R^0 genotype is more common in blacks would be important if D-positive, C-negative units were requested.

anti-e. Agglutination with the antisera indicates that the antigen is present on the red cell; no agglutination indicates the absence of the antigen.

When the phenotype is known, the most probable genotype can be determined by knowing the most common Rh blood group system genes for the race of the person being tested (Table 5-4). In the white population, the four most common genes encountered, in order of frequency from highest to lowest, are CDe (R^1), ce (r), cDE (R^2), and cDe (R^0). In the black population, the order of gene frequency from highest to lowest is cDe (R^0), ce (r), CDe (R^1), and cDE (R^2). The genes Ce (r'), cE (r''), CDE (R^z), and CE (r^y) are not commonly found in either race. If a red cell specimen is typed as D+, C+, E−, c+, e+, the phenotype would be CcDe. When the genotype is inferred in the white population, the combination CDe/ce or R^1r would be the most probable genotype. In the black population, the most probable genotype would be CDe/cDe or R^1R^0 because R^0 allele is more common than the r allele. Table 5-5 lists phenotypes determined by reactions with specific antisera and the most probable genotype based on gene frequency in the population.

Pedigree diagrams illustrate inheritance patterns. In Fig. 5-3, the inheritance of the Rh blood group system is diagrammed to illustrate the concept that the Rh blood group system is inherited as a haplotype. Because the RHD and RHCE loci are close on chromosome 1, it is easy to follow the inheritance of the gene complex using Wiener terminology. A Punnett square, which can predict phenotypes and genotypes, can also be used to illustrate the probability of being D-positive or D-negative (Fig. 5-4).

SECTION 3
ANTIGENS OF THE Rh BLOOD GROUP SYSTEM

D ANTIGEN

Immunogenicity: ability of an antigen to stimulate an immune response.

The D antigen is the most immunogenic antigen in the Rh blood group system. **Immunogenicity** refers to the ability of an antigen to elicit an immune response. As many as 85% of D-negative people receiving a D-positive red blood cell (RBC) transfusion produce an antibody with anti-D specificity.[14] For that reason, a D-negative patient should receive D-negative RBC units. Fig. 5-5 illustrates the variation of the D antigen concentration in different phenotypes.

Because of the high immunogenicity of the D antigen, testing for the presence or absence of the D antigen is included in routine blood typing along with the ABO antigens.

Weak D

Weak D: weak form of the D antigen that requires the indirect antiglobulin test for its detection.

Most red cells can be typed for the D antigen directly with anti-D reagents. Although the antibody to D is typically of the IgG class, reagent manufacturers have developed monoclonal anti-D antisera that can be used concurrently with anti-A and anti-B testing. When the D antigen is weakly expressed on the red cell, its detection requires the indirect antiglobulin test (IAT) (Fig. 5-6). Red cells that are positive for D only by the IAT are referred to as **weak D.** Table 5-6 shows the interpretation of this test, which must always include a control. The D control is a reagent made by manufacturers that consists of all additives

TABLE 5-5 Rh Phenotypes and Genotypes

RESULTS WITH ANTISERA						GENOTYPE		GENOTYPE FREQUENCY	
ANTI-D	ANTI-C	ANTI-E	ANTI-C	ANTI-E	PHENOTYPE	CDE	Rh-hr	WHITE	BLACK
+	+	−	+	+	CcDe	*CDe/ce*	R^1r	**31**	9
						CDe/cDe	R^1R^0	3	**15**
						Ce/cDe	$r'R^0$	<1	2
+	+	−	−	+	CDe	*CDe/CDe*	R^1R^1	**18**	3
						CDe/Ce	R^1r'	2	<1
+	−	+	+	+	cDEe	*cDE/ce*	R^2r	**10**	6
						cDE/cDe	R^2R^0	1	**10**
+	−	+	+	−	cDE	*cDE/cDE*	R^2R^2	2	1
						cDE/cE	R^2r''	<1	<1
+	+	+	+	+	CcDEe	*CDe/cDE*	R^1R^2	**12**	4
						CDe/cE	R^1r''	1	<1
						Ce/cDE	$r'R^2$	1	<1
+	−	−	+	+	cDe	*cDe/ce*	R^0r	3	**23**
						cDe/cDe	R^0R^0	<1	**19**
−	−	−	+	+	ce	*ce/ce*	rr	15	7
−	+	−	+	+	Cce	*Ce/ce*	$r'r$	<1	<1
−	−	+	+	+	cEe	*cE/ce*	$r''r$	<1	<1
−	+	+	+	+	CcEe	*Ce/cE*	$r'r''$	<1	<1

Note. The more common genotypes and genotype frequencies are shown in bold. This information shows the more probable genotypes given Rh antigen phenotype determinations. Depending on the race of the individual, a different genotype of the red cells might be predicted.

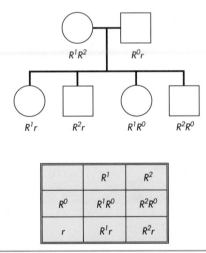

Fig. 5-3 Inheritance of Rh haplotypes. Because the genes coding for the Rh blood group system are very close on the chromosome, Rh antigens are inherited as haplotypes. This inheritance is illustrated in a pedigree chart and in a Punnett square.

except the D antibody. It is used to determine whether agglutination by anti-D at immediate-spin is false positive, which could be due to the reagent additives, such as albumin. The D control tested at the antiglobulin phase determines whether patient cells are already coated with IgG antibodies before testing. Reagent manufacturers specify the use of controls in their package inserts, and it is important to become familiar with these

Fig. 5-4 Inheritance of the D antigen. Predicting the probability of D-positive offspring from a D-negative mother and a heterozygous *(Dd)* father. The *d* gene does not exist and is being used only for illustrative purposes. From this mating, it is shown that 50% of the children could be D-positive.

$$-D- > R^2R^2 > R^1R^1 > R^1r \text{ or } R^0r > R^1r' \text{ or } R^0r'$$

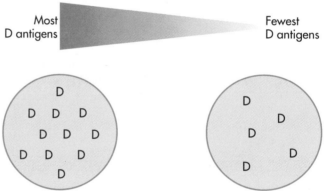

Fig. 5-5 D antigen concentration. The D antigen concentration varies with the antigens inherited at the *RHCE* gene. The D-deletion phenotype has the most D antigen sites. The *C* gene weakens the D antigen expression if inherited on the opposite chromosome. R^2R^2 cells show a higher D expression than R^1R^1 cells. If anti-D was reacted with R^2R^2 cells, they would typically demonstrate a stronger pattern of agglutination.

TABLE 5-6	Weak D Test: Interpretation with Control Results		
	REACTION WITH		
SAMPLE NO.	**ANTI-D**	**CONTROL**	**INTERPRETATION**
1	+	0	D-positive
2	0	0	D-negative
3	+	+	Unable to interpret

Note. The weak D test is an antiglobulin test used to detect the D antigen on the cell. Because the test uses anti-IgG to demonstrate the presence of the D antigen, preexisting IgG on the cell would cause a "false-positive" result, as in sample no. 3. The control must be negative for the presence of IgG for the weak D test to be valid as in sample nos. 1 and 2.

guidelines. Chapter 2 discusses Rh reagents in detail. If the control is positive, additional serologic techniques may be required, which are discussed in Chapter 7.

Older terminology classified weak D antigens as D^u. The IAT used to determine whether a weak form of D is present is still sometimes referred to as the D^u test, although this is incorrect terminology.[14] Newer monoclonal antibody typing reagents for Rh blood

1. Label 2 test tubes: **anti-D** and **Control**. Place one drop of the 2-5% cells suspension of the sample to be tested in each.

Anti-D   Rh control

2. Add one drop of the anti-D into one test tube and 1 drop of the Rh control into the other test tube.
3. Incubate 15-30 minutes.
4. Wash 3X with saline.

Anti-IgG

5. Add 1-2 drops of antiglobulin reagent: IgG or polyspecific (refer to manufacturer's directions).
6. Mix and centrifuge.
7. Gently resuspend and examine for agglutination, grade, and record.
8. Add IgG coated control cells to negative results, spin, and read.

Fig. 5-6 Weak D test procedure. (Modified from Immucor, Norcross, GA.)

group system antigens have enhanced the ability to detect the weaker D antigens without additional IAT testing.

Weaker D expression can result from several different genetic circumstances that are outlined briefly in the following section. Only the first type of weak D requires detection of the D antigen by the IAT.

Weak D: Genetic

Some *RHD* genes code for a weaker expression of the D antigen. This quantitative variation in the *RHD* gene is more common in blacks and is often part of the *cDe (R_0)* haplotype. An IAT using anti-D is usually required to detect this form of D.

Weak D: Position Effect

Weaker expression of the D antigen can be found when the *Ce (r′)* gene is inherited in *trans* to the *RHD* gene (Fig. 5-7). Genes inherited in *trans* are inherited on opposite chromosomes. The *Ce (r′)* gene paired with a *CDe (R^1)* or a *cDe (R^0)* gene weakens the expression of the D antigen. This type of D antigen is usually detected without additional testing by the IAT using anti-D because of the increased sensitivity of monoclonal reagents. The occurrence of the *Ce (r′)* gene is less than 2%.

Weak D: Partial D

Although rare, some individuals who are positive for the D antigen can make an alloantibody that appears to be anti-D after exposure to D-positive red cells. Investigation of this phenomenon revealed that some D-positive cells could be missing parts of the D antigen complex. When these individuals are exposed to the "whole D" antigen, they

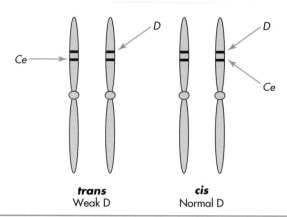

Fig. 5-7 Weak D caused by *Ce* inherited in *trans*. D-antigen expression is weaker when the *D* and *Ce* genes are inherited on the opposite chromosome.

TABLE 5-7	Weak D Summary		
TYPES OF WEAK D EXPRESSION	**DETECTED BY**	**CAN MAKE ANTI-D**	
Genetic, reduced D antigen	Weak D test	No	
Ce in *trans* to *RHD* (example: R^0r')	Monoclonal reagents	No	
Partial D	Most monoclonal reagents and/or weak D test	Yes, antibody to the missing epitope	

Partial D: D antigen that is missing part of its typical antigenic structure.

can make an antibody to the part they are missing. In the past, the **partial D** phenotype was termed *D variant* or *D mosaic*. Lomas et al[15] established nine partial D phenotypes, which are classified by their parts or epitopes.

Red cells of most partial D phenotypes react as strongly with monoclonal antibody anti-D reagents as red cells composed of the complete D antigen. For this reason, partial D phenotypes are infrequently detected. A partial D phenotype should be suspected if a D-positive individual makes an antibody that reacts with D-positive cells but is nonreactive with his or her own cells.[14] In addition, the partial D phenotype should be suspected if two different manufacturers' monoclonal anti-D reagents are used and the interpretation as D-positive or D-negative does not agree. In this circumstance, the clone used to manufacture the reagent may vary in the ability to detect all the epitopes or parts of the D antigen. The types of weak D are summarized in Table 5-7.

Significance of Testing for Weak D

The AABB *Standards* requires testing for weak D on all donor red cells that do not directly agglutinate with anti-D reagents.[16] Weak D–positive units are labeled D-positive and should be transfused only to D-positive recipients. A D control or an autocontrol is an important part of the weak D test because it verifies that a positive result is not due to red cells already coated with antibodies. If red cells are coated with IgG antibodies before testing with anti-D at the antiglobulin phase, the test is invalid, and additional procedures are required to determine the D antigen status of the donor.

Testing for weak D on potential transfusion recipient samples is not required. Many facilities perform only the direct test for the D antigen and do not complete the antiglobulin procedure if the reaction is negative. This policy may be most cost-effective in terms of time and reagents because most D-negative individuals do not test positive for the weak D antigen. Patients are classified as D-negative in this case and transfused with D-negative blood.

The weak D test should not be performed on cells with a positive direct antiglobulin test because false-positive results would occur.

Some facilities test for weak D on recipient samples. If a weak D is detected, D-positive blood is provided. Although unlikely, a patient with a weak D because of the partial D phenotype can theoretically make anti-D. The partial D phenotype is rare and with current monoclonal reagents usually does not require the antiglobulin test for detection.

Weak D testing is also performed on prenatal evaluations and Rh immune globulin (**RhIG**) work-ups. The decision to give RhIG to weak D–positive women during prenatal evaluations varies among institutions. It is unknown if prophylaxis would be successful in the case of a mother with a partial D phenotype with a D-positive infant. This clinical situation is discussed further in Chapter 11. Some debate about these policies exists; however, the important element in weak D testing by the IAT is that the interpretation be made with proper controls to detect cells already sensitized with IgG antibodies.

OTHER Rh BLOOD GROUP SYSTEM ANTIGENS

Antigens in the Rh blood group system other than D, C, E, c, and e are alternate forms or variations produced by the *RHD* and *RHCE* genes. These antigens and corresponding antibodies and their clinical relevance, are outlined in the following section. Table 5-8 provides a summary of less common antigens and antibody characteristics. A more thorough discussion of these rare phenotypes is beyond the scope of this text, and the reader is referred to the Suggested Readings.

Compound Antigens

Examples of **compound antigens** in the Rh blood group system include the following:
* Rh6 (ce or f)
* Rh7 (Ce)
* Rh27 (cE)
* Rh22 (CE)

A compound antigen is the additional antigen product formed when certain genes code for an additional protein. For example, when c and e are inherited as *RHce*, another

> **RhIG:** Rh immune globulin (RhIG), also referred to by the trade name RhoGAM, is purified anti-D prepared from immunized donors and is given to D-negative mothers to prevent the formation of anti-D.

> Weak D typing is a required test for donors who initially are typed as D-negative. Policies regarding typing for weak D in potential transfusion recipients vary among institutions.

> **Compound antigens:** distinct antigens produced when two other antigens are encoded by the same gene.

TABLE 5-8	Summary of Less Common Rh Blood Group System Antigens and Antibodies	
ANTIGEN	**ANTIGEN CHARACTERISTICS**	**ANTIBODY CHARACTERISTICS**
Ce or f	*cis*-product antigen; present when c and e are inherited as a haplotype	Rare antibody; can cause HTR and HDFN; c– or e– blood is f–
Ce or Rh7	*cis*-product antigen; present when C and e are inherited as a haplotype	Anti-Ce is often made by D+ patients who make anti-C
C^w	Low-frequency antigen, found in 2% of whites and rarely in blacks; most C^w+ are also C+	Can be naturally occurring; immune examples can cause HDFN and HTR
C^x	Low (<0.01%) occurrence; C^x+ is C+	Rare, can cause mild HTR and HDFN
V or Ce^s	Found in 30% of blacks and <1% of whites	Often found with other antibodies; can cause HTR but not HDFN
G	Present on most D+ and all C+ cells	Antibody appears to be anti-D and anti-C; can cause HDFN and HTR
Rh29 or total Rh	Present on all red cells except Rh$_{null}$ cells	Anti-total Rh is made by Rh$_{null}$ individuals (amorph and regulator)
RH:17	Present on all red cells except -D- cells (D deletion)	Antibody made by individuals who are -D-
hr^s	e-like antigens (e variants) produced by all Rh genes that make e; antigen hr^s is associated with weak e-antigen typing	Antibodies found when an e+ person makes an apparent anti-e

HDFN, Hemolytic disease of the fetus and newborn; *HTR*, hemolytic transfusion reaction.

TABLE 5-9   Compound Antigens on Rh Proteins

COMPOUND ANTIGEN	Rh PROTEIN	FISHER-RACE/WIENER NOTATION
ce or f	Rhce	Dce (R_0) or ce (r)
Ce or Rh7	RhCe	DCe (R_1) or Ce (r′)
cE or Rh27	RhcE	DcE (R_2) or cE (r″)
CE or Rh22	RhCE	DCE (R_z) or CE (r^y)

epitope called "f" is expressed in addition to the c and e antigens. This epitope can also elicit its own immune response. The f antigen would not be present on the red cell if the person's genotype was *DCe/DcE*, even though the red cells would type positive for both the c and the e antigens. In this case, the *c* and *e* alleles were inherited from the *RHCe* and *RHcE* genes, and f would not be formed. Compound antigens were previously referred to as *cis* products to indicate that the antigens were coded from a haplotype rather than a single gene coding for a single protein.[14] Table 5-9 summarizes the compound antigen combinations.

Antibodies to compound antigens are infrequently encountered. If they are identified, locating antigen-negative units would require the use of common Rh antisera, such as anti-E, anti-C, anti-c, and anti-e. For example, if anti-f were identified, RBC units that are c-negative or e-negative would also be negative for the f antigen. When RBCs are required, units that are negative for one of the antigens creating the compound antigen can be safely transfused.

G Antigens

Genes that code for RhD, RhCe, and RhCE also code for a particular amino acid that results in an antigen called G. Cells that are negative for both the D and the C antigen are negative for the G antigen. Because an antibody to G reacts with cells that are either D-positive or C-positive, the specificity appears to be anti-D and anti-C. In other words, anti-G antibodies mimic the reactions observed with anti-D and anti-C antibodies. In some cases, a D-negative person may receive D–, C+ red cells and appear to produce anti-C as well as anti-D. The antibody produced in this case was most likely anti-G. Distinguishing anti-G, anti-D, and anti-C antibodies requires adsorption and elution procedures.[17] Extensive testing to identify anti-G is not usually necessary. Individuals making anti-G (or what appears to be anti-D or anti-C) should receive red cells that are negative for *both* D and C antigens. Rare cells exist that are negative for D and positive for G *(r^G)*. G is not a compound antigen; G is present when D *or* C is inherited.

UNUSUAL PHENOTYPES

Unusual phenotypes in the Rh blood group system are rarely encountered in routine blood bank testing. Unusual phenotypes include cells that have diminished or undetectable Rh blood group system antigen expression. Understanding the inheritance patterns and cell characteristics of unusual phenotypes provides insight into the genetics and biochemistry of the system. **Null phenotypes** are found in many blood group systems and have led to an understanding of the role of the antigen on the red cell. Serologically, null phenotypes have provided the mechanism to categorize blood group systems.

Null phenotypes: absences of a particular blood group system from the red cell membrane.

D-Deletion Phenotype

Rare Rh phenotypes demonstrate no reactions when the red cells are tested with anti-E, anti-e, anti-C, or anti-c. Genetic material has been deleted or rendered nonfunctional at the *RHCE* site. Red cells that lack C/c or E/e antigens may demonstrate stronger D antigen activity (see Fig. 5-5). Individuals who have the "D-deletion" phenotype may produce an antibody that reacts as a single specificity (anti-Rh17) or separable specificities such as anti-e and anti-C. An individual who produces anti-Rh17 would require D-deleted RBC units if transfusions are necessary. The D-deletion phenotype is written as -D- or D--.

Rh$_{null}$ Phenotype

The Rh$_{null}$ phenotype appears to have no Rh antigens and can be produced from two distinct genetic mechanisms. Cells that type as Rh$_{null}$ have membrane abnormalities that shorten their survival and cause hemolytic anemia of varying severity.[18] Antibodies produced by immunized individuals who lack all Rh antigens may be directed to "total-Rh" (Rh29) or to an individual Rh-antigen specificity. If an anti-Rh29 is detected, Rh$_{null}$ cells are needed for transfusion. Donations from siblings, autologous donations, and donations from the rare donor registry could be potential sources of compatible RBC units.

The inheritance of the Rh$_{null}$ phenotype can result from a **regulator** gene or an amorph gene. A regulator gene, *RHAG* (*Rh associated glycoprotein*), is inherited on chromosome 6 and codes for the thirtieth named blood group system. Although the RHAG blood group system does not carry any Rh system antigens, its presence is essential for the expression of the Rh system antigens. *RHAG* mutations are associated with the absence of expression of Rh antigens.[7] In the regulator type Rh$_{null}$, the Rh genes are inherited but are not expressed. The amorph Rh$_{null}$ phenotype is less well understood. The *RHD* gene is absent, and there is a lack of expression of the *RHCE* gene, causing neither protein to be produced.[19]

> **Regulator gene:** gene inherited at another locus or chromosome that affects the expression of another gene.

Rh$_{mod}$ Phenotype

The Rh$_{mod}$ phenotype is similar to the regulator Rh$_{null}$. In this phenotype, red cells lack most of their Rh antigen expression as a result of the inheritance of a modified *RHAG* gene. Hemolytic anemia is also a characteristic of this phenotype.

SECTION 4
Rh ANTIBODIES

GENERAL CHARACTERISTICS

Rh blood group system antibodies are usually made by exposure to Rh antigens through transfusion or pregnancy. Antibodies to Rh blood group system antigens show similar serologic characteristics. Most antibodies are IgG (IgG$_1$) and bind at 37° C; agglutination is observed by the IAT. Enhancement with high-protein, low-ionic-strength saline (LISS), proteolytic enzymes, and polyethylene glycol (PEG) **potentiators** is useful in identification procedures. Some Rh antibodies may be IgM (anti-E) or found in individuals who never underwent transfusion or were never pregnant (anti-C^w). Stronger reactivity with homozygous antigen expression (dosage) is characteristic of antibodies to C, c, E, and e, although this is not typical of anti-D. Anti-D is typically stronger with R$_2$R$_2$ red cells because these cells have more D antigen sites. Rh antibodies are not associated with complement activation, which would be detected by hemolysis in tube testing or the use of polyspecific antihuman globulin reagent.

> **Potentiators:** reagents added to the serum-cell mixture to enhance antibody uptake during the incubation phase of the indirect antiglobulin test.

When an R$_1$R$_1$ individual makes an anti-E, anti-c often may be present, although possibly weak or undetectable. Because of this association, some workers provide both c-negative and E-negative blood when anti-E is identified. It is recommended that more sensitive methods to detect anti-c be used when anti-E is present.

CLINICAL CONSIDERATIONS

Transfusion Reactions

Antibodies to Rh blood group system antigens can cause hemolytic transfusion reactions. Although antibodies often remain detectable for many years, their reactivity in agglutination procedures can decrease to undetectable levels. Reexposure to the antigen when the antibody has formed produces a rapid secondary immune response. Antigen-negative RBCs should be transfused if antibodies to Rh blood group system antigens are identified or have been previously noted in the patient's history. It is important to check previous records of patients who may be transfused for a history of red cell antibodies that may have developed from previous transfusions or pregnancies. Antibody detection is discussed in more detail in Chapter 7.

Hemolytic Disease of the Fetus and Newborn

HDFN was initially observed in infants of D-negative women with D-positive mates. First pregnancies were usually unaffected. Infants from subsequent pregnancies were often stillborn or severely anemic and jaundiced. The initial pregnancy stimulated the mother to produce anti-D from the exposure to D-positive cells that occurred during birth when the infant's and mother's circulations mixed. Because maternal anti-D antibodies can cross the placenta, fetal red cells in subsequent pregnancies were destroyed by the mother's antibody. RhIG protects D-negative mothers against the production of anti-D after delivery. Anti-C, anti-c, anti-E, and anti-e are not protected by RhIG and can cause HDFN. An important aspect of prevention of HDFN is antibody screening early in pregnancy and the determination of the D antigen status of mothers to ascertain RhIG candidacy. Chapter 11 contains a discussion of HDFN and RhIG.

SECTION 5
LW BLOOD GROUP SYSTEM

RELATIONSHIP TO THE Rh BLOOD GROUP SYSTEM

The LW blood group system is presented in this chapter because of its phenotypic relationship to the Rh blood group system. The antigens and antibodies are similar in serologic properties but are not genetically related. As discussed earlier, the LW antibody, made by guinea pigs and rabbits that were immunized with red cells from rhesus monkeys in early experiments, is similar to the anti-D antibody. Anti-LW reacts strongly with D-positive cells and weakly with D-negative cells. Rh$_{null}$ cells are negative for LW antigens as well. The theory suggesting a precursor relationship between the Rh blood group system and LW antigens has been discounted, although the membrane biochemistry is still being studied.[20] A summary of LW system antigens and antibodies appears in Table 5-10.

The LW locus is mapped to chromosome 19. The LW system alleles are *LW^a*, *LW^b*, and *LW*. LW(a+b−) is the most common phenotype in the population because the *LW^a* gene is of high frequency. The *LW* gene is an amorph, and inheriting two *LW* genes produces the rare LW(a−b−) phenotype. Antibodies to the LW system are clinically significant and rare.

TABLE 5-10	LW Blood Group System	
GENOTYPE	**PHENOTYPE**	**CHARACTERISTICS**
LW^{a}LW^a or *LW^{a}LW*	LW(a+b−)	Most common (97%) LW phenotype
LW^{a}LW^b	LW(a+b+)	3%
LW^{b}LW^b or *LW^{b}LW*	LW(a−b+)	Rare
LWLW	LW(a−b−)	Rare; can make anti-LW, which reacts more strongly with D+ cells

CHAPTER SUMMARY

The major concepts of the Rh blood group system regarding inheritance theories, nomenclature, antigens, and antibodies are summarized in the following table.

Summary of Rh Blood Group System Antigens

Biochemical composition	Polypeptides with no carbohydrate residues
Gene products	416 amino acids that traverse the membrane 12 times
Current genetic theory	Two genes, *RHD* and *RHCE*; alleles include *RHCE, RHCe, RHcE, RHce*
Fisher-Race theory	Three genes; alleles include *D/d, C/c, E/e*
Wiener theory	One gene; alleles include $R^0, R^1, R^2, R^z, r, r', r'', r^y$
Rosenfield/Numeric terminology	Numeric—D = Rh1, C = Rh2, E = Rh3, c = Rh4, e = Rh5
ISBT: standard numeric	Rh blood group system is 004; each antigen has a number as shown in Rosenfield system
Genetic loci	Chromosome 1
Weak D	D antigen that can be detected only by IAT
Compound antigens	ce or f, Ce or Rh7, CE or Rh22, and cE or Rh27
G antigen	Present whenever the D or C antigen is on the red blood cell
Rh$_{null}$ phenotype	Results from an amorph gene or *RHAG* regulator gene; no Rh antigens, abnormal red blood cell membrane

Summary of Rh Blood Group System Antibodies

Antibody production	Red blood cell stimulation through transfusion or pregnancy
Immunoglobulin class	IgG; usually IgG1 and IgG3
In vitro reactions	Binds at 37° C; agglutination observed using IAT
Enhancement	LISS, proteolytic enzymes, albumin, and PEG
Complement binding	No
Clinical significance	Yes; can cause delayed transfusion reactions and HDFN
Dosage	Yes; stronger reactions with homozygous expression

CRITICAL THINKING EXERCISES

EXERCISE 5-1

A transfusion request was received for 4 units of R_2R_2 RBCs for a transfusion recipient from an outside facility. From this request, determine the following:
1. Which Rh blood group system antigens are requested to be negative?
2. Will this blood order request be easy to fill? Why or why not?
3. How many donor units need to be screened to satisfy the request? (Refer to Chapter 3 for review.)
4. What Rh blood group system antibody does this transfusion recipient possess?
5. How would the requested R_2R_2 donor units be written in Fisher-Race and Rosenfield terminology?

EXERCISE 5-2

The following reactions were obtained by testing red cells from a donor unit with Rh blood group system antisera:

	Donor RBC Reaction
Anti-D:	+
Anti-C:	+
Anti-E:	0
Anti-c:	0
Anti-e:	+
Rh control:	0

+, Agglutination; *0*, no agglutination.

1. What Rh antigens does the donor possess?
2. What is the Rh phenotype?
3. Determine the most probable Rh genotype if the donor is white.
4. Is the Rh genotype different in this case if the donor is black?
5. What Rh antibodies could this donor make if he were to be transfused?
6. Is this Rh phenotype rare or common?

EXERCISE 5-3

The following results were obtained from a 65-year-old patient with cancer:

Anti-A	Anti-B	Anti-D	D Control	A$_1$ Cells	B Cells	Interpretation
4+	4+	1+	1+	0	0	AB, D-positive

1. Is the interpretation of the patient's blood type correct?
2. What test should be performed next to solve the Rh typing discrepancy?
3. Should a weak D test be performed if the patient has a positive direct antiglobulin test?
4. If the patient needs a transfusion before the resolution of the discrepancy, what blood type should this patient receive?

EXERCISE 5-4

The following results were obtained from a first-time blood donor:

Anti-A	Anti-B	Anti-D	Weak D	D Control	A$_1$ Cells	B Cells	Interpretation
4+	0	0	2+	0 ✓	0	4+	

1. What is the correct ABO and D typing interpretation for this donor?
2. Discuss the validity of the test.
3. Why is it unnecessary to perform D control with the weak D test?
4. Would the interpretation of this individual's blood type be the same if he were to receive RBCs?

EXERCISE 5-5

A 25-year-old man received 5 units of group O, D-negative RBCs in the ER following a serious car accident. His blood type, which was determined from a sample collected before transfusion, was group O, D-negative. A sample was resubmitted 2 weeks after the accident for pretransfusion testing before orthopedic surgery. The antibody screen was positive, and the antibodies identified were anti-D and anti-C.
1. What are possible explanations for the antibodies identified?
2. What additional testing should be performed to explain the problem?
3. If the blood type of the units he received was correct, what is the probable Rh phenotype of the units that he received?
4. What antigen or antigens should be negative if he needs RBC transfusions in the future?
5. Will it be difficult to obtain these units?

STUDY QUESTIONS

1. The Rh genotype *CDE/cDE* is written in Wiener notation as:
   a. R^0R^1
   b. R^yR^2
   c. R^2R^1
   d. R^zR^2

2. In Rosenfield notation, the phenotype of a donor may be written as Rh:1,−2,−3,4,5. What is the correct phenotype in Fisher-Race (CDE) notation?
   a. cDe
   b. CcDe
   c. CcDE
   d. CDEe

3. Anti-f was identified in a patient. Because commercial antisera are not available, what is the best course of action to locate compatible RBC units?
   a. crossmatch E-negative units
   b. contact the rare donor registry
   c. release O, D-negative units
   d. crossmatch c-negative units

4. A patient's Rh phenotype was determined to be D+, c+, e+, C–, E–. The race of this donor is most likely:
   a. black
   b. white
   c. Asian
   d. Native American

5. The test for the weak D antigen involves:
   a. the IAT
   b. The DAT
   c. anti-D^u typing sera
   d. anti-D antisera with a LISS potentiator

6. The anti-G antibody would be negative with which of the following red cell genotypes?
   a. R_0r
   b. rr
   c. R_2r
   d. $r'r$

7. Results of a weak D test on a patient with a positive direct antiglobulin test would be:
   a. accurate as long as the check cells were positive
   b. unreliable because of immunoglobulins already on the cell
   c. reliable if a high-albumin anti-D was used
   d. false-negative because of antibody neutralization

8. The Rh$_{null}$ phenotype is associated with:
   a. elevated D antigen expression
   b. increased LW antigen expression
   c. the Bombay phenotype
   d. red cell membrane abnormalities

9. The blood group system that was originally identified as the Rh blood group system is now called:
   a. Kell
   b. Lutheran
   c. Lewis
   d. LW

10. A donor tested D-negative using commercial anti-D reagent. The weak D test was positive. How should the RBC unit be labeled?
    a. D-positive
    b. D-negative
    c. D variant
    d. varies with blood bank policy

11. Which offspring is *not* possible from a mother who is R_2r and a father who is R_1r?
    a. *DcE/DcE*
    b. *DCe/DcE*
    c. *DcE/ce*
    d. *ce/ce*

12. Antibodies to the Rh blood group system antigens are usually characterized as:
    a. naturally occurring IgM
    b. immune IgG
    c. immune IgM
    d. naturally occurring IgG and IgM

13. Which of the following genotypes is heterozygous for the C antigen?
    a. R^1r
    b. R^2R^2
    c. R^1R^1
    d. $r'r'$

14. What is the likelihood that two heterozygous D-positive parents will have a D-negative child?
    a. less than 1%
    b. not possible
    c. 25%
    d. 75%

15. Which of the following genotypes could make anti-Ce (Rh7)?
    a. R^2R^2
    b. R^1R^0
    c. R^1R^2
    d. $r'r$

16. Which of the following phenotypes would react with anti-f?
    a. rr
    b. R_1R_1
    c. R_2R_2
    d. R_1R_2

17. A donor is tested with Rh antisera; given the following results, what is the most probable Rh genotype?

	Donor RBC Reaction
Anti-D:	+
Anti-C:	+
Anti-E:	0
Anti-c:	+
Anti-e:	+
Rh control:	0

+, Agglutination; 0, no agglutination.

    a. R_1R_1
    b. R_1r
    c. R_0r
    d. R_2r

18. Anti-D was detected in the serum of a D-positive person. What is a possible explanation?
    a. the antibody is really anti-G
    b. compound antibody was formed
    c. regulator gene failure
    d. missing antigen epitope

19. An antibody to the E antigen was identified in a patient who received multiple transfusions. What is the *most likely* phenotype of the patient's red cells?
    a. R_1R_1
    b. R_2R_2
    c. R_1r
    d. $r'r'$

20. The regulator gene *RHAG*:
    a. is inherited on chromosome 1
    b. is responsible for the Rh_{mod} phenotype
    c. must be inherited to express LW antigens
    d. is responsible for the D-deletion phenotype

REFERENCES

1. Levine P, Stetson RE: An unusual case of intragroup agglutination, *JAMA* 113:126, 1939.
2. Landsteiner K, Wiener AS: An agglutinable factor in human blood recognized by immune sera for rhesus blood, *Proc Soc Exp Biol N Y* 43:223, 1940.
3. Tippett P: A speculative model for the Rh blood groups, *Ann Hum Genet* 50:241, 1986.
4. Colin Y, Cherif-Zahar B, Le Van Kim C, et al: Genetic basis of the RhD-positive and RhD-negative blood group polymorphism as determined by Southern analysis, *Blood* 78:2747, 1991.
5. Mouro I, Colin Y, Cherif-Zahar B, et al: Molecular genetic basis of the human Rhesus blood group system, *Nat Genet* 5:62, 1993.
6. Arge P, Cartron JP: Molecular biology of the Rh antigens, *Blood* 78:551, 1991.
7. Westhoff CM: The Rh blood group system in review: a new face for the next decade, *Transfusion* 44:1663, 2004.
8. Cherif-Zahar B, Bloy C, Le Van Kim C, et al: Molecular cloning and protein structure of a human blood group Rh polypeptide, *Proc Natl Acad Sci U S A* 87:6243, 1990.
9. Daniels G, Lomas-Francis C, Wallace M, et al: Epitopes of Rh D: serology and molecular genetics. In Silberstein LE, editor: *Molecular and functional aspects of blood group antigens*, Bethesda, MD, 1995, AABB.
10. Race RR: The Rh genotypes and Fisher's theory, *Blood* 2:27, 1948.
11. Wiener AS: Genetic theory of the Rh blood types, *Proc Soc Exp Biol Med* 54:316, 1943.
12. Rosenfield RE, Allen FH Jr, Swisher SN, et al: A review of Rh serology and presentation of a new terminology, *Transfusion* 2:287, 1962.

13. Lewis M, Anstee DJ, Bird GWG, et al: Blood group terminology 1990: the ISBT working party on terminology for red cell surface antigens, *Vox Sang* 58:152, 1990.
14. Roback JD, editor: *Technical manual*, ed 17, Bethesda, MD, 2011, AABB.
15. Lomas C, McColl K, Tippett P: Further complexities of the Rh antigen D disclosed by testing category D^{II} cells with monoclonal anti-D, *Transfus Med* 3:67, 1993.
16. Carson TH: *Standards for blood banks and transfusion services*, ed 27, Bethesda, MD, 2011, AABB.
17. Issitt PD: *Applied blood group serology*, ed 3, Miami, FL, 1985, Montgomery Scientific.
18. Schmidt PJ: Hereditary hemolytic anemias and the null blood types, *Arch Intern Med* 139:570, 1979.
19. Cherif-Zahar B, Raynal V, Le Van Kim C, et al: Structure and expression of the RH locus in the Rh-deficiency syndrome, *Blood* 82:656, 1993.
20. Bloy C, Hermand P, Cherif-Zahar B, et al: Comparative analysis by two-dimensional iodopeptide mapping of the RhD protein and LW glycoprotein, *Blood* 75:2245, 1990.

SUGGESTED READINGS

Daniels G, Bromilow I: *Essential guide to blood groups*, ed 2, West Sussex, UK, 2010, Wiley-Blackwell.
Reid ME, Lomas-Francis C: *The blood group antigen facts book*, ed 2, San Diego, 2004, Elsevier Academic Press.

CHAPTER OUTLINE

LEARNING OBJECTIVES

On completion of this chapter, the reader should be able to:

1. Identify the major antigens classified within the other blood group systems.
2. Predict the frequencies of the observed phenotypes and the association of phenotypes with ethnic group diversity.
3. Describe the biochemical characteristics of antigens within each blood group system.
4. Discuss the genetic mechanisms for antigen inheritance in each blood group system. Predict the null phenotypes associated with genetic variations.
5. Compare and contrast the serologic characteristics and clinical relevance of the antibodies associated with each blood group system.

6. Identify unique characteristics of selected blood group systems, their associations with disease, and their biologic functions.
7. Solve complex antibody problems using serologic characteristics of blood group system antibodies.
8. Select compatible donor units for patients with multiple and rare antibodies.
9. Differentiate high-frequency and low-frequency antigens in antibody identification problems.

SECTION 1

WHY STUDY OTHER BLOOD GROUP SYSTEMS?

In addition to the antigens of the ABO and Rh blood group systems, more than 200 unique antigens have been documented on red cells. At the present time, the International Society of Blood Transfusion (ISBT) has defined 30 blood group systems. As previously discussed, the antigens of the ABO and Rh blood group systems are of primary importance in transfusion. The antibodies to ABO and Rh blood group system antigens are capable of effecting a decreased survival of transfused red cells and playing a role in the pathogenesis of hemolytic disease of the fetus and newborn (HDFN). Antigens assigned to other blood group systems can also elicit immune responses in transfusion or pregnancy. Some of these antibodies produced are considered clinically relevant in transfusion medicine. Knowledge of the blood group systems provides the foundation for solving complex antibody problems in a logical and efficient manner.

In traditional terms, the blood group antigen has been considered the target of a red cell alloantibody or autoantibody. The antigen-antibody complex may trigger a process leading to the immune-mediated destruction of red cells. Primary efforts in the blood bank have revolved around problem resolution relating to this pathophysiologic role.

In addition to these pathophysiologic roles, the molecular cloning of blood group genes has provided insight into the primary functional roles of these blood group antigens. More recent studies have linked blood group systems with unique roles in the following physiologic functions related to red cell membranes[1]:

- Molecules that function in transporting water-soluble molecules across the lipid bilayer for intake of nutrients and excretion of waste products
- Molecules that function in the complement pathway
- Molecules that play a role in the ability of cells to adhere to other cells
- Molecules that function as structural proteins to maintain red cell shape and mechanical deformability
- Molecules with suggested enzymatic activities

In addition to serving these physiologic functions, red cell antigens can function as microbial receptors for infection by microorganisms (bacteria, viruses, or protozoan parasites). For example, the Duffy antigens Fy^a and Fy^b serve as the attachment sites for certain malarial parasites. An overview of the relationships of the blood group systems and their unique functional roles is presented in Table 6-1.[1]

ORGANIZATION OF CHAPTER

This chapter highlights the major facts relating to the antigens and antibodies of the other blood group systems. Each blood group system section begins with a box that outlines the major features of each system. The following information is featured:

- ISBT blood group system symbol
- ISBT blood group system number
- Clinical significance of the blood group system antibodies

YES = Antibodies are of clinical significance; reports of decreased red cell survival in vivo (e.g., transfusion reactions and HDFN) are associated with the presence of these antibodies

NO = Antibodies are not of clinical significance; there is no association of decreased red cell survival in vivo (e.g., transfusion reactions and HDFN) with the presence of the antibodies

TABLE 6-1	Functional Roles of the Blood Group Systems
Glycosyltransferases	
ABO, P1PK, Lewis, and H blood group systems	
Structural Relationship to Red Cell	
MNS, Diego, and Gerbich blood group systems	
Transport Proteins	
Rh, Kidd, Diego, Colton, and Kx blood group systems	
Complement Pathway Molecules	
Chido/Rodgers, Cromer, and Knops blood group systems	
Adhesion Molecules	
Lutheran, Xg, Landsteiner-Wiener, and Indian blood group systems	
Microbial Receptors	
MNS, Duffy, P, Lewis, and Cromer blood group systems	
Biologic Receptors	
Duffy, Knops, and Indian blood group systems	

Note. Many of these functional relationships have been predicted based on molecular cloning studies and remain under investigation.

- Immunoglobulin class of most antibodies produced: IgM or IgG immunoglobulin class
- Optimal in vitro antibody binding temperature

 = Antibodies bind at 37° C

 = Antibodies bind at room temperature or lower

- Optimal in vitro reaction method
  RT = Agglutination reactions are observed at room temperature or lower or with a neutral gel card if using gel technology
  AHG = Agglutination reactions are enhanced in indirect antiglobulin tests (IATs) or using the antiglobulin methods of gel technology or solid phase red cell adherence assays (SPRCAs)
- Antibody reactivity with enzyme-treated reagent red cells (ficin or papain)

 = No significant changes in the strength of agglutination reactions are observed with enzyme-treated reagent red cells

 = Agglutination reactions with enzyme-treated reagent red cells are increased in strength (e.g., enhanced)

 = No agglutination is observed with enzyme-treated reagent red cells; the agglutination reactions disappear with enzyme-treated reagent red cells

  VAR = Variable agglutination reactions are observed with enzyme-treated reagent red cells

KELL BLOOD GROUP SYSTEM

ISBT System Symbol	ISBT System Number	Clinical Significance	Antibody Class	Optimal Temperature	Reaction Phase	Effect of Enzymes
KEL	006	YES	IgG		AHG	E → NO EFFECT

CHARACTERISTICS AND BIOCHEMISTRY OF KELL ANTIGENS

Kell Antigens Facts

In 1946, Coombs et al[2] reported the detection of a new blood group antibody in a patient named Kelleher after using their antiglobulin test. This antibody was associated with a case of HDFN, a disease characterized by the decreased survival of fetal red cells because of their sensitization with maternal immunoglobulin G (IgG) antibodies. This antibody, anti-Kell, defined a red cell antigen that was designated the Kell antigen; the Kell blood group system was established. Since its discovery 60 years ago, the Kell blood group system has grown into a complex polymorphism of 32 red cell antigens.[3] Numeric and alphabetic terminologies similar to those of the Rh blood group system have evolved for the Kell blood group system. Any references to the blood group system as an entity are called Kell, whereas appropriate references to the antigens within the system are made through the numeric or alphabetic notations. The original names of the Kell antigens are appropriately used only in an historical context. The correct terminology for the original antigen is K or KEL1 rather than Kell.

Population studies determined that the K (KEL1) antigen has about a 9% frequency in the white population. Its antithetical antigen, k or KEL2 (originally designated as Cellano), possesses a 99.8% frequency in whites and was first reported in 1949.[4] Additional pairs of high-frequency and low-frequency antithetical antigens intrinsic to the Kell blood group system were discovered over the next several years. These antigens were designated Kp^a or KEL3 (originally designated as Penney) and Kp^b or KEL4 (originally designated as Rautenberg).[5,6] The Kp^b (KEL4) antigen possesses a high frequency (99.9%), whereas the Kp^a (KEL3) antigen is rarely expressed in the white population (2%). The Js^a or KEL6 antigen (originally designated as Sutter) and the Js^b or KEL7 antigen (originally known as Matthews) were added to the Kell blood group system as a pair of high-frequency and low-frequency antithetical antigens.[7,8] The Js^a antigen has a 20% frequency in the black population and a 0.1% frequency in whites. At the present time, 32 red cell antigens are assigned to the Kell blood group system, which are summarized in Table 6-2. Similarities to the Rh blood group system include the confinement of Kell antigens to red cells and the presence of detectable antigens on fetal red cells. As a result of this early antigen development, Kell antibodies have been implicated in HDFN cases.

Biochemistry of Kell Antigens

In biochemical terms, the Kell blood group system antigens are located on a glycoprotein that is integral to the red cell membrane.[9] The Kell glycoprotein is covalently linked to another protein, Kx, which defines the Kx blood group system. Special studies of the Kell glycoprotein have revealed that 4000 to 18,000 Kell antigen sites exist per red cell.[10] The biologic role of the Kell glycoprotein has been characterized as a zinc endopeptidase, which is central to zinc binding and catalytic activity.[3]

The Kell antigens are characteristically sensitive to treatment with **sulfhydryl reagents,** such as 2-mercaptoethanol (2-ME), dithiothreitol (DTT), or 2-aminoethylisothiouronium bromide (AET). These reagents reduce the disulfide bonds, which results in a disruption of multiple disulfide bonds in the protein. An antigen with a three-dimensional highly

Red cell antigens classified as high frequency are present in greater than 99% of the population. Red cell antigens classified as low frequency are present in less than 10% of the population.

High-frequency and low-frequency red cell antigens may be inherited together in an antithetical manner, which means on opposite alleles.

K, Kp^a, and Js^a red cell antigens are extremely rare in Asian populations.[12]

Sulfhydryl reagents: reagents that disrupt the disulfide bonds between cysteine amino acid residues in proteins; DTT, 2-ME, and AET function as sulfhydryl reagents.

TABLE 6-2	Summary of Antigens: Kell Blood Group System
Antithetical Antigens: High Frequency and Low Frequency	
K (KEL1) and k (KEL2)	
Kp^a (KEL3), Kp^b (KEL4), and Kp^c (KEL21)	
Js^a (KEL6) and Js^b (KEL7)	
Cote (KEL11) and Wk^a (K17)	
KEL14 and KEL24	
Antithetical Antigens: Low Frequency	
VLAN (KEL25) and VONG (KEL28)	
High-Frequency Antigens	
Ku (KEL5)	
KEL19	
KEL12	
KEL20	
KEL13	
KEL22	
KEL16	
KEL26 (TOU)	
KEL18	
KEL27 (RAZ)	
KALT	
KTIM	
KUCI	
KASH	
KANT	
KELP	
Low-Frequency Antigens	
Ul^a (KEL10)	
KEL23	
KYO	

Modified from Oyen R, Halverson GR, Reid ME: Review: conditions of causing weak expression of Kell system antigens, *Immunohematology* 13:75, 1997.
Note. K8 and K9 are obsolete; K15 (Kx) is no longer included in the Kell system.

folded protein structure is susceptible to any agent that interferes with its tertiary structure. Molecular cloning studies have demonstrated that the Kell glycoprotein possesses an extensively folded disulfide-bonded region. This factor explains Kell antigen sensitivity to disulfide-reducing agents.[11] Treatment of red cells with these sulfhydryl reagents creates red cells that lack Kell antigens. Ethylenediaminetetraacetic acid (EDTA)-glycine acid (EGA, Immucor, Norcross, GA), a reagent that dissociates IgG from red cells, also destroys Kell antigens.[12]

> Kell blood group system red cell antigens are not destroyed when treated with papain or ficin enzymes.

Immunogenicity of Kell Antigens

The K (KEL1) antigen is strongly immunogenic. The immunogenicity of the K antigen ranks second to the D antigen in terms of eliciting an immune response in transfusions. Studies reported that 1 in 10 K-negative individuals who are transfused with K-positive donor red cells develop anti-K in response to transfusion. Other antigens within the Kell blood group system are less immunogenic. Antibodies to these antigens are not commonly observed because of a combination of two factors: antigen frequency and immunogenicity of structure.

K$_0$ or Kell$_{null}$ Phenotype

A red cell phenotype lacking expression of the Kell glycoprotein, and consequently the Kell antigens, was identified by Chown et al[13] in 1957. This null phenotype is designated K$_0$ or Kell$_{null}$ phenotype. The inheritance of two recessive K_0 genes in a homozygote *(K_0K_0)*

results in the null phenotype. These individuals lack all Kell system antigens but express another related antigen, Kx antigen. This antigen is discussed later in this chapter.

The alloantibody stimulated immunologically in K_0 individuals who have received transfusions has been called anti-Ku or anti-KEL5 and is clinically significant for transfusion purposes. Anti-Ku is produced because the Ku antigen is present on all red cells except K_0 cells. Immunized K_0 individuals require transfusion with rare K_0 donor units. Rare donor units can be obtained by contacting the American Rare Donor Program sponsored by the AABB and the American Red Cross.

GENETICS OF KELL BLOOD GROUP SYSTEM

The Kell blood group system gene, *KEL,* is located on chromosome 7. The Kell locus is the site of the different Kell genes that produce the antigens of the Kell blood group system. Five sets of alleles that produce the Kell system's antithetical antigens exist within the Kell locus. These alleles include the following:

- *K* and *k*
- *Kp^a* and *Kp^b*
- *Js^a* and *Js^b*
- *KEL11* and *KEL17 (Wk^a)*
- *KEL14* and *KEL24*
- *VLAN* and *VONG* (both low-frequency antigens)

The high-incidence genes include *k, Kp^b, Js^b,* and *KEL11.* This haplotype is common in all populations. Low-incidence genes include *K, Kp^a, Js^a,* and *KEL17.* The incidence of low-frequency alleles varies among different ethnic groups. The *K, Kp^a,* and *KEL17* alleles are more common in the white population, whereas the *Js^a* allele is more common in the black population.[14] Table 6-3 summarizes the common phenotypes and their frequency distribution of the Kell blood group system.

Other unrelated genetic loci may affect the expression of Kell antigens on red cells. The Kell antigens may be modified by regulator genes on the X chromosome in relation to the Kx blood group system as discussed later in this chapter.

CHARACTERISTICS OF KELL ANTIBODIES

Most Kell system antibodies possess the following characteristics:
- Immunoglobulin class is IgG.
- Antibodies are produced in response to antigen exposure through transfusion or pregnancy.

TABLE 6-3 Common Phenotypes and Frequencies in the Kell Blood Group System

PHENOTYPE	FREQUENCY (%) WHITE	BLACK
K–k+	91	98
K+k–	0.2	Rare
K+k+	8.8	2
Kp(a+b–)	Rare	0
Kp(a–b+)	97.7	100
Kp(a+b+)	2.3	Rare
Js(a+b–)	0	1
Js(a–b+)	100	80
Js(a+b+)	Rare	19

From Reid ME, Lomas-Francis C: *The blood group antigen facts book,* ed 2, San Diego, 2004, Elsevier Academic Press.

- Antibodies agglutinate optimally in the IAT.
- Antibodies usually do not bind complement.
- Antibodies have been associated with hemolytic transfusion reactions and HDFN.
- Enzyme treatment of red cells shows no enhancement or depression of antibody reactivity.
- Depressed reactivity of anti-K is observed in some low-ionic-strength solution (LISS) reagents.

Anti-K is the most commonly observed antibody of the Kell blood group system in the transfusion service. Most examples of anti-K are IgG and react well in IATs. Despite its low frequency (9%), the K antigen's high degree of immunogenicity is responsible for the occurrence of the antibody in a patient population. Examples of IgM anti-K elicited from exposure to some bacteria may also be present in a patient population.[3]

Antibodies to k, Kp^b, and Js^b are not commonly detected because individuals who lack these high-incidence antigens are scarce. An antibody to one of these antigens should be considered when patient serum reacts with most or all panel cells in antibody identification studies. Anti-k and anti-Kp^b production is associated with the white population, whereas anti-Js^b is associated with the black population. Sources of compatible donor red cell units are difficult to obtain when dealing with an antibody to a high-frequency antigen. Suitable donors often may be obtained from the patient's siblings or the American Rare Donor Program.

Antibody production to the Kp^a and Js^a antigens is also infrequent in a patient population because both antigens possess low frequencies. Donor units possessing these antigens are uncommon; exposure to these antigens by transfusion recipients is minimal.

> The association of certain antibodies and race can assist in the resolution of antibody identification. For example, anti-Js^b is associated with the black population.

> Few examples of non–red cell–stimulated anti-K were reported in healthy male donors with no transfusion history. In other examples, a microbial infection was implicated as the immunizing agent.[12]

SECTION 3

Kx BLOOD GROUP SYSTEM

ISBT system symbol: **XK**
ISBT system number: **019**

Kx ANTIGEN AND ITS RELATIONSHIP TO KELL BLOOD GROUP SYSTEM

As previously discussed in the genetics section, the autosomal gene responsible for the production of the Kell glycoprotein is located on chromosome 7. Another gene, assigned to the X chromosome and designated as *XK1,* encodes a protein that carries the Kx antigen. Kx has been assigned to the Kx blood group system. A discussion of this blood group system is included here because the absence of Kx antigen in the McLeod phenotype (discussed in the next section) weakens the expression of Kell antigens.

Although the Kx antigen is genetically independent of the Kell antigens, it possesses a phenotypic relationship to the Kell blood group system. Red cells with normal Kell phenotypes carry trace amounts of Kx antigen. Red cells from K_0 individuals possess elevated levels of Kx antigen.

McLEOD PHENOTYPE

When the *XK1* gene is not inherited, Kx antigen is not expressed on the red cells. The absence of Kx antigen from red cells and a concurrent reduced expression of the Kell blood group system antigens are characteristically associated with a red cell abnormality known as the McLeod phenotype. Individuals with the McLeod phenotype have red cell morphologic and functional abnormalities characterized by decreased red cell survival (Fig. 6-1). The McLeod phenotype is very rare and is seen almost exclusively in males as a result of the X chromosome–borne gene. The Kx antigen, the McLeod phenotype, and the K_0 phenotype are summarized in Table 6-4.

Fig. 6-1 McLeod phenotype: morphologic and functional red cell abnormalities. Individuals expressing the McLeod phenotype have decreased red cell survival with increased hematologic **acanthocytosis** and **reticulocytosis**.

Acanthocytosis: presence of abnormal red cells with spurlike projections in the circulating blood.

Reticulocytosis: increase in the number of reticulocytes in the circulating blood.

TABLE 6-4	Summary of Kell Blood Group System Phenotypes			
	ANTIGEN EXPRESSION			NORMAL RED CELL
PHENOTYPE	**KELL**	**Kx**	**POSSIBLE SERUM ANTIBODIES?**	**MORPHOLOGY?**
Common	Normal	Weak	Kell alloantibodies	Yes
K_0	None	↑↑↑	Anti-Ku	Yes
McLeod	↓↓↓	None	Anti-KL (anti-Kx and anti-Km)	Acanthocytes
DTT-treated	None	↑	Not applicable	Not applicable

Modified from Reid ME, Lomas-Francis C: *The blood group antigen facts book,* ed 2, San Diego, 2004, Elsevier Academic Press.
↓↓↓, Marked reduction; ↑↑↑, marked increase; ↑, slight increase.

McLEOD SYNDROME

The McLeod phenotype is just one phenomenon attributed to the McLeod syndrome. Individuals with McLeod syndrome, in addition to having red cell abnormalities, may possess associated defects of muscular and neurologic origins. Elevated levels of creatine kinase accompany the syndrome. The correlation of depressed Kell antigens and these defects currently is undetermined. The X-linked disorder of **chronic granulomatous disease** is occasionally associated with McLeod syndrome. In this disorder, the normal functional properties of phagocytic white blood cells are impaired. The phagocytes are able to engulf but not kill microorganisms. Because of this functional defect, patients possess an increased susceptibility to infections. A genetic deletion of chromosomal material encompassing both genetic loci on the X chromosome accounts for the association of the McLeod phenotype and chronic granulomatous disease.

Chronic granulomatous disease: inherited disorder in which the phagocytic white blood cells are able to engulf but not kill certain microorganisms.

SECTION 4
DUFFY BLOOD GROUP SYSTEM

ISBT System Symbol	ISBT System Number	Clinical Significance	Antibody Class	Optimal Temperature	Reaction Phase	Effect of Enzymes
FY	008	YES	IgG		AHG	Ⓔ

CHARACTERISTICS AND BIOCHEMISTRY OF DUFFY ANTIGENS

Duffy Antigens Facts

The Duffy blood group system was first described in 1950 when a previously unrecognized antibody was discovered in the serum of a hemophiliac who received multiple transfusions, Mr. Duffy.[15] The antigen that defined this antibody was called Fy^a(FY1). Its antithetical antigen, Fy^b(FY2), was described the following year.[16] When phenotypic studies of the Fy^a and Fy^b antigens were performed, investigators observed that whites commonly had phenotypes Fy(a+b+), Fy(a–b+), or Fy(a+b–). Sanger et al[17] reported in 1955 that most blacks lacked both Fy^a and Fy^b antigens and had the phenotype Fy(a–b–). The Fy(a–b–) phenotype is rare among whites.

Common phenotypes and frequencies of the Duffy antigens are presented in Table 6-5, which shows that phenotype frequencies differ significantly between whites and blacks. A white Australian woman with the rare Fy(a–b–) phenotype was the first to produce anti-Fy3, which reacted with all Fy(a+) and Fy(b+) red cells.[18] This Duffy antigen was called Fy3. Additional antigens (Fy5 and Fy6) have been assigned to the system, which now includes five antigens. Duffy antigens are well developed at birth and detectable on fetal red cells. As with the Kell blood group system antigens, the Duffy antigens have not been identified on granulocytes, lymphocytes, monocytes, or platelets. The Fy^a and Fy^b antigens are considered of greatest importance for transfusion purposes. The antigens in this blood group system are summarized in Table 6-6.

Biochemistry of Duffy Antigens

The Duffy antigens have been mapped to a glycoprotein of the red cell membrane.[19] Molecular studies of the Duffy glycoprotein determined that the glycoprotein spans the lipid bilayer of the membrane multiple times. The Fy^a, Fy^b, and Fy6 antigens are susceptible to proteolytic degradation by the enzymes papain and ficin. When red cells are treated with papain or ficin, these antigens are destroyed.

In 1993, Horuk et al[20] identified the Duffy glycoprotein as an erythrocyte receptor for numerous proinflammatory **chemokines**. These chemokines are involved in the activation

Chemokines: group of cytokines involved in the activation of white blood cells during migration across the endothelium.

TABLE 6-5	Common Phenotypes and Frequencies in the Duffy Blood Group System

	PHENOTYPE		FREQUENCY (%)	
REACTIONS WITH ANTI-Fy^a	REACTIONS WITH ANTI-Fy^b	INTERPRETATION	WHITE	BLACK
+	0	Fy(a+b–)	17	9
0	+	Fy(a–b+)	34	22
+	+	Fy(a+b+)	49*	1
0	0	Fy(a–b–)	Rare	68†

From Reid ME, Lomas-Francis C: *The blood group antigen facts book*, ed 2, San Diego, 2004, Elsevier Academic Press.
*Most common phenotype in the white population.
†Most common phenotype in the black population.

TABLE 6-6	Summary of Antigens and Their Characteristics in the Duffy Blood Group System
Fy^a and Fy^b	Antithetical antigens Expressed on cord blood cells Sensitive to ficin or papain treatment Receptors for *Plasmodium vivax* and *Plasmodium knowlesi*
Fy3	Expressed on cord blood cells Resistant to ficin or papain treatment Red cells that are Fy(a–b–) are also Fy:-3
Fy5	Expressed on cord blood cells Resistant to ficin or papain treatment Common in whites Altered expression in Rh$_{null}$ phenotype Possible antigen interaction between Duffy and Rh proteins
Fy6	Expressed on cord blood cells Red cells that are Fy(a–b–) are also Fy:-6 Sensitive to ficin or papain treatment Antigen has been defined by murine monoclonal antibodies; no human anti-Fy6 has been described

Note: Fy4 is obsolete in this system.

of white blood cells. In this functional role, the Duffy glycoprotein is capable of binding molecules responsible for cell-to-cell communication. Research suggests that the Duffy glycoprotein functions as a biologic sponge for these excess chemokines.

> Fy^a and Fy^b antigens are destroyed with enzymes. Their corresponding antibodies do not react with enzyme-treated red cells.

GENETICS OF DUFFY BLOOD GROUP SYSTEM

In 1968, Donahue et al[21] showed that the Duffy gene, *DARC*, was located on chromosome 1. Their report marked the first assignment of a human gene to a specific chromosome. The Duffy blood group system locus is **syntenic** with the Rh blood group system locus and consists of the following alleles:

> **Syntenic:** genetic term referring to genes closely situated on the same chromosome without being linked

- *Fy^a* and *Fy^b*, which are codominant alleles that produce Fy^a and Fy^b antigens, respectively
- *Fy^x* allele, which encodes a weakened Fy^b antigen
- *Fy* allele, which encodes no identifiable Duffy antigen

The genetic mechanisms for the remaining Duffy blood group system antigens are not completely understood at this time.

> *Fy* allele produces no Duffy glycoprotein on the red cell. *FyFy* homozygotes have the phenotype Fy(a–b–). This phenotype is found in 70% of African Americans and 100% of Gambians.[12]

CHARACTERISTICS OF DUFFY ANTIBODIES

Discussion of Duffy antibodies is limited to anti-Fy^a and anti-Fy^b. Common characteristics of anti-Fy^a and anti-Fy^b include the following:

- The antibodies are stimulated by antigen exposure through transfusion or pregnancy.
- Agglutination reactions are best observed in IATs.
- Immunoglobulin class is IgG.
- The antibodies usually do not bind complement.
- The antibodies possess clinical significance in transfusion and are an uncommon cause of HDFN.
- Anti-Fy^a and anti-Fy^b are nonreactive with enzyme-treated cells because the antigens are degraded by these enzymes.
- Weaker examples of Duffy antibodies demonstrate stronger agglutination reactions with the homozygous expression of antigen [Fy(a–b+) or Fy(a+b–)] versus the heterozygous expression of antigen [Fy(a+b+)]; antibodies are detecting dosage of antigen expression.
- Anti-Fy^a is more commonly observed than anti-Fy^b.

DUFFY SYSTEM AND MALARIA

Most African and American blacks are resistant to infection from certain forms of malarial parasites. Miller et al[22] first made the connection between malaria and the Duffy blood group system in 1975. These investigators showed that Fy(a−b−) red cells were not invaded by *Plasmodium knowlesi* parasites. Later observations confirmed that *P. knowlesi* and *Plasmodium vivax* invaded Fy(a+) or Fy(b+) red cells, but Fy(a−b−) red cells were resistant to infection. The Duffy antigens serve as biologic receptor molecules to assist the attachment of the merozoite to the red cell. The high incidence of the Fy(a−b−) phenotype in the West African population supports the hypothesis that this phenotype offered a selective evolutionary advantage for resistance to *P. vivax* infection. However, resistance to *Plasmodium falciparum* is not a characteristic of the Fy(a−b−) phenotype.

> *Fy* allele provides a genetic selective advantage in geographic areas where *P. vivax* is endemic.

SECTION 5
KIDD BLOOD GROUP SYSTEM

ISBT System Symbol	ISBT System Number	Clinical Significance	Antibody Class	Optimal Temperature	Reaction Phase	Effect of Enzymes
JK	009	**YES**	IgG		AHG	E ↑

CHARACTERISTICS AND BIOCHEMISTRY OF KIDD ANTIGENS

Kidd Antigens Facts

In contrast to the polymorphism of the Rh and Kell blood group systems, the Kidd blood group system is relatively uncomplicated at both the serologic and the genetic levels. The unique characteristic of the Kidd blood group system arises from the challenge for the transfusion service personnel to detect Kidd alloantibodies in vitro. The Kidd antibodies are often linked to extravascular hemolysis in delayed hemolytic transfusion reactions, where removal of antibody-sensitized red cells is facilitated by the reticuloendothelial system.

Three antigens—Jk^a, Jk^b, and Jk3—define the Kidd blood group system. The original reports of the antibodies to Jk^a and Jk^b appeared in the early 1950s,[23,24] followed by the discovery of the Jk(a−b−) phenotype, or the Kidd null phenotype.[25] Individuals with this null phenotype are usually from the Far East and Pacific Island areas and may produce an antibody, anti-Jk3, that is reactive serologically as an inseparable combination of anti-Jk^a and anti-Jk^b. This unique antibody defined an antigen specified as Jk3. The Jk3 antigen is present whenever Jk^a or Jk^b antigens are also produced. This antigen is analogous to Fy3 antigen in that Fy3 antigen is present on Fy(a+) and Fy(b+) red cells. Kidd antigens develop early in fetal life and are detectable on fetal red cells. In general, the Kidd antigens do not rank high in terms of red cell immunogenicity. The Kidd antigens are not denatured after exposure to routine proteolytic enzyme reagents. The common phenotypes and frequencies of the Kidd antigens are presented in Table 6-7.

Biochemistry of Kidd Antigens

Heaton and McLoughlin[26] reported the first evidence clarifying the biochemical structure of the Kidd antigens in 1982. These investigators showed that Jk(a−b−) red cells were more resistant to lysis in the presence of 2 M urea than red cells possessing either the Jk^a or Jk^b antigens. Red cells of normal Kidd phenotypes swell and lyse rapidly on exposure to 2 M urea. From these observations, they suggested that the molecule expressing the Kidd antigens was a urea transporter because the absence of the Kidd antigens resulted in a defect in urea transport. More recently, it was reported that the Kidd blood group and urea transport function of human erythrocytes were carried by the same protein.[27]

TABLE 6-7	Common Phenotypes and Frequencies in the Kidd Blood Group System			
	PHENOTYPE		FREQUENCY (%)	
REACTIONS WITH ANTI-Jk^a	REACTIONS WITH ANTI-Jk^b	INTERPRETATION	WHITES	BLACKS
+	0	Jk(a+b−)	26.3	51.1*
0	+	Jk(a−b+)	23.4	8.1
+	+	Jk(a+b+)	50.3†	40.8
0	0	Jk(a−b−)	Rare	Rare

From Reid ME, Lomas-Francis C: *The blood group antigen facts book,* ed 2, San Diego, 2004, Elsevier Academic Press.
*Most common phenotype in the black population.
†Most common phenotype in the white population.

From a practical perspective, screening methods based on the property of resistance to 2 M urea can be used to identify rare Jk(a−b−) donor units.

GENETICS OF KIDD BLOOD GROUP SYSTEM

The Kidd blood group system has been assigned to a genetic locus, *JK*, located on chromosome 18. Characteristics of the alleles within the locus include the following:
- *Jk^a* allele encodes the Jk^a and Jk3 antigens and is codominant with the *Jk^b* allele.
- *Jk^b* allele encodes the Jk^b and Jk3 antigens and is codominant with the *Jk^a* allele.
- *Jk* allele is a silent allele that produces neither Jk^a nor Jk^b antigens; it is a common allele in Polynesians, Filipinos, and Chinese; the *JkJk* genotype results in a Jk(a−b−) phenotype.
- Jk(a−b−) phenotype can also be derived by the action of a dominant suppressor gene, *In(Jk)*.

CHARACTERISTICS OF KIDD ANTIBODIES

As previously mentioned, the alloantibodies produced in response to Kidd antigen exposure are of clinical significance for transfusion recipients. Their importance lies in their characteristic weak reactivity in vitro combined with the capacity to effect severe red cell destruction in vivo. After immune stimulation, antibody titers increase and may quickly decrease to undetectable levels. Delayed hemolytic transfusion reactions and extravascular hemolysis are commonly associated with the antibodies of this blood group system. In addition, rare examples of Kidd antibodies capable of the activation and binding of complement proteins may cause intravascular red cell destruction in a transfusion reaction. A patient's previous records should be consulted before selecting donor units to reduce the incidence of these transfusion reactions.

Common characteristics of anti-Jk^a and anti-Jk^b include the following:
- The immunoglobulin class is IgG.
- Agglutination reactions are best observed by the IAT.
- The antibodies show dosage of Kidd antigens on red cells; weak examples of antibodies demonstrate stronger agglutination reactions with the homozygous expression of antigen [Jk(a−b+) or Jk(a+b−)] versus the heterozygous expression of antigen [Jk(a+b+)].
- Some antibodies may bind complement.
- The antibodies are produced in response to antigen exposure through transfusion or pregnancy.
- The antibodies usually appear in combination with multiple antibodies in the sera of individuals who have formed other red cell antibodies.
- Antibody detection is aided with enzyme reagents, LISS, and polyethylene glycol (PEG).
- The antibodies do not store well; antibody reactivity quickly declines in vitro.

TABLE 6-8	Characteristics of Antibodies in the Kell, Duffy, and Kidd Blood Group Systems		
CHARACTERISTIC	**KELL SYSTEM**	**DUFFY SYSTEM**	**KIDD SYSTEM**
Red cell stimulated	Yes	Yes	Yes; weak antibody
IgG	Yes	Yes	Yes
Reactive with AHG	Yes	Yes	Yes
Effect of enzymes	No effect	No reactivity	Enhanced
Clinical significance	Yes	Yes	Yes
Unique features	Anti-K most common Anti-Js^b more common in blacks Anti-Kp^b more common in whites		Bind complement Common cause of delayed hemolytic transfusion reactions

Because antibodies to the Kell, Duffy, and Kidd blood group antigens are of great clinical significance, their recognition in antibody identification testing is vital to ensure that patients receive antigen-negative donor red cell units when necessary. Each of these blood group systems shares similar antibody characteristics. Table 6-8 compares the important characteristics of these system antibodies.

SECTION 6
LUTHERAN BLOOD GROUP SYSTEM

ISBT System Symbol	ISBT System Number	Clinical Significance	Antibody Class	Optimal Temperature	Reaction Phase	Effect of Enzymes
LU	005	Lu^b **YES**	IgG and IgM		RT (Lu^a)	**E** →
		Lu^a **NO**			AHG (Lu^b)	

CHARACTERISTICS AND BIOCHEMISTRY OF LUTHERAN ANTIGENS

Lutheran Antigens Facts

The Lutheran blood group system comprises 20 antigens. The Auberger antigens, Au^a and Au^b, first reported in 1961 and 1989, respectively, were added more recently to the Lutheran system and assigned to LU18 and LU19.[28] Lutheran antigens have not been found on lymphocytes, granulocytes, monocytes, or platelets. In addition, Lutheran antigens are weakly expressed on cord blood cells. Most Lutheran antigens are of high incidence; corresponding red cell alloantibodies are infrequently encountered in the transfusion service.

The two primary antigens of this system include the antithetical antigens, Lu^a (LU1) and Lu^b (LU2). Antibodies to these antigens are occasionally observed in patient samples. Lu^a (LU1) and Lu^b (LU2) antigens are resistant to ficin and papain treatment of red cells. Individuals in most populations have the Lu(a−b+) phenotype (Table 6-9).

| TABLE 6-9 | Common Phenotypes and Frequencies in the Lutheran Blood Group System | | |

| | PHENOTYPE | | |
REACTIONS WITH ANTI-Lu^a	REACTIONS WITH ANTI-Lu^b	INTERPRETATION	FREQUENCY (%): MOST POPULATIONS
+	0	Lu(a+b−)	0.2
0	+	Lu(a−b+)	92.4
+	+	Lu(a+b+)	7.4
0	0	Lu(a−b−)	Rare

From Reid ME, Lomas-Francis C: *The blood group antigen facts book*, ed 2, San Diego, 2004, Elsevier Academic Press.

The Lu$_{null}$ phenotype, Lu(a−b−), rarely occurs and may manifest itself in any of the following three unique genetic mechanisms:

* Recessive: only true Lu$_{null}$ phenotype; homozygosity for a rare recessive amorph, *Lu*, at the *LU* locus
* Dominant inhibitor or In(Lu) phenotype: heterozygosity for a rare dominant inhibitor gene, *In(Lu)*, that is not located at the *LU* locus
* X-linked suppressor gene: inherited in a recessive manner

Biochemistry of Lutheran Antigens

In biochemical studies using monoclonal antibodies, the Lutheran antigens were located on a membrane glycoprotein.[29] The biologic importance of the Lutheran glycoproteins may be linked to adhesion properties and the mediation of intracellular signaling.[3]

GENETICS OF LUTHERAN BLOOD GROUP SYSTEM

The *LU* locus has been assigned to chromosome 19 and is linked to the *Se* (secretor) locus. The *H, Le,* and *LW* genetic loci are also located on chromosome 19. The *Lu^a* and *Lu^b* codominant alleles genetically encode the production of the low-frequency antigen Lu^a and the high-frequency antigen Lu^b.

CHARACTERISTICS OF LUTHERAN ANTIBODIES

Important serologic characteristics of the Lutheran antibodies are outlined as follows.

Anti-Lu^a

* Anti-Lu^a may be present without immune red cell stimulation.
* Immunoglobulin classes are IgM and IgG.
* Optimal in vitro agglutination reactions are observed at room temperature.
* Anti-Lu^a has a characteristic mixed-field pattern of agglutination; small agglutinates are surrounded by unagglutinated free red cells.
* It has no clinical significance in transfusion; mild cases of HDFN have been reported.

Anti-Lu^b

* Anti-Lu^b is a rare antibody because of the antigen's high incidence.
* Immunoglobulin class is IgG.
* Most examples of anti-Lu^b agglutinate at the antiglobulin phase.
* Some examples of anti-Lu^b show a mixed-field agglutination pattern.
* Anti-Lu^b has been associated with transfusion reactions and mild cases of HDFN.

SECTION 7
LEWIS BLOOD GROUP SYSTEM

ISBT System Symbol	ISBT System Number	Clinical Significance	Antibody Class	Optimal Temperature	Reaction Phase	Effect of Enzymes
LE	007	**NO**	IgM		RT AHG	E ↑

CHARACTERISTICS AND BIOCHEMISTRY OF LEWIS ANTIGENS

Lewis Antigens Facts

The Lewis antigens, in contrast to other blood group antigens, are manufactured by tissue cells and secreted into body fluids.[30] Lewis antigens are found primarily in secretions and plasma and are adsorbed onto the red cell membrane. In contrast to the antigens of the Kell, Duffy, and Kidd blood group systems, the Lewis antigens are not integral to the red cell membrane. The development of the Lewis antigen structure begins in the first week after birth and may continue for 6 years. The Lewis system is similar to the ABO system in that the antigen development depends on three sets of independently inherited genes. Lewis genes encode a glycosyltransferase that adds a sugar to an antigen precursor structure. The Lewis antigen system is not particularly relevant from a clinical standpoint because Lewis antibodies do not usually cause in vivo red cell destruction. The antibodies are common, however, and an understanding of antigen genetics and biochemistry is helpful in the discernment of the serologic characteristics. Frequency distributions of the Lewis antigens appear in Table 6-10.

Biochemistry of Lewis Antigens

The product of the Lewis gene is L-fucosyltransferase, which adds L-fucose to the number 4 carbon of N-acetylglucosamine of type 1 precursor structures. The structure acquires Le^a antigen specificity and is adsorbed onto the red cell membrane, which creates the Le(a+) phenotype. If type 1 H structures are also present in the secretions, the Lewis transferase adds L-fucose to this structure. This resulting product, Le^b, is adsorbed preferentially over the Le^a glycoprotein onto the red cell membrane. As discussed in Chapter 4, the difference between type 1 and type 2 structures is the linkage between the carbons of D-galactose and N-acetylglucosamine on the H precursor chain. In type 2 H chains, the number 4 carbon is unavailable for fucose attachment; type 2 chains never express Lewis antigen activity.

TABLE 6-10 Lewis System Phenotypes and Frequencies

	PHENOTYPE		FREQUENCY (%)	
REACTIONS WITH ANTI-Le^a	REACTIONS WITH ANTI-Le^b	INTERPRETATION	WHITES	BLACKS
+	0	Le(a+b−)	22	23
0	+	Le(a−b+)	72	55
0	0	Le(a−b−)	6	22
+	+	Le(a+b+)	Rare	Rare

From Roback JD: *Technical manual*, ed 17, Bethesda, MD, 2011, AABB.

Newborn red cells possess the Le(a–b–) phenotype. As the Lewis antigens begin to develop, the cells may type as Le(a+b+) until the transition to Le(a–b+) is complete. Reliable Lewis phenotyping may be impossible until about 6 years of age. During pregnancy, Lewis antigens are greatly reduced on red cells.[3]

INHERITANCE OF LEWIS SYSTEM ANTIGENS

The Lewis system depends on three genes to produce the Lewis antigen structures: *H, Se* (secretor), and *Le* (Lewis). The *H, Se,* and *Le* gene products are glycosyltransferases called *FUT1, FUT2,* and *FUT3*. The *Se* gene enables the *H* gene transferase to act in the secretions. The *le, h,* and *se* genes are amorphs and produce no detectable products. If a *Le* gene is inherited, Le[a] antigens are found in the secretions and are adsorbed onto the red cells, regardless of the secretor status. If the *Se* gene is inherited in addition to the *Le* gene, the Lewis transferase converts the available H soluble structure to a Le[b] antigen, and the red cells adsorbs Le[b] instead of Le[a]. This concept is illustrated in Fig. 6-2. If the gene inherited from both parents is *le*, no antigen structure is present on the red cells.

A summary of Lewis inheritance and biochemistry concepts is provided in Table 6-11. Table 6-12 summarizes the genes, plasma products, and red cell phenotypes that arise from the *Le, Se,* and *H* genes.

> The Le[b] antigen is the receptor for *Helicobacter pylori,* a gram-negative bacterium associated with gastritis, peptic ulcer disease, gastric carcinoma, and the Norwalk virus.[12]

TABLE 6-11	Summary of Lewis Inheritance and Biochemistry Concepts

- Le[a] and Le[b] are *not* alleles
- Le(a–b+) red cell phenotype arises from the inheritance of an *Le, Se,* and *H* gene
- Individuals who have a phenotype of Le(a+b–) are not secretors with the exception of the Bombay phenotype
- Bombay phenotype *(hh)* cannot express the Le[b] antigen
- A person can be a nonsecretor *(sese)* and still secrete Le[a] into body fluids
- Lewis antigens found in the secretions are glycoproteins
- Lewis antigens found in plasma are glycolipids
- Red cells adsorb only glycolipids, not glycoproteins, onto the membrane
- Adult red cells with a phenotype of Le(a+b+) are very rare

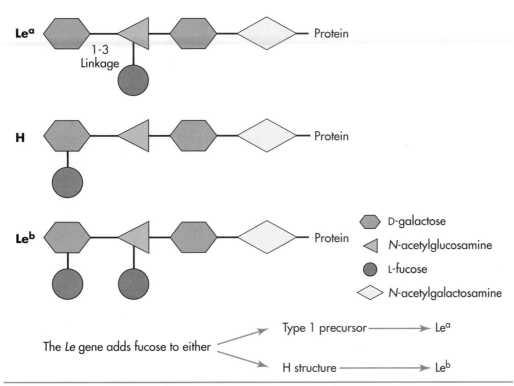

Fig. 6-2 Formation of the Lewis antigens.

TABLE 6-12	Lewis Genes and Red Cell Phenotypes	
GENES PRESENT	**ANTIGENS IN SECRETIONS**	**RED CELL PHENOTYPE**
Le sese H	Le^a	Le(a+b−)
Le Se H	Le^a Le^b H	Le(a−b+)
lele sese H	None	Le(a−b−)
lele Se H	H	Le(a−b−)
Le sese hh	Le^a	Le(a+b−)
Le Se hh	Le^a	Le(a+b−)
lele sese hh	None	Le(a−b−)
lele Se hh	None	Le(a−b−)

CHARACTERISTICS OF LEWIS ANTIBODIES

Lewis antibodies occur almost exclusively in the serum of Le(a−b−) individuals, usually without known red cell stimulus.[30] Le(a−b+) individuals do not produce anti-Le^a, and it is rare to find anti-Le^b in an Le(a+b−) individual. Anti-Le^a or anti-Le^b can be found in an Le(a−b−) individual. Lewis antibodies are IgM and have no clinical significance. If a donor unit of Lewis antigen–positive blood was transfused to a patient with a Lewis antibody, the Le^a or Le^b antigens in the donor plasma would readily neutralize Lewis antibodies. For this reason, it is exceedingly rare for Lewis antibodies to cause decreased survival of transfused Le(a+) or Le(b+) cells. Phenotyping donor blood for the presence of Lewis antigens when a recipient has an anti-Lewis antibody is unnecessary. Crossmatching for compatibility using anti-IgG antihuman globulin, with or without prewarming, provides a good indication of transfusion safety.[31] Avoiding room temperature reactions in the antibody screen or antibody identification panel also avoids anti–Lewis antibody reactivity. Lewis antibodies have not been implicated in HDFN because the antibodies do not cross the placenta, and the antigens are not well developed at birth. Anti-Le^a and anti-Le^b are found during and immediately after pregnancy more often than would be expected.

Serologic Characteristics

Lewis system antibodies can be challenging to identify because the reactions can have a wide temperature range. The challenges include the following:
- Agglutination is observed at immediate spin, 37° C, and the antiglobulin phase.
- Agglutination is often fragile and easily dispersed.
- Enzymes enhance anti-Le^b antibody reactivity.
- Hemolysis is sometimes seen in vitro, especially if fresh serum is used, because anti-Le^a efficiently binds complement.
- Neutralization techniques using commercially prepared Lewis substance may be helpful to confirm the presence of a Lewis antibody or eliminate the reactions to identify other antibodies mixed in the serum.

> Neutralization is an antibody identification technique that combines a soluble antigen with antibody in vitro. If the patient's serum contains the antibody, the soluble antigen makes the antibody inactive.

SECTION 8

I BLOOD GROUP SYSTEM AND i ANTIGEN

ISBT System Symbol	ISBT System Number	Clinical Significance	Antibody Class	Optimal Temperature	Reaction Phase	Effect of Enzymes
I	027	NO	IgM		RT	E ↑

I AND i ANTIGENS FACTS

The I blood group system is composed of one antigen named I, which was assigned to a blood group system in 2002. The product of the *I* gene is *n*-acetylglucosaminyltransferase and is the branching transferase. The i antigen remains in Ii Blood Group Collection 207. The gene for the production of the i antigen has not been identified and is formed from the sequential action of multiple gene products encoding glycosyltransferases. I and i are not antithetical antigens.[3] The i antigen is expressed on newborn and cord blood cells, whereas the I antigen is expressed on adult cells. Anti-I is a commonly encountered auto-antibody with optimal reactivity at colder temperatures. The antibody has no clinical significance because it does not elicit red cell destruction during transfusion or pregnancy. However, this antibody often causes a great deal of confusion in serologic testing.

> Red cell antigens that have not been assigned to a blood group system are classified in blood group collections. The blood group collections contain two or more antigens that are related serologically, biochemically, or genetically. However, these antigens do not fit the criteria for a blood group system.

BIOCHEMISTRY OF I AND i ANTIGENS

The I and i antigens exist on the precursor A, B, and H oligosaccharide chains at a position closer to the red cell membrane. The I antigen is associated with branched chains, and the i antigen is associated with linear chains (Fig. 6-3). The I and i antigens are present on both glycolipid and glycoprotein structures on the red cell membrane. They also can be found as soluble glycoprotein antigens in plasma and in body secretions such as human milk and amniotic fluid.

The I antigen is not well developed at birth; linear chains of the oligosaccharide precursor chain are found predominantly in newborns. As the straight chains develop into branched chains through the action of the branching transferase, the i antigen converts to the I-antigen structure over a 2-year period. Adult red cells possess a strong expression of I antigen and trace amounts of i antigen. Conversely, cord cells possess a strong expression of i antigen and a weak expression of I antigen.

> Autoanti-I can interfere with ABO serum testing and compatibility testing. The frequency of alloanti-I is rare.

> Autoanti-i is an uncommon cold agglutinin that reacts strongly with cord blood cells or adult red cells.

SEROLOGIC CHARACTERISTICS OF AUTOANTI-I

Anti-I is usually found as a cold-reacting, **clinically insignificant** IgM autoantibody. Most individuals possess an autoanti-I detectable at 4° C. Anti-I is often detected when samples are tested at room temperature. Anti-I varies in its reactivity with different adult red cells because the branching oligosaccharide chain structures vary.[30] Because anti-I binds complement, polyspecific antiglobulin reagents may detect the C3d component attached to the red cell. When anti-I is detected, efforts to avoid its reactivity are often accomplished with **prewarming techniques.** This procedure is discussed further in Chapter 7. The use of enzyme reagents in antibody detection enhances anti-I reactivity.

Anti-I also reacts as a compound antibody. It is often found as an anti-IH and exhibits stronger agglutination, with red cells having greater numbers of H antigens, such as group O and group A_2 cells. This antibody is also clinically insignificant. When crossmatching a group A individual, this specificity is noted if agglutination reactions are stronger with panel and screening reagent red cells than with group A donor units.

Clinically insignificant: antibody that does not shorten the survival of transfused red cells or has been associated with HDFN.

Prewarming techniques: patient serum and test cells are prewarmed separately before combining to prevent reactions of cold antibodies binding at room temperature and activating complement.

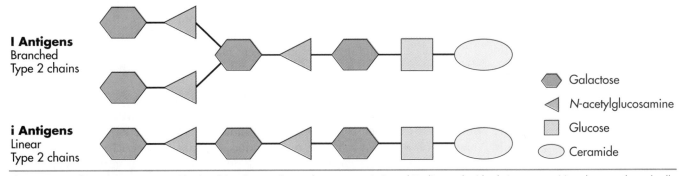

Fig. 6-3 I and i antigen structures. The I and i antigens exist on the precursor A, B, and H oligosaccharide chains at a position closer to the red cell membrane. The I antigen is associated with branched chains, and the i antigen is associated with linear chains.

DISEASE ASSOCIATION

Cold hemagglutinin disease:
autoimmune hemolytic anemia
produced by an autoantibody that
reacts best in colder temperatures
(<37°C).

Strong autoanti-I is associated with *Mycoplasma pneumoniae* infections and **cold hemagglutinin disease.** Anti-i is associated with infectious mononucleosis, lymphoproliferative disease, and occasionally cold hemagglutinin disease. In these situations, if transfusion becomes necessary, finding serologically compatible blood may be more difficult. I-negative or i-negative donor units are not required. Serologic techniques to evaluate these antibodies are discussed further in Chapter 7.

SECTION 9

P1PK BLOOD GROUP SYSTEM, GLOBOSIDE BLOOD GROUP SYSTEM, AND GLOBOSIDE BLOOD GROUP COLLECTION

P1 ANTIGEN

ISBT System Symbol	ISBT System Number	Clinical Significance	Antibody Class	Optimal Temperature	Reaction Phase	Effect of Enzymes
P1PK	003	NO	IgM		RT	E ↑

P ANTIGEN

ISBT System Symbol	ISBT System Number	Clinical Significance	Antibody Class	Optimal Temperature	Reaction Phase	Effect of Enzyme
GLOB	028	YES	IgM and IgG		RT AHG	E ↑

P1PK AND GLOB BLOOD GROUP SYSTEM ANTIGENS FACTS

The P1PK blood group system includes two antigens, P1 and P^k, which include the phenotypes P_1 and P_2 and the null phenotype p. The P antigen in the GLOB (globoside) blood group system is also involved in these phenotypes because P^k is the precursor of the P antigen. These blood group antigens are structurally related to the ABH antigens and exist as glycoproteins and glycolipids. The antigens are formed by the action of glycosyltransferases, and the P1 antigen is present in soluble form in some secretions. Three antigens (P1, P, and P^k) produce five distinct phenotypes: P_1, P_2, p, P_1^k, and P_2^k. These phenotypes and their corresponding antigens in the P system are shown in Table 6-13. Table 6-14 summarizes the antigen and antibody characteristics. The LKE antigen is assigned to the GLOB collections and is associated with the P1, P^k, and P antigens.

The P_1 and P_2 phenotypes
account for greater than 99%
of donors.[12]

The most common phenotypes in the P1PK blood group system are P_1 and P_2, analogous to the A_1 and A_2 phenotypes in the ABH system. Individuals with the P_1 phenotype have both P and P1 antigens on their red cells. Individuals with the P_2 phenotype express only P antigen on their red cells and may produce an anti-P1. The P1 antigen is poorly developed at birth and is variably expressed on adult cells. The antigen expression decreases on storage of the red cells. The P1 antigen exists in a soluble form and can be detected in plasma and **hydatid cyst fluid.**

Hydatid cyst fluid: fluid
obtained from a cyst of the dog
tapeworm.

TABLE 6-13	P1PK and GLOB Blood Group Systems Phenotypes, Antigens, and Frequencies

		FREQUENCIES (%)	
PHENOTYPE	ANTIGENS	BLACKS	WHITES
P_1	P1 P P^k	94	79
P_2	P P^k	6	21
P_1^k	P1 P^k	Very rare	Very rare
P_2^k	P^k	Very rare	Very rare
p	—	Very rare	Very rare

TABLE 6-14	P1PK and GLOB Blood Group Systems Antigen and Antibody Characteristics

PHENOTYPE	ANTIGEN CHARACTERISTICS	POSSIBLE ANTIBODIES	ALLOANTIBODY CHARACTERISTICS
P_1	Red cells express P, P1, and P^k antigens P1antigen is not well developed at birth Most common phenotype	None	Not applicable
P_2	Lacks P1 antigen but expresses P and P^k antigens Second most common phenotype	Anti-P1	IgM; room temperature; not clinically significant Variable reactions with adult cells
P_1^k	Red cells express P1 and P^k antigens Very rare phenotype	Anti-P	Clinically significant; associated with spontaneous abortions (rare)
P_2^k	Red cells express only P^k antigens Very rare phenotype	Anti-P and anti-P1	Anti-P and anti-P1 characteristics
p	Null phenotype of system Negative for P, P1, and P^k antigens Very rare phenotype	Anti-PP1P^k (Tj^a)	Hemolytic; clinically significant; can be separated into three specificities

P, P^k, and LKE antigens are high-frequency antigens. Their relevance in routine testing is uncommon because antibodies to these antigens are very rare. The P^k antigen was thought to be expressed only by the P^k phenotype until the discovery that all red cells except P cells express P^k.[3] LKE-negative cells have a stronger expression of the P^k antigen.

BIOCHEMISTRY

Expression of the P^k, P, and P1 antigens proceeds through the stepwise addition of sugars to lactosylceramide. The P^k antigen is first synthesized through the addition of the carbohydrate galactose by galactosyltransferase 1. The P^k antigen serves as the substrate for *N*-acetylgalactosaminyltransferase 1, which adds *N*-acetylgalactosamine to the terminal

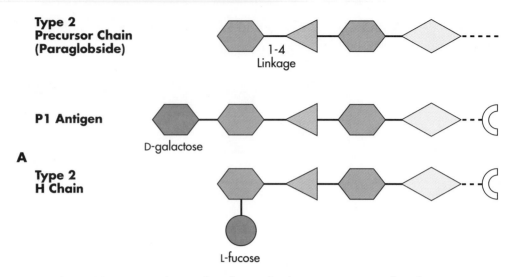

The type 2 precursor chain is the substrate for the P1 antigen as well as the H antigen.

The P antigen structure is similar to the P^k structure; the addition of N-acetylgalactosamine changes P^k to P.

Fig. 6-4 P1PK and GLOB system antigen structures. **A,** P1 antigen. **B,** P^k and P antigen structure.

galactose to make the P antigen. The P1 antigen is formed by the addition of galactose to the paragloboside precursor chain. The formation of the P1PK and GLOB blood group antigens is shown in Fig. 6-4.

P1PK AND GLOB BLOOD GROUP SYSTEM ANTIBODIES

Anti-P1

Anti-P1 is frequently encountered in the serum of P$_2$ individuals and does not require red cell immune stimulation. This antibody is an IgM cold-reactive agglutinin enhanced with enzymes. Commercially available P1 substance can be used to neutralize the antibody to confirm the antibody presence or eliminate the reactions.

Anti-P1 rarely decreases red cell survival. Providing P1-positive red cells is acceptable if compatible at the antiglobulin phase.[32] If reactions are interfering with the crossmatch, avoiding the immediate spin reading usually eliminates the antibody reactions.

Other alloantibodies in these systems are rarely encountered and are summarized in Table 6-14.

Autoanti-P

Paroxysmal cold hemoglobinuria: rare autoimmune disorder characterized by hemolysis and hematuria associated with exposure to cold.

Biphasic hemolysin: antibody, such as the Donath-Landsteiner antibody, that requires a period of cold and warm incubations to bind complement with resulting hemolysis.

Autoanti-P is associated with an immune hemolytic anemia called **paroxysmal cold hemoglobinuria** (PCH). Autoanti-P is an IgG antibody known as the Donath-Landsteiner antibody. This **biphasic hemolysin** binds to P-positive (P$_1$ or P$_2$) red cells at lower temperatures in the extremities. Complement is attached, which effects hemolysis when the red cells are subsequently warmed to 37° C. This rare autoantibody may

Incubation	Result

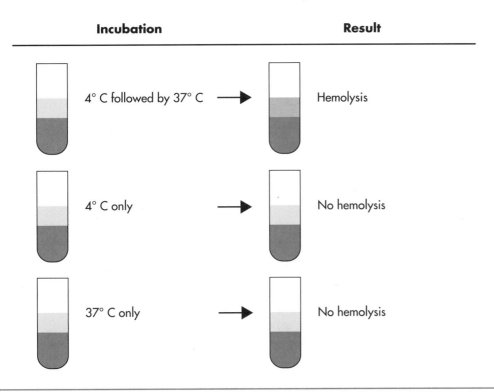

Fig. 6-5 Donath-Landsteiner test. After the patient's freshly drawn serum and red cells are incubated, complement binds only at lower temperatures and causes hemolysis when the tube is warmed to 37°C.

appear transiently in children after viral infections and in adults with tertiary syphilis. The autoantibody reacts weakly or not at all in routine in vitro test methods and requires the Donath-Landsteiner test for confirmation. A summary of this test appears in Fig. 6-5. Another autoantibody that has been implicated in PCH is anti-Pr.

Patients with autoanti-P may have a weak positive direct antiglobulin test because of complement coating. If transfusion becomes necessary, P-negative blood is not required. However, the red blood cell unit may be administered through a **blood warmer.**[33] Patients should be kept warm at all times.

Blood warmer: medical device that prewarms donor blood to 37° C before transfusion.

Anti-PP1P^K

Individuals with the null phenotype (p phenotype) can make an antibody with anti-PP1P^k specificity. This antibody was originally referred to as anti-Tj^a before it became associated with the P system. It can be separated into three antibodies and often exhibits hemolysis in vitro. Anti-PP1P^k is a clinically significant antibody, and red cells from donors who are also "p" are required if transfusion becomes necessary.[34]

SECTION 10
MNS BLOOD GROUP SYSTEM

M AND N ANTIGENS

ISBT System Symbol	ISBT System Number	Clinical Significance	Antibody Class	Optimal Temperature	Reaction Phase	Effect of Enzymes
MNS	002	NO	IgM		RT AHG	Ⓔ

S AND s ANTIGENS

ISBT System Symbol	ISBT System Number	Clinical Significance	Antibody Class	Optimal Temperature	Reaction Phase	Effect of Enzymes
MNS	002	**YES**	IgG		AHG	VAR

The MNS system includes 46 antigens that are expressed primarily on red cells.[12] Molecular genetics have provided insight into the genetic nature of the various MNS system antigens, many of which result from crossing over, gene recombination, and substitutions. This section limits the discussion of the MNS antigens and antibodies to M (MNS1) N (MNS2), S (MNS3), s (MNS4), and U (MNS5).

GENETICS AND BIOCHEMISTRY

The two genes that encode the MNS system antigens are located on chromosome 4. Because of their proximity, they are usually inherited as a haplotype. One gene codes for M or N, and the other codes for S or s. The most frequently inherited haplotype is Ns, followed by Ms, MS, and NS.

The genes *GYPA* and *GYPB* code for **glycophorin** A (GPA) and glycophorin B (GPB), respectively. GPA codes for the M and N antigens, and GPB codes for S and s antigens.

The structures that carry the MNS blood group system antigens are glycoproteins; because most of the sugars carry **sialic acid** structures, the membrane structures are called sialoglycoproteins.[35] The MN sialoglycoprotein (GPA) and the Ss sialoglycoprotein (GPB) structures are similar but distinct. The amino acid sequence makes each a unique structure; Fig. 6-6 compares the antigen structures.

GPA: M and N Antigens

Characteristics of M and N antigens include the following:
- GPA consists of 131 amino acids, with 72 outside the cell membrane.
- M and N antigens differ at positions 1 and 5; the first and fifth amino acid residues for the M antigen structure are serine and glycine, respectively, whereas the N antigen structure has leucine and glutamic acid at positions 1 and 5, respectively.
- Inheriting M or N in the homozygous state [(M+N–) or (M–N+)] greatly enhances the strength of the antigen expression.

GPB: S, s, and U Antigens

Characteristics of S, s, and U antigens include the following:
- GPB consists of 72 amino acids, with 43 outside the cell membrane.
- S and s antigens differ at amino acid position 29; S antigen has methionine at that position, whereas s antigen has threonine.
- The U antigen is located near the membrane and is always present when S or s is inherited.
- Absence of or altered GPB expression would result in red cells phenotyping as S–s–U–.

GPB carries the same first 26 amino acid sequence as the N antigen of the GPA structure. Inheriting S or s provides antigenic activity similar to N called the "N" antigen. This N-like structure may prevent N-negative individuals from forming an anti-N antibody.[34] However, anti-N formed by N-negative individuals and reagent anti-N do not react with "N" because there are too few antigen copies to support agglutination.[36]

ANTIBODIES OF MNS BLOOD GROUP SYSTEM

Antibodies to the antigens included in the MNS system vary in their clinical significance and serologic properties. They are summarized in Table 6-15.

Glycophorin: glycoprotein that projects through the red cell membrane and carries many blood group antigens.

Sialic acid: constituents of the sugars attached to proteins on red cells that lend a negative charge to the red cell membrane.

Fig. 6-6 MN and Ss sialoglycoprotein structural comparison. *COOH,* Carboxy terminal; *Gly,* glycine; *Leu,* leucine; *Glu,* glutamic acid; *Met,* methionine; *NH₂,* Amino terminal; *1,* amino acid 1; *131,* amino acid 131; *Ser,* serine; *Thr,* threonine.

TABLE 6-15	Antibody Characteristics in the MNS System			
ANTIBODY	IMMUNOGLOBULIN CLASS	CLINICALLY SIGNIFICANT	EFFECT OF FICIN	CHARACTERISTICS
M	IgM*	No	Removed	Rarely reported to cause HDFN or HTR; stronger reactions with cells from homozygote
N	IgM	No	Removed	Weak, cold reactive
S	IgG	Yes	Variable	
s	IgG	Yes	Variable	
U	IgG	Yes	Resistant	Reacts with all S+ or s+ red cells; U-negative cells are found only in blacks

HDFN, Hemolytic disease of the fetus and newborn; *HTR,* hemolytic transfusion reaction.
*Sometimes can be whole or partially IgG.[30]

Anti-M

Examples of IgM and IgG forms of anti-M have been reported. Anti-M occurs naturally and is considered a clinically insignificant antibody.[30] Examples of anti-M that react at the antiglobulin phase after a prewarming procedure should be considered clinically significant. Anti-M is rarely implicated in HDFN.

TABLE 6-16	Phenotype Frequencies in MNS System	
	PHENOTYPE FREQUENCIES (%)	
ANTIGEN	WHITES	BLACKS
M+	78	74
N+	72	75
S+	55	31
s+	89	93
U+	99.9	99

From Reid ME, Lomas-Francis C: *The blood group antigen facts book*, ed 2, San Diego, 2004, Elsevier Academic Press.

Anti-M may demonstrates variable reactions with different manufacturers' panel or screening cells because of the pH of the preservative.[37] Some examples of anti-M react better at a pH of 6.5. Anti-M demonstrates marked dosage because agglutination reactions are stronger with homozygous expressions of the antigen (e.g., M+N– reagent red cells have a stronger reaction than M+N+ reagent red cells).

Anti-N

Anti-N is a rarely encountered IgM cold-reacting antibody that is not usually clinically significant. Examples of an N-like antibody have been found more frequently in dialysis patients exposed to formaldehyde-sterilized dialyzer membranes. This anti-N–like antibody is also not clinically significant and may be a result of an altered N-antigen structure on the red cells.[37]

Anti-S, Anti-s, and Anti-U

Anti-S, anti-s, and anti-U are clinically significant IgG antibodies that can cause decreased red cell survival and HDFN. It is not difficult to find compatible blood for patients who have made anti-S or anti-s. Table 6-16 shows the frequency of S and s antigens in the population. The U antigen is a high-incidence antigen, occurring in more than 99% of the population. Anti-U is rare but should be considered when serum from a previously transfused or pregnant black person contains an antibody to a high-incidence antigen. The probability of anti-U existence can be established by showing that the person is S– and s–. U-negative blood can be found in less than 1% of the black population and is not found in white donors. The Rare Donor Registry may need to be contacted if a patient with an anti-U needs a transfusion.

> Anti-M is commonly observed. Anti-N is rare. Most anti-M and anti-N are not clinically significant. When M or N antibodies reactive at 37° C are detected, antigen-negative or compatible red cells should be provided.[12]

SECTION 11

MISCELLANEOUS BLOOD GROUP SYSTEMS

This section addresses the blood groups that are less commonly encountered in routine transfusion medicine. In many of these systems, the clinical significance of the antibodies associated with the system is unknown or not well documented because of the scarcity of examples. Antibodies to the antigens in these systems are infrequent because most are of either high frequency or low frequency, and others are of low immunogenicity. Table 6-17 summarizes these systems or collections. Low-frequency antigens that do not belong to a collection or system are not included. The use of molecular techniques has added to the knowledge of genetics and antigen products and in some instances has altered their classification.

TABLE 6-17 Miscellaneous Blood Groups

NAME	ANTIGEN SYMBOL	ISBT NO.	ANTIGENS	CHARACTERISTICS
Diego	Di, Wr	010	Di^a Di^b Wr^a **Wr^b**	Di^a is more common in South American Indians; anti-Wr^a is commonly found with other antibodies
Cartwright	Yt	011	**Yt^a** Yt^b	Variably sensitive to enzymes; sensitive to DTT
Xg	Xg	012	Xg^a	Inherited on X chromosome; frequency varies with sex
Scianna	SC	013	**SC:1** SC:2 **SC:3**	
Dombrock	Do	014	Do^a Do^b **Gy^a Hy Jo^a**	Hy phenotype is found only in blacks; anti-Do^a and anti-Do^b antibodies are rarely found as a single specificity
Colton	Co	015	Co^a **Co^b Co3**	Anti-Co^b is rarely found as a single specificity
Chido/ Rodgers	Ch/Rg	017	**Ch Rg**	Antigens are sensitive to enzymes and found in plasma; antibodies have HTLA characteristics
Gerbich	Ge	020	**Ge2 Ge3 Ge4** Wb Ls^a An^a Dah	All antigens except for Ge4 are sensitive to enzymes
Cromer	Cr	021	**Cr^a Tc^a** Tc^b Tc^c **Dr^a Es^a IFC WES^a** WES^b **UMC**	Antigen is also found in plasma; located on decay-accelerating factor
Knops	Kn	022	**Kn^a** Kn^b **McC^a Sl^a Yk^a**	Antigen depression in SLE, PNH, and AIDS; antigens are weakened by ficin treatment; antibodies have HTLA characteristics
Cost	Cs	205	**Cs^a** Cs^b	Part of a blood group collection rather than a system
Vel	Vel	901.001	**Vel**	Variable antigen expression on red cells; both IgG and IgM antibodies are associated with hemolytic reactions; antibodies react best with enzyme-treated red cells
JMH	JMH	026	**JMH**	Autoanti-JMH is often found in elderly patients with absent or weak antigen expression; antibodies have HTLA characteristics; antigens are sensitive to enzymes and DTT
Sd^a	Sd^a	901.012	**Sd^a**	Antigen found in guinea pig and human urine; antibodies are typically weak and agglutination is mixed field; reduction of Sd^a expression during pregnancy

Note. Items in boldface indicate antigens of high incidence.
AIDS, Acquired immunodeficiency syndrome; *DTT,* dithiothreitol; *HTLA,* high-titer, low-avidity;
PNH, paroxysmal nocturnal hemoglobinuria; *SLE,* systemic lupus erythematosus.

CHAPTER SUMMARY

Appreciating the unique characteristics of each blood group system is helpful in understanding the serologic and clinical features of the associated antibodies. The clinical significance of the systems is summarized in the following table. With the exception of the ABO system, antibodies that are IgM are usually not clinically significant and react at room temperature, whereas antibodies that are IgG require the antiglobulin test and are clinically significant.

Summary of Clinical Significance of Blood Group Systems[3]

Clinical significance	Blood group system alloantibodies
Clinically significant	ABO, Rh, Kell, Kidd; Duffy; S, s, and U, Lutheran (Lu^b)
Usually clinically insignificant	I, Lewis, M, N, P1, Lutheran (Lu^a)

Modified from Reid ME, Lomas-Francis C: *The blood group antigen facts book,* ed 2, San Diego, 2004, Elsevier Academic Press.

Being familiar with the antigen and antibody characteristics of each blood group system is essential in performing pretransfusion testing, which is introduced in the next section. The following table serves as a quick reference for the important concepts described in this chapter.

System	Antigens	Frequency White	Frequency Black	Reactions Phase	Reactions Enzyme	Class	Comments
Kell	K	9	2	AHG	→	IgG	Antigens in the Kell system are destroyed by DTT
	k	99.9	99.8	AHG	→	IgG	
	Kp^a	2	<1	AHG	→	IgG	
	Kp^b	99.9	>99.9	AHG	→	IgG	
	Js^a	<1	20	AHG	→	IgG	
	Js^b	>99.9	99	AHG	→	IgG	
Duffy	Fy^a	66	10	AHG	⊘	IgG	Fy(a−b−) is protective against malaria
	Fy^b	83	23	AHG	⊘	IgG	
Kidd	Jk^a	77	91	AHG	↑	IgG	Associated with delayed transfusion reactions
	Jk^b	73	49	AHG	↑	IgG	
Lutheran	Lu^a	7.6	5.3	RT	→	IgM	May exhibit mixed-field reactions
	Lu^b	99.8	99.9	AHG	→	IgG	
Lewis	Le^a	22	23	RT	↑	IgM	Lewis antigens are found in plasma and red cells
	Le^b	72	55	RT	↑	IgM	Le^b arises from *H, Le,* and *Se* genes
I	I	>99.9	>99.9	RT	↑	IgM	Frequently found as a cold autoantibody
	i	<1	<1	RT	↑	IgM	I is negative on cord cells
P1PK	P1	79	94	RT	↑	IgM	
MNS	M	78	74	RT	⊘	IgM	Antigens M and N show dosage
	N	72	75	RT	⊘	IgM	
	S	55	31	AHG	var	IgG	S−s− are also U-negative
	s	89	93	AHG	var	IgG	

CRITICAL THINKING EXERCISES

EXERCISE 6-1

The blood bank received a call requesting 2 units of "Kell-negative" red blood cells for a patient with anti-K. Discuss why this request is incorrect. What should the request have stated?

EXERCISE 6-2

List the red cell antibodies with serologic reactivity that is usually enhanced with enzyme-treated panel cells.

EXERCISE 6-3

A patient has a history of the following alloantibodies: anti-S, anti-Le^b, and anti-Jk^a. Which of these antibodies are clinically significant? How would you test for compatible red cell donor units? How would enzyme-treated panel cells react?

EXERCISE 6-4

A patient has a history of a previously identified autoanti-I. The current sample is nonreactive with screening cells when tested at room temperature. What are the implications of this result in a current request for the transfusion of 2 units of red cells?

EXERCISE 6-5

Explain how you would differentiate a Donath-Landsteiner antibody from a cold autoantibody.

EXERCISE 6-6

An anti-Js^b is detected in a prenatal sample. Is this antibody clinically significant? What is the most probable race of this patient? What reagents would be helpful in the work-up of this antibody?

EXERCISE 6-7

A physician requests donor red blood cell units that are phenotypically matched for a very young sickle cell patient. Her phenotype is D+, C−, E−, c+, e+, K, S−, s+, M−, N+; Le(a−b−); Fy(a−b−); Jk(a+b−).

Which donor population (race) would you test to find a close match? Which antigens are not important to match because of the corresponding antibody's clinical significance?

EXERCISE 6-8

A patient has a phenotype of Le(a−b+). Is this patient a secretor or a nonsecretor? What genes are responsible for conferring Le^a and Le^b antigens on the red cells?

EXERCISE 6-9

A patient was admitted for surgery with a history of a previous anti-U. You are directed to test this patient's siblings because U-negative donor units are rare. No commercial antiserum is available for testing. What other antisera could you use to determine the phenotype of the patient's siblings?

EXERCISE 6-10

Does a patient with an anti-Vel present a problem for provision of compatible donor units? How would Vel-negative units be located?

EXERCISE 6-11

What are the Xg blood group system phenotypes of the male and female offspring from the mating of an Xg(a+) male and an Xg(a−) female?

STUDY QUESTIONS

1. Which blood group system possesses the Js^b and Kp^a antigens?
   a. Duffy
   b. Lutheran
   c. Kell
   d. Kidd

2. An antibody commonly associated with delayed transfusion reactions is:
   a. anti-Lu^a
   b. anti-S
   c. anti-Jk^b
   d. anti-M

3. Which phenotype is associated with a resistance to *Plasmodium vivax*?
   a. Fy(a–b–)
   b. Jk(a–b–)
   c. Le(a–b–)
   d. Lu(a–b–)

4. Enzyme-treated reagent red cells used in antibody identification enhance all of the following antibodies *except:*
   a. anti-M
   b. anti-Le^a
   c. anti-Jk^b
   d. anti-I

5. Which of these antibodies are typically IgM?
   a. anti-K
   b. anti-S
   c. anti-U
   d. anti-N
   e. anti-Le^b
   f. anti-Jk^b
   g. anti-P1

6. Which of the following reagents destroys the Kell system antigens?
   a. ficin
   b. albumin
   c. PEG
   d. DTT

7. Glycophorin A and glycophorin B possess antigen sites for which blood group system?
   a. Duffy
   b. Kidd
   c. Lewis
   d. MNS

8. Select the antibody that is characteristically clinically insignificant:
   a. anti-Kp^b
   b. anti-S
   c. anti-Le^b
   d. anti-Fy^a

9. The McLeod phenotype is associated with:
   a. Rh_{null} phenotype
   b. K_0 phenotype
   c. U-negative phenotype
   d. absence of Kx antigens

10. Typing as Lu(a–b–) would be considered:
    a. rare in whites but not blacks
    b. rare in blacks but not whites
    c. rare in all populations
    d. common in all populations

11. Cold autoantibodies are usually of which specificity?
    a. I
    b. M
    c. P1
    d. S

12. Individuals with the p phenotype can make:
    a. anti-P2
    b. anti-p
    c. anti-P
    d. anti-Tj^a

13. Alleles within the Lewis system include:
    a. *Le, le*
    b. *Le^a, Le^b*
    c. *Le, Se, H*
    d. *Le, Le*

14. Which of the following antibodies requires the antiglobulin test for in vitro detection?
    a. anti-M
    b. anti-P₁
    c. anti-U
    d. anti-I

15. What procedure would help to distinguish between an anti-Fyᵃ and anti-Jkᵃ in an antibody mixture?
    a. lowering the pH of the patient's serum
    b. using a thiol reagent
    c. testing at colder temperatures
    d. testing ficin-treated panel cells

16. Anti-K:
    a. agglutinates in IAT phases of the antibody screen
    b. is usually of the IgM antibody class
    c. does not agglutinate with K+k+ panel cells
    d. loses reactivity in enzyme phases

17. Which of the following antigens is poorly expressed on cord blood cells?
    a. K
    b. M
    c. Leᵇ
    d. D

18. Reagent antibody screening cells may not detect antibodies directed against low-incidence antigens. Which antibody is most likely to go undetected?
    a. Vel
    b. S
    c. Kpᵃ
    d. K

19. Select the disease commonly associated with the McLeod phenotype:
    a. infectious mononucleosis
    b. chronic granulomatous disease
    c. Hodgkin's disease
    d. PCH

20. Which set of antibodies could you possibly find in a patient with no history of transfusion or pregnancy?
    a. anti-I, anti-S, and anti-P1
    b. anti-M, anti-c, and anti-B
    c. anti-A, anti-I, and anti-D
    d. anti-B, anti-I, and anti-Leᵃ

21. What is the most likely Lewis phenotype of a nonsecretor?
    a. Le(a−b−)
    b. Le(a+b+)
    c. Le(a+b−)
    d. Le(a−b+)

22. Anti-N is identified in a white patient who requires a blood transfusion. If 10 donor red cell units were tested, how many of these units would most likely be negative for the N antigen?
    a. 0
    b. 3
    c. 7
    d. 10

23. Which of the following antibodies can be neutralized by pooled human urine?
    a. anti-Csᵃ
    b. anti-Sdᵃ
    c. anti-Ch
    d. anti-Vel

24. The red cells of a donor have a phenotype of U-negative. What red cell antibody would not react with these red cells?
    a. anti-M
    b. anti-S
    c. anti-P1
    d. anti-K

25. Chronic granulomatous disease is associated with a depression of the antigens in the _____ blood group system.
    a. Duffy
    b. Kidd
    c. P
    d. Kell

REFERENCES

1. Lublin DM: Functional roles of blood group antigens. In Silberstein LE, editor: *Molecular and functional aspects of blood group antigens*, Bethesda, MD, 1995, AABB.
2. Coombs RR, Mourant AE, Race RR: In vivo isosensitization of red cells in babies with hemolytic disease, *Lancet* 1:264, 1946.
3. Reid ME, Lomas-Francis C: *The blood group antigen facts book*, ed 2, San Diego, 2004, Elsevier Academic Press.
4. Levine P, Backer M, Wigod M, et al: A new human hereditary blood property (Cellano) present in 99.8% of all bloods, *Science* 109:464, 1949.
5. Allen FH, Lewis SJ: Kp^a (Penney), a new antigen in the Kell blood group system, *Vox Sang* 2:81, 1957.
6. Allen FH, Lewis SJ, Fudenberg HH: Studies of anti-Kp^b, a new alloantibody in the Kell blood group system, *Vox Sang* 3:1, 1958.
7. Gibett ER: Js, a "new" blood group system antigen found in Negroes, *Nature* 181:1221, 1958.
8. Walker RH, Argall CI, Steane EA, et al: Anti-Js^b, the expected antithetical antibody of the Sutter blood group system, *Nature* 197:295, 1963.
9. Marsh WL, Redman CM: The Kell blood group system: a review, *Transfusion* 30:158, 1990.
10. Parsons SF, Judson PA, Anstee DJ: Monoclonal antibodies against Kell glycoprotein: serology, immunochemistry, and quantitation of antigen sites, *Transfus Med* 3:137, 1993.
11. Lee S, Zambas ED, Marsh WL, et al: Molecular cloning and primary structure of Kell blood group protein, *Proc Natl Acad Sci U S A* 88:6353, 1991.
12. Roback JD: *Technical manual*, ed 17, Bethesda, MD, 2011, AABB.
13. Chown F, Lewis M, Kaita H: A new Kell blood group phenotype, *Nature* 180:711, 1957.
14. Issitt PD, Antsee DJ: *Applied blood group serology*, ed 4, Durham, NC, 1998, Montgomery Scientific.
15. Cutbush M, Mollison PL, Parker DM: A new human blood group, *Nature* 165:188, 1950.
16. Ikin EW, Mourant AE, Pettenkoffer JH, et al: Discovery of the expected haemagglutinin, anti-Fy^b, *Nature* 168:1077, 1951.
17. Sanger R, Race RR, Jack J: The Duffy blood groups of New York Negroes: the phenotype Fy(a−b−), *Br J Haematol* 1:370, 1955.
18. Albrey 'A, Vincent EE, Hutchinson J, et al: A new antibody, anti-Fy3, in the Duffy blood group system, *Vox Sang* 20:29, 1971.
19. Moore S, Woodrow CF, McClelland DB: Isolation of membrane components associated with human red cell antigens Rh(D), (c), (E) and Fy, *Nature* 295:529, 1982.
20. Horuk R, Chitnis CE, Darbonne WC, et al: A receptor for the malarial parasite *Plasmodium vivax*: the erythrocyte chemokine receptor, *Science* 261:1182, 1993.
21. Donahue RP, Bias WB, Renwick JH, et al: Probable assignment of the Duffy blood group locus to chromosome 1 in man, *Proc Natl Acad Sci U S A* 61:949, 1968.
22. Miller LH, Mason SJ, Dvorak JA, et al: Erythrocyte receptors for *(Plasmodium knowlesi)* malaria: Duffy blood group determinants, *Science* 189:561, 1975.
23. Allen FH, Diamond LK, Niedziela B: A new blood group antigen, *Nature* 167:482, 1951.
24. Plaut G, Ikin EW, Mourant AE, et al: A new blood group antibody, anti-Jk^b, *Nature* 171:431, 1953.
25. Pinkerton FJ, Mermod LE, Liles BA, et al: The phenotype Jk(a−b−) in the Kidd blood group system, *Vox Sang* 4:155, 1959.
26. Heaton DC, McLoughlin K: Jk(a−b−) RBCs resist urea lysis, *Transfusion* 28:197, 1982.
27. Olivès B, Mattei MG, Huet M, et al: Kidd blood group and urea transport function of human erythrocytes are carried by the same protein, *J Biol Chem* 270:15607, 1995.
28. Zelinski T, Kaita H, Coghlan G, et al: Assignment of the Auberger red cell antigen polymorphism to the Lutheran blood group system: genetic justification, *Vox Sang* 61:275, 1991.
29. Parsons SF, Mallinson G, Holmes CH, et al: The Lutheran blood group glycoprotein, another member of the immunoglobulin superfamily, is widely expressed in human tissues and is developmentally regulated in human liver, *Proc Natl Acad Sci U S A* 92:5496, 1995.
30. Harmening DM: *Modern blood banking and transfusion practices*, ed 3, Philadelphia, 1994, FA Davis.
31. Waheed A, Kennedy MS, Gerhan S: Transfusion significance of Lewis system antibodies: report on a nationwide survey, *Transfusion* 21:542, 1981.
32. Anstall HB, Blaylock RC: The P blood group system: biochemistry, genetics and clinical significance. In Moulds JM, Woods LL, editors: *Blood groups: P, I, Sd^a and Pr*, Arlington, VA, 1991, AABB.
33. Mollison PL, Engelfriet CP, Contreras M: *Blood transfusion in clinical medicine*, ed 9, Oxford, UK, 1993, Blackwell Scientific.
34. Anstall HB, Urie PM: Transfusion therapy in special clinical situations. In Anstall HB, Urie PM: *A manual of hemotherapy*, New York, 1986, John Wiley & Sons.
35. Stroup M, Treacy M: *Blood group antigens and antibodies*, Raritan, NJ, 1982, Ortho Diagnostics.
36. Issitt P: *Applied blood group serology*, ed 3, Miami, 1985, Montgomery Scientific.

37. Holliman SM: The MN blood group system: distribution, serology and genetics. In Unger PJ, Laird-Fryer B, editors: *Blood group systems: MN and Gerbich*, Arlington, VA, 1989, AABB.

SUGGESTED READINGS

Poole J, Daniels G: Blood group antibodies and their significance in transfusion medicine, *Transfus Med Rev* 21:58, 2007.

7

Antibody Detection and Identification

CHAPTER OUTLINE

LEARNING OBJECTIVES

On completion of this chapter, the reader should be able to:

1. Define atypical or unexpected antibodies, and explain how they are formed.
2. Evaluate antibody screen and direct antiglobulin test (DAT) reactions to predict the most likely category of antibody problem.
3. Compare and contrast autocontrol and DAT.
4. Explain why patient information including transfusion or pregnancy history, age, race, and diagnosis helps in the process of antibody identification.
5. Describe the reagent red cell panel and antigram with regard to antigen configuration and ABO type.
6. Analyze the phase of reactions to determine the potential clinical significance of an antibody.
7. Correlate the reaction strength of an antibody to the dosage of an antigen and how it can be a clue to antibody resolution.
8. Interpret panel reactions using the process of "ruling out."
9. Explain the "rule of three" with regard to antibody identification.
10. List methods that can be used when identifying multiple antibodies in a serum sample.
11. Differentiate warm autoantibody reactions from an antibody to a high-frequency antigen.
12. Explain the importance of a control when performing antibody neutralization.
13. Discuss the use of and the potential problems with the prewarm procedure.
14. Apply methods to enhance the serologic reactions of weak IgG antibodies.
15. Explain the process of identifying the specificity of a cold autoantibody and techniques to avoid cold autoantibody reactivity.
16. Describe the process and limitations of adsorption techniques as they apply to warm and cold autoantibodies.
17. Illustrate the elution procedure, and list the methods and application of this test.

The detection of an "atypical" or "unexpected" antibody in the screen of a patient or donor initiates the identification process, which can seem like detective work. The terms atypical and unexpected refer to antibodies other than ABO blood group system antibodies. These unexpected antibodies can be made in response to a transfusion of red cells or exposure to fetal cells during pregnancy or delivery. Because these antibodies are directed to a non–self-antigen, they are called alloantibodies. Autoantibodies are antibodies, usually formed by a disease process or medication, made to a person's own red cells. Determining the specificity of antibodies, or antibody identification, necessitates the knowledge of blood group system antigen and antibody characteristics outlined in previous chapters and an understanding of the reagents used to enhance or eliminate reactions. Clues are often subtle and elusive, and the process must be methodical and accurate. Except for a simple antibody with one specificity, each sample is often unique and may necessitate several different approaches to reach a conclusive identification. Proficiency and confidence in antibody resolution come from experience and an understanding of basic theoretical concepts involved in the process. It is also important to review the unique blood group antigen and antibody characteristics discussed in Chapters 5 and 6. This chapter outlines the theory behind problem-solving techniques.

SECTION 1

ANTIBODY DETECTION

ANTIBODY SCREEN

The antibody screen determines whether an antibody to a red cell antigen has been made. Antibody screens are performed to detect antibodies in the following people:
- Patients requiring transfusion
- Women who are pregnant or following delivery
- Patients with suspected transfusion reactions
- Blood and plasma donors

The antibody screen involves incubating the patient's serum or plasma with screening cells at 37° C and performing an indirect antiglobulin test (IAT) for the detection of IgG antibodies. Antibody screening cells are group "O" reagent red cells. These cells are tested with the patient's serum to determine whether an unexpected antibody exists. Fig. 7-1 is an example of an antigram for a two-cell screen. An antigram lists the antigens present in the reagent red cell suspension. A reaction to one or both of the screen cells demonstrates the presence of an atypical antibody. Some workers prefer the three-cell screen because it provides a D-negative cell and homozygous cells for the Duffy and Kidd blood groups. The most common clinically significant antibodies react with a two-cell or three-cell screen. Initial conclusions regarding the type of antibody can often be made when the antibody screen is complete. A summary of typical screen results with the tentative interpretations is listed in Fig. 7-2. Careful attention to the antibody screen results can save time when proceeding to the panel. The screen provides the initial clues that begin the antibody identification process.

Equally important as the detection of clinically significant antibodies is the recognition of false-positive reactions and the potential causes. Reactions that appear to be agglutination but are not can cause unnecessary testing and delay if transfusions are needed. False-positive reactions can be caused by rouleaux, antibodies to preservatives, fibrin, contamination of the sample, and presence of cryoprecipitate from frozen samples.

> The procedure for the antibody screen and other procedures discussed in this chapter are included in the *Laboratory Manual* that accompanies this textbook.

Cell	Rh							MNSs				P₁	Lewis		Lutheran		Kell		Duffy		Kidd				
	D	C	E	c	e	f	Cᵂ	M	N	S	s	P₁	Leᵃ	Leᵇ	Luᵃ	Luᵇ	K	k	Fyᵃ	Fyᵇ	Jkᵃ	Jkᵇ			
I R1R1 (56)	+	+	0	0	+	0	0	+	+	0	+	0	+	0	0	+	+	+	+	0	+	+			
II R2R2 (89)	+	0	+	+	0	0	0	0	+	+	0	+	0	+	0	+	0	+	0	+	+	0			

Fig. 7-1 Screening cell antigram.

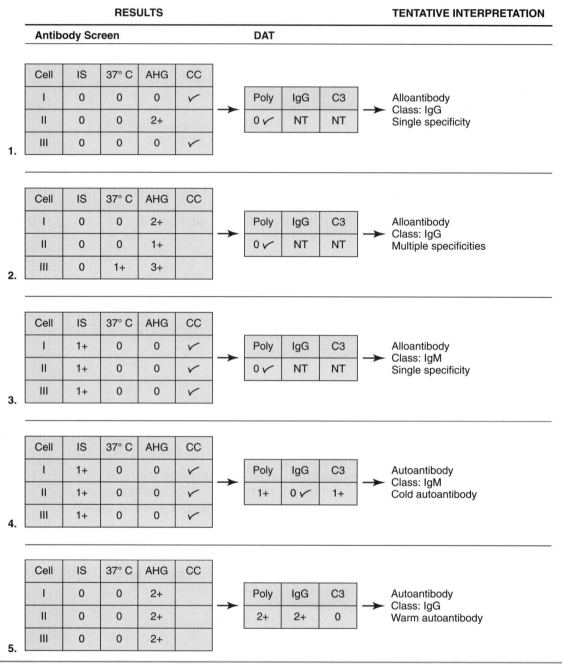

RESULTS   **TENTATIVE INTERPRETATION**

Antibody Screen   **DAT**

1.

Cell	IS	37° C	AHG	CC
I	0	0	0	✓
II	0	0	2+	
III	0	0	0	✓

Poly	IgG	C3
0 ✓	NT	NT

Alloantibody
Class: IgG
Single specificity

2.

Cell	IS	37° C	AHG	CC
I	0	0	2+	
II	0	0	1+	
III	0	1+	3+	

Poly	IgG	C3
0 ✓	NT	NT

Alloantibody
Class: IgG
Multiple specificities

3.

Cell	IS	37° C	AHG	CC
I	1+	0	0	✓
II	1+	0	0	✓
III	1+	0	0	✓

Poly	IgG	C3
0 ✓	NT	NT

Alloantibody
Class: IgM
Single specificity

4.

Cell	IS	37° C	AHG	CC
I	1+	0	0	✓
II	1+	0	0	✓
III	1+	0	0	✓

Poly	IgG	C3
1+	0 ✓	1+

Autoantibody
Class: IgM
Cold autoantibody

5.

Cell	IS	37° C	AHG	CC
I	0	0	2+	
II	0	0	2+	
III	0	0	2+	

Poly	IgG	C3
2+	2+	0

Autoantibody
Class: IgG
Warm autoantibody

Fig. 7-2   Screen interpretations. Tentative interpretations that can be made after testing of the antibody screen and direct antiglobulin test. *IS,* Immediate-spin; *37° C,* 37° C incubation; *AHG,* antihuman globulin; *CC,* check cells; ✓, check cells agglutinate; *NT,* not tested; *Poly,* polyspecific antiglobulin reagent; *C3,* anticomplement reagent.

> A positive antibody screen occurs as a result of prior exposure to red cell antigens from pregnancy or transfusions.

Polyethylene glycol (PEG) can cause false-positive reactions if the reactions are read at 37° C. Before extensive work-ups are initiated, investigating the patient's diagnosis, reviewing methodologies, and obtaining a new sample are recommended.

AUTOCONTROL AND DIRECT ANTIGLOBULIN TEST

An autocontrol tests the patient's serum with his or her own red cells and includes the potentiator used in the antibody screen or panel. It is usually incubated with the antibody identification panel and read at the same phases appropriate for the potentiator. The direct antiglobulin test (DAT) is performed on the patient's cells without serum and potentiator or an incubation step. The differences and uses for both tests are explained later in this chapter. Testing an autocontrol routinely with the screen is optional; most workers prefer to perform a DAT only if the screen is positive.[1] The autocontrol and DAT provide useful information in determining whether the patient's antibody is directed against his or her red cells or against transfused cells, in the case of a recent transfusion.

POTENTIATORS

Potentiators are commonly used in both antibody screening and identification procedures to increase the speed and sensitivity of the antibody attachment to the red cell antigen. Chapter 2 explains the theory of each type of enhancement medium—low-ionic-strength saline (LISS), bovine serum albumin (BSA), polyethylene glycol (PEG), and proteolytic enzymes. Alternative methods such as solid phase and gel technology are increasingly being incorporated in routine screening and antibody identification procedures. Each method has limitations and advantages, which are explained in this section. Selection of potentiators and laboratory methods for antibody detection and identification is usually based on the patient population, workload, and degree of expertise in the laboratory.

LISS is a commonly used potentiator with the screen because it speeds the agglutination, is economical, and provides good sensitivity. LISS testing also has several disadvantages. Increasing serum in the test alters the ionic strength of a LISS procedure, decreasing the sensitivity of the test system. LISS also has been reported by many individuals to enhance cold autoantibodies, especially if the tubes are centrifuged at immediate-spin and microscopic evaluations are performed.

Another potentiator, although less frequently used in routine antibody detection and identification, is 22% BSA, which works well in enhancing the binding of Rh blood group system antibodies. For optimal results, increased incubation time is necessary. BSA reduces the repulsion between cells but does not shorten the incubation time. It does not enhance warm autoantibodies, which is beneficial in working with samples from patients with autoantibodies in their serum.

PEG increases the sensitivity of detection and identification and often detects the presence of antibodies not found with BSA or LISS. Antibodies generally considered of little clinical significance (IgM in nature) do not react well or at all with this potentiator. PEG has been observed to enhance warm autoantibodies, which is an important consideration when using this potentiator.

Proteolytic enzymes (ficin or papain) are not usually used as potentiators in the screen because they eliminate some antigens from the red cells. Enzymes can be used as additional tools for investigating complex antibody problems, but they should never be the sole method. Enzymes may enhance the reactions of one antibody in a mixture of antibodies or abolish the reactions, which lends important information in the solution of the problem. Enzymes enhance cold and warm autoantibodies. The use of enzymes is discussed in further detail later in this chapter.

Gel technology, also sometimes referred to as column agglutination, and solid-phase red cell adherence (SPRCA) techniques are sensitive alternatives to tube testing for the screen that can be automated. In contrast to tube testing using LISS, the only phase that is observed is the antiglobulin phase, avoiding the detection of antibodies of the IgM class. The theory and methodology of these alternative techniques are described in more detail in Chapters 2 and 9.

The uses and limitations of LISS, BSA, PEG, and enzyme potentiators along with gel technology and SPRCA techniques are outlined in Table 7-1. Appreciating the differences and limitations of the potentiators and methods helps the technologist select the most appropriate one for the antibody involved.

PATIENT HISTORY

Before beginning antibody identification procedures, it is essential to obtain a complete transfusion and pregnancy history. Transfusions within the last 3 months present the possibility of a mixed red cell population and recent antibody stimulation. The patient

TABLE 7-1	Comparison of Potentiators and Methods	
POTENTIATOR	**USE**	**LIMITATIONS**
Low-ionic-strength saline (LISS)	Sensitive, economical, and allows for shorter incubation time	Enhances cold autoantibodies Some weak anti-K antibodies may be missed Equal parts of plasma/serum and LISS is important
Bovine serum albumin (BSA)	Affects second stage of agglutination Does not enhance warm autoantibodies	Needs longer incubation Not sensitive for most antibodies except in Rh blood group system
Polyethylene glycol (PEG)	Shows increased sensitivity	Enhances warm autoantibodies Recommend using anti-IgG AHG, not anti-IgG, -C3d AHG No 37° C readings May require extra wash
Enzymes: ficin, papain	Eliminates reactivity of Fy^a, Fy^b, M, and N antigens; S and s antigens are variable Enhances Rh, JK, LE, P1 antibodies	Enhances cold and warm autoantibodies Should not be used as the only method
Gel technology	Avoids cold reactive antibodies Shows increased sensitivity Can be automated	Enhances warm autoantibodies Weak anti-K maybe missed owing to LISS-suspended red cells
Solid phase (SPRCA)	Avoids cold reactive antibodies Shows increased sensitivity Can be automated	Enhances warm autoantibodies Weak anti-K may be missed owing to LISS potentiators Manual method may be difficult to read

AHG, Antihuman globulin.

may not be aware of red cell antibodies. This information might not have been transferred if the patient moved to a different hospital. Communicating with previous medical facilities where the patient may have undergone transfusion is often helpful.

The diagnosis, race, and age of the patient should also be noted because this information offers additional clues to the nature of the antibody problem. Some diseases are associated with the development of certain antibodies. For example, a patient with systemic lupus erythematosus or carcinoma is frequently associated with a warm autoantibody, whereas pneumonia may result in a cold autoimmune process. Patients with sickle cell disease can have both multiple antibodies and autoantibodies. Generally, autoantibodies are rarely encountered in patients younger than 50 years old or in healthy blood donors. Some antibodies are associated only with certain races because of the frequency of antigens in certain populations.

> A patient's transfusion and pregnancy history can provide important clues to the antibodies made to red cell antigens.

SECTION 2

ANTIBODY IDENTIFICATION

INITIAL PANEL

Testing the serum or plasma against a panel of reagent red cells usually follows the detection of the antibody in the screen. A panel, similar to the screening cells, consists

TABLE 7-2	Key to Reactions and Abbreviations
Key to Reactions	
0	No agglutination or hemolysis
+ w	Very tiny agglutinates; cloudy background
1 +	Small agglutinates; cloudy background
2 +	Medium agglutinates; clear background
3 +	Several large agglutinates; clear background
4 +	One solid agglutinate
H	Hemolysis
✓	Check cells agglutinate
NT	Not tested
Key to Abbreviations	
IS	Immediate spin
RT	Room temperature
IAT	Indirect antiglobulin test
AHG	Antihuman globulin
DAT	Direct antiglobulin test
Poly	Polyspecific antiglobulin reagent
CC	Check cells
LISS	Low-ionic-strength saline
PEG	Polyethylene glycol
37	37° C incubation

of group O reagent red cells with phenotypes for most common antigen specificities. Manufacturers prepare panels with various antigen configurations, which may include 10, 11, 15, 16, or 20 cells, which can be thought of as extended antibody screens. Panels are usually initially tested using the same potentiators used in the screen. The use of an autocontrol with the panel is recommended, especially if it is not routinely tested with the screen. Some variation exists among transfusion services and reference laboratories regarding antibody identification procedures. This chapter follows the most widely accepted procedures and provides brief discussions regarding alternative methods.

The panel "map" or antigram is unique to each panel lot number and is used to record and interpret the results. It is important to grade reactions consistently while following specific laboratory guidelines; procedure manuals often represent this as the "key." This key allows more accurate interpretation and the ability of another technologist to review or perform additional testing. The key used for the antibody problems presented in this chapter is shown in Table 7-2.

After results are recorded for each phase and negative reactions can be confirmed with check cells (IgG-sensitized reagent red cells), the panel can be interpreted. The interpretation guidelines in Table 7-3 outline important concepts in evaluating antibody screen results. These guidelines can be used in the examples of antibody problems that follow.

PANEL INTERPRETATION: SINGLE ANTIBODY SPECIFICITY

Refer to Panels 7-1 and 7-2 for the following discussion of interpreting a single antibody.

TABLE 7-3   Guidelines for Interpretation of a Panel

LOOK AT	RESULT	INTERPRETATION
Autocontrol	Negative	Alloantibody
	Positive	Autoantibody or drug interaction Delayed transfusion reaction; transfused cells are sensitized with antibody
Phases	Room temperature or immediate-spin	Cold or IgM antibody
	37° C reactions	May be cold (IgM) if reactions started at room temperature May be warm (IgG) if reactions are not seen at room temperature but noticed at AHG
	AHG	Warm or IgG antibody; clinically significant
Reaction strength	Single strength	Probably one antibody specificity
	Varying strengths	More than one antibody or one antibody showing dosage
Ruling out	Negative reactions	If no reaction was observed, the antibody to the antigen on the panel was probably not present If the antigen on the panel is heterozygous, the antibody may be showing dosage; rule out carefully
	Positive reactions	*Never* rule out using positive reactions
Matching the pattern	Single antibody	If the specificity is a single antibody, the pattern matches one of the antigen columns
	Multiple antibodies	When more than one antibody is present, it is difficult to match a pattern unless the phases or reaction strengths are unique
Rule of three	Three positives	Is the suspected antibody reactive with at least three panel cells that are antigen positive?
	Three negatives	Is the suspected antibody negative with at least three panel cells that do not possess the antigen?
Phenotype of the patient	Negative	If the patient does not possess the antigen, it is possible to make the antibody
	Positive	Transfused red cells are present if patient received a unit of RBCs within 120 days Suspected antibody is incorrect

AHG, Antihuman globulin; *RBCs,* red blood cells.

Panel 7-1   Single Antibody Specificity

Cell	D	C	E	c	e	f	Cʷ	M	N	S	s	P₁	Leᵃ	Leᵇ	Luᵃ	Luᵇ	K	k	Fyᵃ	Fyᵇ	Jkᵃ	Jkᵇ	IS	37	AHG	CC
1 R1R1 (51)	+	+	0	0	+	0	0	+	+	+	0	+	0	+	0	+	+	+	0	+	+	0	0	0	2+	
2 R1R1* (32)	+	+	0	0	+	0	+	+	0	0	+	+	+	0	+	0	+	0	+	0	+	+	+	0	0	0	✓
3 R2R2* (64)	+	0	+	+	0	0	0	0	+	0	+	+	+	0	0	+	+	+	0	0	+	+	0	0	2+	
4 r'r* (75)	0	+	0	+	+	+	0	+	0	+	+	+	0	+	0	+	0	+	+	0	+	+	0	0	0	✓
5 r"r* (87)	0	0	+	+	+	+	0	+	+	+	+	+	0	+	0	+	0	+	+	0	+	0	0	0	0	✓
6 rr* (98)	0	0	0	+	+	+	0	+	+	+	+	+	+	0	0	+	0	+	+	0	+	+	0	0	0	✓
7 rr* (76)	0	0	0	+	+	+	0	+	0	+	0	0	0	+	0	+	+	0	+	+	0	+	0	0	3+	
8 rr* (53)	0	0	0	+	+	+	0	+	0	+	+	+	0	0	0	+	0	+	0	+	0	+	0	0	0	✓
9 rr* (23)	0	0	0	+	+	+	0	+	+	+	+	0	+	0	0	+	0	+	+	+	+	0	0	0	0	✓
10 R1R1* (34)	+	+	0	0	+	0	+	0	+	+	0	+	0	+	0	+	0	+	0	+	+	0	0	0	0	✓
Autocontrol: patient's red cells and patient serum																							0	0	0	✓

*Use negative reactions to rule out.
+, Antigen present; 0, antigen absent.

Panel 7-2 Ruling Out and Determining a Specificity

Cell	D	C	E	c	e	f	Cʷ	M	N	S	s	P₁	Leᵃ	Leᵇ	Luᵃ	Luᵇ	K	k	Fyᵃ	Fyᵇ	Jkᵃ	Jkᵇ	IS	37	AHG	CC
	Rh							MNSs				P₁	Lewis		Lutheran		Kell		Duffy		Kidd		LISS			
1 R1R1 (51)	+	+	0	0	+	0	0	+	+	+	0	+	0	+	0	+	+	+	0	+	+	0	0	0	2+	
2 R1R1 (32)	+	+	0	0	+	0	+	+	0	0	+	+	0	+	0	+	0	+	0	+	+	+	0	0	0	✓
3 R2R2 (64)	+	0	+	+	0	0	0	0	+	0	+	+	+	0	0	+	+	+	0	0	+	+	0	0	2+	
4 r'r (75)	0	+	0	+	+	+	0	+	0	+	+	+	0	+	0	+	0	+	+	0	+	+	0	0	0	✓
5 r"r (87)	0	0	+	+	+	+	0	+	+	+	+	+	0	+	0	+	0	+	+	0	+	0	0	0	0	✓
6 rr (98)	0	0	0	+	+	+	0	+	+	+	+	+	+	0	0	+	0	+	+	0	+	+	0	0	0	✓
7 rr (76)	0	0	0	+	+	+	0	+	0	+	0	0	0	+	0	+	+	0	+	+	0	+	0	0	3+	
8 rr (53)	0	0	0	+	+	+	0	+	+	+	+	+	0	0	0	+	0	+	0	+	0	+	0	0	0	✓
9 rr (23)	0	0	0	+	+	+	0	+	+	+	+	0	+	0	0	+	0	+	+	+	+	0	0	0	0	✓
10 R1R1 (34)	+	+	0	0	+	0	+	0	+	+	0	+	0	+	0	+	0	+	0	+	+	0	0	0	0	✓
Patient cells																							0	0	0	✓

Interpretation: Anti-K and anti-Luᵃ are not crossed out. Anti-K matches the reaction pattern. Three positive cells and three negative cells are demonstrating, "satisfying the rule of 3." Note that cell 7 is homozygous for the *K* gene. The reaction is stronger (showing dosage) with this panel cell as compared with cells 1 and 3.
+, Antigen present, *0*, antigen absent.

Autocontrol

The autocontrol determines whether alloantibody or autoantibody specificity exists. The autocontrol is a suspension of the patient's red cells with the patient's serum. It is incubated with the panel and read at the same phases as the panel. The autocontrol is typically included at the end of the panel, indicated on the panel as "patient cells." If the autocontrol is positive and the DAT is negative, the potentiator may be causing false-positive results. In that case, the panel should be repeated using a different type of potentiator or no enhancement solution. Usually a positive autocontrol or positive DAT indicates an autoantibody or an antibody produced against recently transfused red cells. Autoantibodies are of the cold or warm type, depending on the optimal reaction temperature; they are discussed in greater detail later in this chapter. Panel 7-1 has a negative autocontrol, which indicates an alloantibody exists only in the serum and not on the patient's red cells.

> The autocontrol and DAT help determine if an autoantibody or alloantibody is present.

Phases

The phase or reaction temperature at which agglutination appears is an indication that the antibody is IgG or IgM. IgM antibodies typically react at room temperature or on immediate-spin. IgM antibodies such as anti-Leᵃ, anti-Leᵇ, anti-M, anti-N, anti-I, and anti-P1 should be suspected if immediate-spin reactions are detected. IgG antibodies react at the antiglobulin phase. Reactions at different phases may indicate more than one antibody and a combination of IgG and IgM antibodies. The example in Panel 7-1 illustrates an IgG antibody.

> The phase of the reaction helps determine if an IgG or IgM antibody is present.

Reaction Strength

The strength of the antibody reaction is a clue to the number of antibodies present. Reactions of varying strengths suggest more than one antibody. In this panel, all reactions are fairly strong and of similar strength. Antibodies such as anti-K, anti-D, anti-E, anti-e, anti-c, and anti-C are commonly stronger than anti-Fyᵃ, anti-Fyᵇ, anti-Jkᵃ, anti-Jkᵇ, anti-S, and anti-s. The strength of the reaction also varies with the antigen "dosage." If a panel cell is homozygous, a stronger reaction may be noticed. In some cases, weak antibodies may not even react with heterozygous antigen expression.

> Dosage may be present if antibody reactions vary in strength or if antibody reactions are "missing."

Ruling Out

Panel cells that give negative reactions (0) with all tested phases can be used to **rule out** antibodies. This process is illustrated in Panel 7-2. Begin with the first negative panel cell

> **Rule out:** to eliminate the possibility that an antibody exists in the serum based on its nonreactivity with a particular antigen.

reaction, which is cell 2. Looking across the panel, place a line through the antigen specificity that is positive (+) on the panel. If an antigen-antibody reaction did not occur, the antibody did not react with the antigen on the panel cell, and it can be eliminated as a possible antibody. Panel cells that are heterozygous, particularly in the Duffy, Kidd, and MNS system, should *not* be crossed out because the antibody might have been too weak to react. Continue ruling out using the panel cells that gave a negative reaction. The process of ruling out has narrowed the antibody possibilities down to anti-K and anti-Lu^a.

Matching the Pattern

The next step in panel interpretation is to look at the reactions that are positive and match the pattern. When a single antibody is present, the pattern of reactions observed matches one of the antigen columns. In this example, agglutination was observed with cells 1, 3, and 7, and the antigen K is present on these cells. Therefore, the antibody identity is anti-K. The other potential antibody specificity is not ruled out; Lu^a is a low-frequency antigen (<2% of the population). Because the antigens are rare in the population, the probability of producing an antibody to them is low. For this reason, they can be ruled out without further testing. Additional antigens that are of low frequency in the population that are sometimes listed on panels are V, C^W, Kp^a, and Js^b. Antibodies to these antigens are also typically ruled out but may be considered if the patient has been multiply transfused or has an incompatible **crossmatch**. (The crossmatch is discussed in Chapter 8.) A "special antigen typing" column is often found on panel antigrams that may also provide clues, if reactions do not fall within the patterns of the more commonly found antibodies.

> **Crossmatch:** part of compatibility testing where the donor's red cells are combined with the patient's serum to determine the serologic compatibility between donor and patient.

Low-Incidence (Frequency) Antigens			
Lu^a	Kp^a	V	VS
C^w	Wr^a	Js^a	Co^b

Rule of Three

Identifying antibodies involves performing tests and making a conclusion based on reaction patterns. To make a scientific conclusion, these reactions must be statistically greater than the reactions in a random event. The *p* **value**, or probability value, must be 0.05 or less for identification to be considered valid.[2] To obtain this probability, at least three antigen-positive red cells that react and three antigen-negative red cells that do not react should be observed. In this example, three antigen-positive cells and seven antigen-negative cells were observed. Therefore the **"rule of three"** has been met. If there were not enough cells in this panel to determine sufficient probability, additional cells from another panel would be selected for testing.

> ***p* value:** probability value; value that provides a confidence limit for a particular event.

> **Rule of three:** confirming the presence of an antibody by demonstrating three cells that are positive and three that are negative.

Patient's Phenotype

Individuals do not make alloantibodies to antigens they possess (self-antigens). Another way to confirm antibody identification is to test the patient's red cells to ensure they are negative for the antigen corresponding to the identified antibody. Testing red cells should be performed only if no recent transfusions have occurred. Red cells from transfused donor units may remain in the circulation for 3 months and may cause misleading and incorrect results if different cell populations are present. The accurate phenotype of a recently transfused patient would necessitate **cell separation** techniques to separate transfused and autologous red cells. Cell separation techniques can be found in the methods section of the *AABB Technical Manual*. In laboratories with access to molecular methods, it is possible to determine the genotype of the recipient who has been multiply transfused.[3]

> **Cell separation:** technique used to separate transfused cells from autologous or patient cells.

MULTIPLE ANTIBODIES

When patients have more than one antibody, additional techniques are needed to resolve the problem. Panels 7-3, 7-4, and 7-5 illustrate an approach to multiple antibody identification.

Panel 7-3 Multiple Antibodies

Cell	D	C	E	c	e	f	Cw	M	N	S	s	P1	Lea	Leb	Lua	Lub	K	k	Fya	Fyb	Jka	Jkb	IS	37	AHG	CC
1 R1R1 (51)	+	+	0	0	+	0	0	+	+	+	0	+	0	+	0	+	+	+	0	+	+	0	0	0	0	✔
2 R1R1 (32)	+	+	0	0	+	0	+	+	0	0	+	+	0	+	0	+	0	+	0	+	+	+	0	0	0	✔
3 R2R2 (64)	+	0	+	+	0	0	0	0	+	0	+	+	+	0	0	+	+	+	0	0	+	+	0	0	3+	
4 r'r (75)	0	+	0	+	+	+	0	+	0	+	+	0	+	0	0	+	0	+	+	0	+	+	0	0	2+	
5 r"r (87)	0	0	+	+	+	+	0	+	+	+	+	+	0	+	0	+	0	+	+	+	0	+	0	0	3+	
6 rr (98)	0	0	0	+	+	+	0	+	+	+	+	+	0	+	0	+	0	+	+	0	+	+	0	0	2+	
7 rr (76)	0	0	0	+	+	+	0	+	0	+	0	0	0	+	0	+	+	0	+	+	0	+	0	0	1+	
8 rr (53)	0	0	0	+	+	+	0	+	0	+	+	0	0	+	0	+	0	+	0	+	0	+	0	0	0	✔
9 rr (23)	0	0	0	+	+	+	0	+	+	+	+	0	0	+	0	+	0	+	+	+	+	0	0	0	1+	
10 R1R1 (34)	+	+	0	0	+	0	+	0	+	+	0	+	0	+	0	+	0	+	0	+	+	+	0	0	0	✔
Patient cells		0																	0				0	0	0	✔

Interpretation: Anti-Fy^a and anti-E.
+, Antigen present; 0, antigen absent.

Panel 7-4 Selected Cell Panel

Cell	D	C	E	c	e	f	Cw	M	N	S	s	P1	Lea	Leb	Lua	Lub	K	k	Fya	Fyb	Jka	Jkb	IS	37	AHG
1 r"r (22)	0	+	0	+	+	0	0	+	+	+	0	+	0	+	0	+	+	+	0	+	+	0			
2 R1R1 (72)	+	+	0	0	+	0	+	+	0	0	+	+	0	+	0	+	0	+	0	+	+	+			
3 R2R2 (45)	+	0	(+)	+	0	0	0	0	+	0	+	+	+	0	0	+	+	+	(0)	0	+	+	0	0	3+
4 r"r (28)	0	0	+	+	+	+	0	+	0	+	+	+	0	+	0	+	0	+	0	+	+	+			
5 rr (88)	0	0	0	+	+	+	0	+	+	+	+	+	0	+	0	+	0	+	0	0	+	0			
6 rr (38)	0	0	0	+	+	+	0	+	+	+	+	+	+	0	0	+	0	+	+	+	+	0			
7 rr (74)	0	0	0	+	+	+	0	+	0	+	0	0	0	+	0	+	+	0	+	+	0	+			
8 rr (21)	0	0	0	+	+	+	0	+	0	+	+	+	0	+	0	+	0	+	0	+	0	+			
9 rr (67)	0	0	0	+	+	+	0	+	+	+	0	+	0	+	0	+	0	+	+	+	+	0			
10 R2R2 (92)	+	0	(+)	+	0	0	0	0	+	+	0	+	0	+	0	+	+	0	(0)	+	+	+	0	0	3+

Interpretation: Selected cells for determining that an anti-E was present in the serum along with the anti-Fy^a.
+, Antigen present; 0, antigen absent.

Panel 7-5 Ficin-Treated Panel

Cell	D	C	E	c	e	f	Cw	M	N	S	s	P1	Lea	Leb	Lua	Lub	K	k	Fya	Fyb	Jka	Jkb	37	AHG	CC	Ficin AHG	Ficin CC	
1 R1R1 (51)	+	+	0	0	+	0	0	+	+	+	0	+	0	+	0	+	+	+	0	+	+	0	0	0	✔	0	✔	
2 R1R1 (32)	+	+	0	0	+	0	+	+	0	0	+	+	0	+	0	+	0	+	0	+	+	+	0	0	✔	0	✔	
3 R2R2 (64)	+	0	(+)	+	0	0	0	0	+	0	+	+	+	0	0	+	+	+	0	0	+	+	0	3+		(3+)		
4 r'r (75)	0	+	0	+	+	+	0	+	0	+	+	0	+	0	0	+	0	+	+	0	+	+	0	2+		0	✔	←
5 r"r (87)	0	0	(+)	+	+	+	0	+	+	+	+	+	0	+	0	+	0	+	+	+	0	+	0	2+		(3+)		
6 rr (98)	0	0	0	+	+	+	0	+	+	+	+	+	0	+	0	+	0	+	+	0	+	+	0	2+		0	✔	←
7 rr (76)	0	0	0	+	+	+	0	+	0	+	0	0	0	+	0	+	+	0	+	+	0	+	0	1+		0	✔	←
8 rr (53)	0	0	0	+	+	+	0	+	0	+	+	0	0	+	0	+	0	+	0	+	0	+	0	0	✔	0	✔	
9 rr (23)	0	0	0	+	+	+	0	+	+	+	+	0	0	+	0	+	0	+	+	+	+	0	0	1+		0	✔	←
10 R1R1 (34)	+	+	0	0	+	0	+	0	+	+	0	+	0	+	0	+	0	+	0	+	+	0	0	0	✔	0	✔	
Patient cells																							0	0	✔	0	✔	

Interpretation: ←arrow shows where Ficin treatment of panel cells removed the Fy^a antigen, causing the antibody to no longer react with the panel cells. The treated panel more clearly shows the anti-E antibody.
+, Antigen present; 0, antigen absent.

Following the guidelines outlined in Table 7-3, several conclusions can be made:

- The autocontrol is negative; an alloantibody should be suspected.
- Reactions only at the antihuman globulin (AHG) phase suggest an IgG antibody.
- The reaction strength is variable, which suggests more than one antibody.
- Anti-E and anti-Fy^a cannot be ruled out after crossing out antigens that did not react with the antibody.
- Matching the pattern is more difficult when more than one antibody specificity exists.
- Under the rule of three, two E-positive panel cells were reactive, and four E-negative panel cells were nonreactive; six Fy(a+) panel cells reacted, and four Fy(a–) panel cells were nonreactive; and one panel cell (cell 5) is positive for *both* E and Fy^a, which cannot be included. Therefore, two more E-positive panel cells that are Fy(a–) need to be tested.
- The phenotype shows the patient is E-negative and Fy(a–), providing additional support that these antibodies could be present.

Multiple Antibody Resolution

Selected cells are often used to complete the requirements for the "rule of three" to confirm the antibody specificities that are initially suspected. Cells may be "selected" from other panels without running the entire panel. In this example, Panel 7-4 shows another panel that can be used to select additional E-positive, Fy(a–) cells. Panel cells 3 and 10 are E-positive and Fy(a–). If the same panel manufacturer is used to select more cells, it is important to check that the "donor number or code" is not the same as the panel cell used in the original panel. This number is usually indicated in the first column of the panel. The donor codes for the selected cells used in this example are 45 and 92, which are not the same as the original cells. If the number were the same, it would mean that the same panel cell is being repeated. It is also important to remember that the screening cells that were initially tested may provide additional selected cells.

Additional Techniques

Proteolytic enzymes can be used to eliminate or enhance antibody activity. The Fy^a, Fy^b, S, M, and N antigenic activity is eliminated using enzyme methods. However, the antibodies to antigens of the Rh, Kidd, and Lewis systems are greatly enhanced using enzymes in the test system (Table 7-4). Enzymes act by removing the sialic acid residues from the red cell membrane, eliminating some red cell antigens while exposing others. Two procedures can be used for enzyme treatment, as follows:

- **One-stage enzyme technique:** simultaneous incubation of test serum, enzyme (papain), and red cells is performed.
- **Two-stage enzyme technique:** panel or screening cells are pretreated with enzymes (ficin or papain), washed, and used without other enhancement media in the antiglobulin test. Enzyme-treated red cells can be prepared before use and are also available commercially.

After enzyme treatment, red cells are retested with the serum to determine whether the antibody (or mixture of antibodies) is still reacting. In the example shown in Panel 7-5, the following conclusions can be made:

- If there is no agglutination after enzyme treatment, it can be concluded that the antibody was specific for one of the antigens removed by enzymes. Panel cells 4, 6, 7, and 9 were not reactive after ficin treatment because the anti-Fy^a reactivity was eliminated.

Selected cells: cells chosen from another panel to confirm or eliminate the possibility of an antibody.

One-stage enzyme technique: antibody identification technique that requires the addition of the enzyme to the cell and serum mixture.

Two-stage enzyme technique: treatment of the red cells with an enzyme before the addition of the serum.

Enzymes should never be used as the only enhancement medium.

TABLE 7-4	Enzyme Treatment Summary
BLOOD GROUP	**REACTIVITY WITH ENZYMES**
Rh, P1, I, Kidd, Lewis	Enhanced
M, N, S, Duffy	Destroyed (S and s variable)
Kell	Unaffected

- Cell 5 could be used to confirm the anti-E specificity. The Fy^a antigen was eliminated with ficin, and the anti-E reaction remained.

When using an enzyme-treated cell, observing agglutination only at the AHG phase is recommended to avoid false-positive reactions. Because enzymes denature some antigens, it should not be used as the only antibody detection or identification method.

ANTIBODIES TO HIGH-FREQUENCY ANTIGENS

An antibody to high-frequency antigens (i.e., antigens with a high incidence) presents another type of identification challenge. If an antigen occurs in the population at a 98% or greater frequency, it is considered high frequency or high incidence. Typical reaction patterns are illustrated in Panel 7-6. By using the panel interpretation guidelines (see Table 7-3), the following conclusions can be made to give direction for additional testing:

Panel 7-6 Antibody to a High-Frequency Antigen

Cell	Rh							MNSs				P$_1$	Lewis		Lutheran		Kell		Duffy		Kidd		LISS			
	D	C	E	c	e	f	C^w	M	N	S	s	P$_1$	Le^a	Le^b	Lu^a	Lu^b	K	k	Fy^a	Fy^b	Jk^a	Jk^b	IS	37	AHG	CC
1 R1R1 (51)	+	+	0	0	+	0	0	+	+	+	0	+	0	+	0	+	+	+	0	+	+	0	0	0	3+	
2 R1R1 (32)	+	+	0	0	+	0	+	+	0	0	+	+	0	+	0	+	0	+	0	+	+	+	0	0	3+	
3 R2R2 (64)	+	0	+	+	0	0	0	0	+	0	+	+	+	0	0	+	+	+	0	0	+	+	0	0	3+	
4 r'r (75)	0	+	0	+	+	+	0	+	0	+	+	+	0	+	0	+	0	+	+	0	+	+	0	0	2+	
5 r''r (87)	0	0	+	+	+	+	0	+	+	+	+	+	0	+	0	+	0	+	+	0	+	0	0	0	2+	
6 rr (98)	0	0	0	+	+	+	0	+	+	+	+	+	+	0	0	+	0	+	+	0	+	+	0	0	2+	
7 rr (76)	0	0	0	+	+	+	0	+	0	+	0	0	0	+	0	+	+	(0)	+	+	0	+	0	0	0	✓
8 rr (53)	0	0	0	+	+	+	0	+	0	+	+	+	0	0	0	+	0	+	0	+	0	+	0	0	2+	
9 rr (23)	0	0	0	+	+	+	0	+	+	+	+	0	+	0	0	+	0	+	+	+	+	0	0	0	2+	
10 R1R1 (34)	+	+	0	0	+	0	+	0	+	+	0	+	0	+	0	+	0	+	0	+	+	0	0	0	3+	
Patient cells			0																	0			0	0	0	✓

Interpretation: Anti-k.
+, Antigen present; 0, antigen absent.

- The autocontrol is negative; therefore, an alloantibody should be suspected.
- The phases show that the reactions are occurring only at the AHG phase, which suggests an IgG antibody.
- The reaction strengths are the same, which suggest a single specificity.
- Because only one negative cell exists on the panel, using it to rule out eliminates the possibility of anti-c anti-e, anti-f, anti-M, anti-S, anti-Le^b, anti-Lu^b, anti-K, and anti-Jk^b, which therefore can be ruled out. Antibodies that are not ruled out are anti-D, anti-C, anti-E, anti-C^w, anti-N, anti-s, anti-P1, anti-Le^a, anti-Lu^a, anti-k, and anti-Jk^a and are therefore possible antibodies in the sample. Because the antigens Fy^a and Fy^b are heterozygous on panel cell 7, they should not be used to rule out potential antibodies to these antigens.
- In matching the pattern, anti-k fits the pattern under the k-antigen column when looking across at the potential specificities; because it was not ruled out, the tentative antibody identification is an anti-k.
- Under the rule of three, two additional k-negative cells need to be "selected" from other panels and tested to conclude that an anti-k exists.
- The frequency of being negative for the k antigen is less than 1 in 500; therefore, if the patient is k-negative, the specificity is probably anti-k.

Additional Testing

Although the antibody specificity determined in Panel 7-6 is probably an anti-k after testing the two additional k-negative selected cells, the antibodies that were not ruled out still need to be investigated. Additional k-negative selected cells should be tested. Phenotyping the patient cells for the antigens corresponding to the antibodies not ruled out could also be done because k-negative panel cells are not common.

Eliminating the antigen reactivity by dithiothreitol (DTT) treatment is another approach to working with anti-k.[3] DTT is a reagent that can be used to denature the Kell system antigens on red cells. It works by disrupting the tertiary structure of proteins, which makes them unable to bind with the specific antibody. Treating k-positive cells with DTT, followed by retesting, would eliminate the anti-k agglutination. Potential antibodies "underlying" the anti-k could then be investigated. The use of DTT is not a routine procedure in most transfusion services. It is most useful when antibodies to the high-frequency Kell system antigens are suspected: k, Kp^b, and Js^b DTT treatment of panel cells is not necessary when identifying anti-K, -Kp^a and Js^a.

Additional clues when working with antibodies to high-frequency antigens are summarized in Table 7-5. The potential of multiple antibodies underlying the high-frequency antibody adds to the challenge. Rare reagent red cells used to identify an antibody to a high-incidence antigen and rule out underlying antibodies are not commonly found on panels. Samples may need to be referred to an immunohematology reference laboratory, where an inventory of frozen rare blood cells and rare antisera is available for further testing.

High-Titer, Low-Avidity Antibodies

Some antibodies to high-incidence antigens may have the characteristic "high-titer, low-avidity" (HTLA) reaction pattern. These antibodies are typically weak (low avidity) and can often be diluted out to relatively high titer despite the weak reaction strengths. HTLA antibodies react at the AHG phase, are inconsistent, and are not usually enhanced with other potentiators such as PEG, increased incubation time, or the addition of more serum. They have not been implicated in causing transfusion reactions or hemolytic disease of the fetus and newborn (HDFN). It is not important to identify the specificity of the HTLA antibody. Clinically significant antibodies may be masked by the HTLA reactions.

TABLE 7-5	Clues for Identifying High-Frequency Antibodies
CLUE	**ANTIBODIES AFFECTED**
Room temperature reactions	I, H, P, P1, $PP1P^k$
Negative with ficin-treated cells	Ch, Rg, JMH
Negative with DTT-treated cells	JMH, Yt^a, Js^b, Kp^b, k, LW
Weakened with DTT-treated cells	Lu^b, Do^b, Kn^a
Weak reactions at AHG	Lu^b, Ch, Rg, Cs^a, Kn^a, McC^a, Sl^a, JMH, Sd^a
Negative or weak on cord blood cells	Sd^a, Ch, Rg, Lu^b, I, Vel, Le^a, Le^b
Stronger on cord blood cells	i, LW
Variable expression on RBCs	Lu^b, Kn^a, Sl^a, I, P_1, Sd^a, Ch, Rg, McC^a, JMH, Vel
Race association: black	U, Js^b, Sl^a, At^a, Hy, Tc^a, Cr^a
Race association: white	Kp^b, Lan
Mixed field and refractile microscopically	Sd^a
High-titer, low-avidity antibodies	Ch, Rg, Yk^a Cs^a JMH,* Kn^a McC^a

DTT, Dithiothreitol; *AHG,* antihuman globulin; *RBCs,* red blood cells.
*JMH can be an autoantibody; occurs in older patients.

TABLE 7-6	Characteristics of High-Titer, Low-Avidity Antibodies

Inconsistent reactions that are sometimes not reproducible
Usually not clinically significant
Often found with other antibodies
Variable reactions among panel cells
Not usually enhanced with polyethylene glycol, low-ionic-strength saline, or enzymes
Nonreactive with autologous cells
Weak reactions at antiglobulin phase, often only microscopic
Reactions may be weaker on older red cells
Titration and inhibition may be useful techniques in classification and identification of these
   antibodies

Table 7-6 summarizes some characteristics of the different HTLA antibodies and provides clues for investigation and identification.[4]

ANTIBODIES TO LOW-FREQUENCY ANTIGENS

Patients who make antibodies to multiple antigen specificities often make antibodies to antigens of low incidence. Antibodies to low-incidence antigens can also sometimes occur alone and may be suspected when the screen is negative and the crossmatch is positive. A panel with only one reactive panel cell suggests this type of antibody. Identification of the antibody is limited to the available panel cells and should never be a reason to delay transfusion. The "special type" column found on panels can be used to find additional selected cells for identification. An "extended cell profile" is often available from most reagent manufacturers; it lists in greater detail the less common specificities found on panel cells.

Antibodies to low-incidence antigens include anti-C^w, anti-Wr^a, anti-V, anti-VS, anti-Co^b, anti-Kp^a, anti-Js^a, and anti-Lu^a. When blood is needed, crossmatching for compatibility through the AHG phase is acceptable. Using reagent antisera to screen RBC units for transfusion is not necessary, and in most labs antisera is not available. If an antibody to a low-frequency antigen is identified in a pregnant woman, testing the serum against the father's red cells can predict the possibility of incompatibility with the fetus (assuming the parents are ABO compatible). Titration studies to determine an increase in titer during pregnancy can be performed using the father's cells.

ENHANCING WEAK IgG ANTIBODIES

Weak IgG antibodies are sometimes difficult to identify because the reaction patterns may not fit probable specificities. Repeating the panel with a different enhancement medium, increasing the serum-to-cell ratio, or increasing the incubation time may be necessary. Panel 7-7 illustrates this concept. The antibody (anti-c) reacted only with homozygous cells in the panel tested with LISS. Repeating the panel using PEG enhanced the anti-c reactions significantly. If the serum-to-cell ratio or incubation time is altered to enhance reaction strength, the package inserts for the enhancement media should be reviewed for specific limitations. Reagent red cells from different manufacturers may also give variable results because of preservatives and slight differences in the pH of the red cell suspension. If this is suspected, washing the panel cells once before use may eliminate the problem. Using panel cells before the expiration date is very important because some antigens deteriorate with storage. Obtaining a fresher sample from the patient may also enhance the antibody activity. Determining the identity of weak reacting antibodies is especially important if the patient has been recently transfused because a new antibody may be developing and can be initially very weak. Fig. 7-3 summarizes approaches for resolving a weak antibody.

Panel 7-7   Polyethylene Glycol (PEG) Enhancement

Cell	D	C	E	c	e	f	Cw	M	N	S	s	P1	Lea	Leb	Lua	Lub	K	k	Fya	Fyb	Jka	Jkb	37	AHG	CC	AHG	CC
			Rh						MNSs			P1	Lewis		Lutheran		Kell		Duffy		Kidd			LISS		PEG	
1 R1R1 (51)	+	+	0	0	+	0	0	+	+	+	0	+	0	+	0	+	+	+	0	+	+	0	0	0	✔	0	✔
2 R1R1 (32)	+	+	0	0	+	0	+	+	0	0	+	+	0	+	0	+	0	+	0	+	+	+	0	0	✔	0	✔
3 R2R2 (64)	+	0	+	+	0	0	0	0	+	0	+	+	+	0	0	+	+	+	0	0	+	+	0	1+		2+	
4 r'r (75)	0	+	0	+	+	+	0	+	0	+	+	+	0	+	0	+	0	+	+	0	+	+	0	0	✔	(2+)	
5 r"r (87)	0	0	+	+	+	+	0	+	+	+	+	+	0	+	0	+	0	+	+	0	+	0	0	+w		2+	
6 rr (98)	0	0	0	+	+	+	0	+	+	+	+	+	+	0	0	+	0	+	+	0	+	+	0	+w		2+	
7 rr (76)	0	0	0	+	+	+	0	+	0	+	0	0	0	+	0	+	+	0	+	+	0	+	0	1+		2+	
8 rr (53)	0	0	0	+	+	+	0	+	0	+	+	+	0	0	0	+	0	+	0	+	0	+	0	1+		2+	
9 rr (23)	0	0	0	+	+	+	0	+	+	+	+	0	+	0	0	+	0	+	+	+	+	0	0	1+		2+	
10 R1R1 (34)	+	+	0	0	+	0	+	0	+	+	0	+	0	+	0	+	0	+	0	+	+	0	0	0	✔	0	✔
Patient cells																							0	0	✔	0	✔

Interpretation: Anti-c, which may have been misidentified without PEG enhancement.
+, Antigen present; 0, antigen absent.

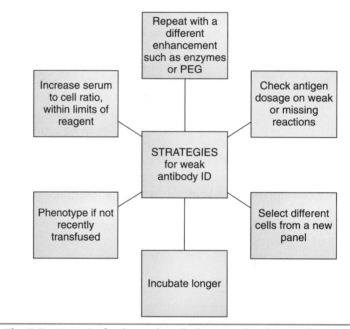

Fig. 7-3   Strategies for the weak antibody or one that does not fit a pattern.

COLD ALLOANTIBODIES

"Cold" or IgM antibodies typically react at immediate-spin, room temperature, and sometimes 37° C phases. These antibodies are usually clinically insignificant in that they do not cause red cell destruction if antigen-positive RBC units are transfused. When the crossmatch is performed, the antibody activity often has to be avoided to find serologically compatible blood.

The specificities of the cold-reacting alloantibodies are anti-P1, anti-M, anti-N, anti-Lea, and anti-Leb. The antibody is usually identified by noting reactions at immediate-spin that may not carry through to the AHG phase, although 37° C reactions are sometimes seen. Panel 7-8 is an example of a "typical" anti-Leb identification panel. Antibodies to P1, M, and N sometimes do not react with all antigen-positive cells because variability often exists in antigen strength. Anti-M and anti-N demonstrate dosage. Anti-P1 reactions vary greatly with the age of the cells used and may not always react with all P1-positive panel cells. To enhance weak reactions or reactions not fitting the expected pattern, incubation at or below room temperature is recommended. Once the antibody is identified, techniques to avoid the reactivity are used to identify underlying clinically significant antibodies and perform a crossmatch.

Panel 7-8 Cold-Reacting Alloantibody																									
	Rh							MNSs				P₁	Lewis		Lutheran		Kell		Duffy		Kidd		LISS			
Cell	D	C	E	c	e	f	Cʷ	M	N	S	s	P₁	Leᵃ	Leᵇ	Luᵃ	Luᵇ	K	k	Fyᵃ	Fyᵇ	Jkᵃ	Jkᵇ	IS	37	AHG	CC
1 R1R1 (51)	+	+	0	0	+	0	0	+	+	+	0	+	0	+	0	+	+	+	0	+	+	0	2+	1+	+w	
2 R1R1 (32)	+	+	0	0	+	0	+	+	0	0	+	+	0	+	0	+	0	+	0	+	+	+	2+	1+	+w	
3 R2R2 (64)	+	0	+	+	0	0	0	0	+	0	+	+	+	0	0	+	+	+	0	0	+	+	0	0	0	✓
4 r′r (75)	0	+	0	+	+	+	0	+	0	+	+	+	0	+	0	+	0	+	+	0	+	+	2+	1+	+w	
5 r″r (87)	0	0	+	+	+	+	0	+	+	+	+	+	0	+	0	+	0	+	0	+	0	+	1+	1+	+w	
6 rr (98)	0	0	0	+	+	+	0	+	+	+	+	+	+	0	0	+	0	+	+	0	+	+	0	0	0	✓
7 rr (76)	0	0	0	+	+	+	0	+	0	+	0	0	0	+	0	+	+	+	0	+	+	0	2+	1+	+w	
8 rr (53)	0	0	0	+	+	+	0	+	0	+	+	+	0	0	0	+	0	+	0	+	0	+	0	0	0	✓
9 rr (23)	0	0	0	+	+	+	0	+	+	+	+	0	+	0	0	+	0	+	+	+	+	0	0	0	0	✓
10 R1R1 (34)	+	+	0	0	+	0	+	0	+	+	0	+	0	+	0	+	0	+	0	+	+	0	1+	1+	+w	
Patient cells																							0	0	0	✓

Reactions are the strongest at IS; therefore a cold-reacting IgM antibody should be suspected, and ruling out should be done at this phase. Interpretation: anti-Leᵇ.
+, Antigen present; 0, antigen absent.

Neutralization techniques are useful procedures for working with certain antibodies to determine if clinically significant antibodies are being masked by their reactions. Soluble forms of Lewis, P1, Sdᵃ, Ch, and Rg antigens can be added to serum to inhibit the reactivity of the antibody. Lewis and P1 substance is available commercially. Sdᵃ substance is found in urine from Sdᵃ-positive individuals. Chido and Rogers antigens are found in plasma from individuals positive for these antigens or a pool of several plasma sources. It is important when performing a neutralization procedure that controls be tested along with the neutralized serum. The control indicates that the negative reactions after neutralization are due to the elimination of antibody reactivity and not simply dilution. An example of potential outcomes of the neutralization technique along with the control is illustrated in Table 7-7.

TABLE 7-7 Neutralization of Anti-Leᵇ			
SELECTED CELLS USED FOR TESTING	CONTROL: SERUM + SALINE	NEUTRALIZATION: SERUM + LEWIS SUBSTANCE	INTERPRETATION
1. Le(a–b+)	1+	0	Lewis antibody was neutralized
2. Le(a–b+)	1+	1+	Lewis antibody was not neutralized or diluted
3. Le(a–b+)	0	0	Antibody was probably diluted

Note. This table illustrates the importance of the control when performing neutralization.
1+, Small agglutinates, clear background; 0, no agglutination or hemolysis.

SECTION 3

AUTOANTIBODIES

The first section of this chapter explained the detection and identification process involving alloantibodies. As previously discussed, the initial investigation of an antibody includes a DAT or autocontrol that, if positive, could be caused by a cold autoantibody, warm autoantibody, drug mechanism, HDFN, or a delayed transfusion reaction. (See the summary in Table 7-8.)

This section describes the techniques used in investigating the DAT and serum reactions caused by cold and warm autoantibodies. Recognizing the presence of an autoantibody and determining if there are clinically significant underlying alloantibodies is the principal focus in this investigation. The specificity of cold and warm autoantibodies is usually not relevant because autoantibodies are reactive with all reagent red cells, donor red cells, and autologous cells, regardless of the antigens present. Detecting and identifying underlying alloantibodies masked by the autoantibody is the chief focus of the investigation. To accomplish this, serologic techniques to avoid interference of the autoantibody or to remove the autoantibody from the serum by **adsorption** are discussed. The clinical manifestations and transfusion support for patients with autoimmune disease are discussed in Chapter 15.

The first clue to an autoantibody is a positive DAT and/or autocontrol along with serum antibodies that are reactive with most or all reagent red cells tested. The patient diagnosis, age, and transfusion and medication history are important to determine the classification and direction of an autoantibody investigation. Also, performing a DAT on a clotted specimen may result in a false-positive complement reaction with anti-C3 and polyspecific AHG reagent. Samples collected in ethylenediamine tetraacetic acid (EDTA) anticoagulant are preferred for performing a DAT to avoid unnecessary testing.

Adsorption: the attachment of antibody to red cell antigens and subsequent removal from the serum.

Detecting and identifying underlying alloantibodies masked by an autoantibody is the primary concern when performing a work up of an autoantibody.

COLD AUTOANTIBODIES

Recognizing the presence of a cold autoantibody is the first step in beginning the investigation. Cold autoantibodies can have reactions at several phases, and each example may be different in the reaction strength and phase noted. As illustrated in Example 4 in Fig. 7-2, the "typical" cold autoantibody is initially observed demonstrating reactions at room temperature, and the DAT is often positive owing to C3.

Panel 7-9 illustrates further the nonspecificity of the reactions, phases, and fairly consistent reaction strengths. Complement-coated patient red cells and panel cells that react at room temperature are the most significant clues in recognizing a cold autoantibody. Although the use of gel technology, solid phase, and PEG do not routinely test at the room temperature phase, cold autoantibodies can attach at room temperature and still demonstrate reactions at AHG. Sometimes the cold antibody may not be detected in the

TABLE 7-8	Interpreting a Positive Direct Antiglobulin Test		
ASSOCIATED WITH	**SPECIFICITY**	**SERUM ANTIBODY**	
Transfusion reaction	IgG	Specific alloantibody	
Warm autoimmune disease	IgG (C3)	Reacts with all cells at antihuman globulin phase	
Cold autoimmune disease; pneumonia	C3	Reacts with all cells at colder temperatures	
Drug interaction	IgG (C3)	Serum may be nonreactive	
Clot tube stored at 4° C	C3	None	
HDFN; maternal antibodies on infant's RBCs	IgG	Alloantibody or ABO antibody from mother on blood cells	

HDFN, Hemolytic disease of the fetus and newborn; *RBCs,* red blood cells.

screen but may become apparent because of an ABO discrepancy in non–group O patients. Patients may have a history of mild anemia, *Mycoplasma pneumoniae* infection, or infectious mononucleosis. Hemolytic cold antibodies found in cold agglutinin syndrome may necessitate transfusion support. Serologic manifestations of cold autoantibodies can be very variable, which contributes to the difficulty in problem resolution.

Panel 7-9 Cold Autoantibody

Cell	D	C	E	c	e	f	Cw	M	N	S	s	P1	Lea	Leb	Lua	Lub	K	k	Fya	Fyb	Jka	Jkb	IS	37	AHG	CC
			Rh							MNSs		P1	Lewis		Lutheran		Kell		Duffy		Kidd				LISS	
1 R1R1 (51)	+	+	0	0	+	0	0	+	+	+	0	+	0	+	0	+	+	+	+	0	+	0	2+	1+	+w	
2 R1R1 (32)	+	+	0	0	+	0	+	+	0	0	+	+	0	+	0	+	0	+	0	+	+	+	2+	1+	1+	
3 R2R2 (64)	+	0	+	+	0	0	0	0	+	0	+	+	+	0	0	+	+	+	0	0	+	+	2+	1+	+w	
4 r'r (75)	0	+	0	+	+	+	0	+	0	+	+	+	0	+	0	+	0	+	+	0	+	+	2+	1+	+w	
5 r''r (87)	0	0	+	+	+	+	0	+	+	+	+	+	0	+	0	+	0	+	+	0	+	0	1+	1+	+w	
6 rr (98)	0	0	0	+	+	+	0	+	+	+	+	+	0	0	0	+	0	+	+	0	+	+	1+	1+	+w	
7 rr (76)	0	0	0	+	+	+	0	+	0	+	0	0	0	+	0	+	+	0	+	+	0	+	1+	1+	+w	
8 rr (53)	0	0	0	+	+	+	0	+	0	+	+	+	0	0	0	+	0	+	0	+	0	+	2+	1+	+w	
9 rr (23)	0	0	0	+	+	+	0	+	+	+	+	0	+	0	0	+	0	+	+	+	+	0	2+	1+	1+	
10 R1R1 (34)	+	+	0	0	+	0	+	0	+	+	0	+	0	+	0	+	0	+	0	+	+	0	1+	1+	+w	
Patient cells																							2+	1+	1+	

+, Antigen present; *0*, antigen absent.

Determining the specificity of the cold autoantibody is helpful to ascertain that additional techniques are reliable. Locating RBC donor units that are negative for the antigen corresponding to the cold antibody is not necessary.

Specificity

Sometimes antibody reactivity that does not fit a particular pattern is attributed to a cold autoantibody. Proceeding with techniques to avoid a suspected cold antibody that was not really there can cause misleading interpretations. Some practitioners advocate establishing the presence of a cold autoantibody before continuing.[5] A "cold panel" is a set of selected reagent red cells that aids in determining the presence of a suspected cold autoantibody (Fig. 7-4). The most common cold autoantibody specificities are anti-I, anti-H, and anti-IH. The I antigen is not well developed at birth; therefore cord blood cells (I-negative) can be useful in determining the specificity. Hospitals with neonatal units usually have access to group O cord samples, which can be used for this purpose. Some manufacturers also have these available on panels. Autoanti-IH and anti-H are more

A		SC I	SC II	AC	Cord	Cord	A₁	A₂	Group O
	4° C	3+	3+	3+	0	0	NT	NT	individual with anti-I

B		SC I	SC II	AC	Cord	Cord	A₁	A₂	Group A
	4° C	3+	3+	3+	1+	1+	1+	2+	individual with cold anti-IH

Fig. 7-4 Mini-cold panel.

commonly found in the serum of group A_1 and A_1B individuals because their red cells have the least amount of H antigen. Differentiating between anti-I, anti-H, and anti-IH is not necessary but can be accomplished by adding A_1 and A_2 cells to the panel.

Avoiding Cold Autoantibody Reactivity

After it has been determined that a cold autoantibody is present and potentially the cause of the reactivity, serologic techniques that *avoid* the reactivity to determine the presence of an underlying alloantibody should be selected. This section outlines the reasons for this approach, as follows:

- *Avoid anticomplement in the AHG test:* The use of anti-IgG antiglobulin reagent rather than polyspecific reagent may help eliminate the cold autoantibody reactions at the AHG phase because this reagent does not detect the attachment of complement. Many laboratories routinely use this reagent for this reason.[5]
- *Eliminate the IS and 37 reading:* By not reading at immediate-spin and the 37° C reaction phase, the attachment of cold autoantibodies can be avoided. Some laboratories do this routinely to avoid detection of cold autoantibodies in testing.
- *Avoid LISS enhancement:* Using 22% BSA as an enhancement instead of LISS avoids some cold autoantibodies that are enhanced by LISS. If albumin is used, an extended incubation is suggested.
- *Perform prewarm technique:* If the procedures listed in the preceding section still do not eliminate a cold autoantibody that is carrying through to the AHG phase, the prewarm technique may be necessary. Fig. 7-5 outlines this technique. Warming the serum and cell suspension to 37° C in separate tubes avoids the antibody attachments that occur at or below room temperature. This technique should be used with care because it can lessen the strength of clinically significant alloantibodies that may be masked by the cold autoantibody.[6] Washing with warm saline after the 37° C incubation and before adding anti-IgG is not recommended because it can remove clinically significant antibodies from the cells, causing antibodies to be missed.[7] In addition, anti-IgG should not be warmed. Because enhancement media are not used, sensitivity is decreased in the prewarmed procedure.[8]

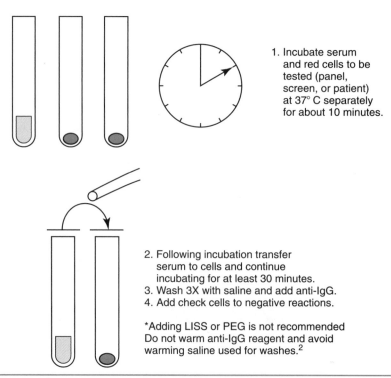

1. Incubate serum and red cells to be tested (panel, screen, or patient) at 37° C separately for about 10 minutes.

2. Following incubation transfer serum to cells and continue incubating for at least 30 minutes.
3. Wash 3X with saline and add anti-IgG.
4. Add check cells to negative reactions.

*Adding LISS or PEG is not recommended
Do not warm anti-IgG reagent and avoid warming saline used for washes.[2]

Fig. 7-5   Prewarm technique. (Modified from Immucor, Norcross, GA.)

TABLE 7-9 Adsorption Techniques

ADSORPTION TECHNIQUE	DESCRIPTION	LIMITATIONS
Rabbit erythrocyte stroma (RESt)	Removes cold (IgM) antibodies, particularly anti-I specificities	May adsorb anti-B and other IgM antibodies[9]
Cold autoadsorption	Patient red cells are used to remove cold autoantibodies to determine if allotransfused antibodies are present	Do not use if recently transfused
Warm autoadsorption	Patient red cells are used to remove warm autoantibodies to determine if alloantibodies are present	Do not use if recently transfused
Differential (allogeneic) adsorption	Uses known phenotyped red cells to separate specificities: • warm autoantibodies from alloantibodies • alloantibodies with several specificities	May adsorb a high-frequency alloantibody

TABLE 7-10 Typical Warm Autoantibody Characteristics

TESTS	RESULTS
Screen and panel	All screen cells, panel cells, and crossmatches reactive at antihuman globulin phase
Direct antiglobulin test	Positive because of IgG on red cells; C3 may also be on red cells
Eluate	Usually reactive with all reagent red cells tested
Hb/Hct	Low Hb/Hct, usually requiring transfusion support, may be chronic or acute
Compatibility test	Determine if there is an underlying alloantibody before transfusion

Hb/Hct, Hemoglobin/hematocrit.

Adsorption Techniques

If the cold autoantibody still persists after implementing the aforementioned techniques, the cold antibody needs to be adsorbed from the serum. If the patient has not been transfused in the last 3 months, an **autoadsorption** can be performed. If the patient has been transfused, the use of **allogeneic** red cells or **rabbit erythrocyte stroma** (RESt, Immucor, Norcross, GA) adsorption is necessary.[2] Table 7-9 compares the adsorption techniques. After the cold autoantibody is adsorbed, the adsorbed serum is retested with a panel to determine whether underlying alloantibodies exist in the serum.

WARM AUTOANTIBODIES

Warm autoantibodies are more common than cold autoantibodies. Similar to cold autoantibodies, the clinical significance and serologic manifestations can vary greatly. Warm autoimmune hemolytic anemia (WAIHA) can be idiopathic with no underlying disease process, or it may be a result of a pathologic disorder or medications used to treat various diseases. The patient diagnosis, medication history, and transfusion history are important in determining whether a warm autoantibody has been detected and what the best approach is to resolving the problem.

The initial antibody screen and DAT results commonly found in a patient with a warm autoantibody are found in example 5 of Fig. 7-2. A typical panel may react as shown in Panel 7-10. Reactions are usually seen with most panel cells and autocontrol and screening cells. The DAT demonstrates that the patient's cells are usually coated with IgG antibodies. Complement also can sometimes be detected. The typical initial serologic and clinical description of a warm autoantibody is outlined in Table 7-10. Because warm autoantibodies react best with LISS, PEG, and enzymes, retesting with 22% albumin as an enhancement may eliminate some or all of the reactivity.

Autoadsorption: attachment of the patient's antibodies to the patient's own red cells and subsequent removal from the serum.

Allogeneic adsorption: use of blood from a genetically different individual, such as reagent or donor cells that have been phenotyped for common red cell antigens, to remove alloantibodies and autoantibodies.

Rabbit erythrocyte stroma: red cell membranes from rabbits used for adsorption of IgM antibodies such as I.

Panel 7-10　Warm Autoantibody

Cell	D	C	E	c	e	f	Cw	M	N	S	s	P1	Lea	Leb	Lua	Lub	K	k	Fya	Fyb	Jka	Jkb	IS	37	AHG	CC
1 R1R1 (51)	+	+	0	0	+	0	0	+	+	+	0	+	0	+	0	+	+	+	0	+	+	0	0	0	3+	
2 R1R1 (32)	+	+	0	0	+	0	+	+	0	0	+	+	0	+	0	+	0	+	0	+	+	+	0	0	3+	
3 R2R2 (64)	+	0	+	+	0	0	0	0	+	0	+	+	+	0	0	+	+	+	0	0	+	+	0	0	3+	
4 r'r (75)	0	+	0	+	+	+	0	+	0	+	+	+	0	+	0	+	0	+	+	0	+	+	0	0	3+	
5 r''r (87)	0	0	+	+	+	+	0	+	+	+	+	+	0	+	0	+	0	+	+	0	+	0	0	0	3+	
6 rr (98)	0	0	0	+	+	+	0	+	+	+	+	+	+	0	0	+	0	+	+	0	+	+	0	0	3+	
7 rr (76)	0	0	0	+	+	+	0	+	0	+	0	0	0	+	0	+	+	0	+	+	0	+	0	0	3+	
8 rr (53)	0	0	0	+	+	+	0	+	0	+	+	+	0	0	0	+	0	+	0	+	0	+	0	0	3+	
9 rr (23)	0	0	0	+	+	+	0	+	+	+	+	0	+	0	0	+	0	+	+	+	+	0	0	0	3+	
10 R1R1 (34)	+	+	0	0	+	0	+	0	+	+	0	+	0	+	0	+	0	+	0	+	+	0	0	0	3+	
Patient cells																							0	0	3+	

Interpretation: an autoantibody is typically reactive at the AHG phase with all panel cells and the autocontrol. A similar reaction strength is usually observed with panel cells, screen cells, and crossmatches.

+, Antigen present; 0, antigen absent.

The goal in testing a sample with a suspected warm autoantibody is to determine whether an underlying alloantibody exists. Although laboratories may have limited resources to perform autoantibody work-ups, understanding the theory of the procedures is important. This section describes some of the procedures used when working with a warm autoantibody.

Specificity

The specificity of a warm autoantibody is sometimes directed to the Rh blood group system, especially to the "e" antigen. When this occurs, the patient's serum appears to be anti-e, although the patient's red cells are e-positive and have a positive DAT. In the case of an autoantibody with anti-e specificity, testing e-negative panel cells can be performed to determine whether an underlying specificity exists. Crossmatching e-negative units provides serologically compatible blood. If chronic hemolysis exists, providing e-negative blood might increase the red cell survival.[2]

Medications sometimes induce the formation of antibodies and may cause autoimmune mechanisms and serologic manifestations similar to autoimmune disease. Drug mechanisms are classified as drug-dependent and drug-independent, depending on whether interference is detected serologically. In a drug-dependent mechanism, the DAT is positive, but the serum is nonreactive with screen and panel cells. Reactions occur in vitro only by adding the drug to the test.[2] In a drug-independent mechanism, the DAT and screen and panel cells are positive and resemble a warm autoantibody in vitro. Classification of drug interactions by serologic techniques is typically beyond the scope of most laboratories.[10] Understanding the mechanisms and recognizing the drugs associated with a positive DAT and serum antibodies is helpful in testing and reporting results. This knowledge often is helpful to physicians, who may want to reconsider certain medications that may be causing cell destruction and serologic problems. Drug mechanisms are summarized in Table 7-11, and a more comprehensive list of drugs associated with a positive DAT and warm autoantibodies can be found in the *AABB Technical Manual*.[2]

Elution

Eluate: antibody removed from red cells to be used for antibody identification.

It is often helpful to identify the specificity of the IgG that is attached to red cells when the DAT is positive. To identify the antibody, the IgG attached to the red cells is dissociated and placed into a solution to test the specificity. This process is called an elution, and the recovered antibody is an **eluate** (Fig. 7-6). Various elution methods are listed in

TABLE 7-11 Drug Mechanisms Associated with a Positive Direct Antiglobulin Test

CATEGORY	MECHANISM	DESCRIPTION	ASSOCIATED DRUGS
Drug-independent	Unknown	Drug causes autoimmune process that resolves itself when the drug is discontinued Appears serologically like a warm autoantibody	Fludarabine, methyldopa
Drug-dependent	Nonimmune protein adsorption	Drug causes modification of red cell membrane, causing proteins to attach Demonstrated by antibodies that react in the presence of the drug	Cephalosporin, cefotetan, ceftriaxone, nonsteroidal antiinflammatory drugs
	Covalently binds to RBC membrane proteins	Drug attaches to red cell membrane; antibody to the drug causes red cell clearance by macrophages Demonstrated by treating cells with drug in vitro	Penicillin, cefotetan

RBC, Red blood cell.

TABLE 7-12 Elution Methods

METHOD	ANTIBODY REMOVAL	BENEFITS	LIMITATIONS
Glycine acid	Lower pH	Rapid and sensitive; commercially available	
Heat Freeze-thaw	Physical	Rapid; effective for ABO antibodies; inexpensive	Not sensitive for antibodies other than ABO
Ether Methylene chloride Chloroform	Organic solvent	Sensitive; inexpensive	Hazardous, carcinogenic, or flammable

Fig. 7-6 Principle of the elution technique.

Table 7-12. Acid elutions are the most commonly used because of their availability in a commercially prepared kit and reliability in antibody recovery. The acid elution reduces the pH, which results in antibody disassociation from the red cell membrane. Organic solvents denature antigens by dissolving the red cell lipid bilayer.[2] Heat produces conformational changes to red cells and antibody molecules. The freeze-thaw elution method lyses red cells to disrupt antigen-antibody bonds. Freeze-thaw and heat elution should be used only when testing for ABO antibodies on red cells because their sensitivity is limited. Elution methods work by disturbing the antigen and antibody bond, allowing the antibody to be removed from the red cell membrane.

In preparing an eluate, the cells are initially washed several times to remove antibody that may be in the serum from the test system. Antibodies that may be in the serum should not be confused with the antibody attached to the red cells. To ensure this washing is done adequately, the "last wash" saline is tested with screening cells. If washing is sufficient, results of this test should be negative. When the eluate is prepared, it is tested against panel cells or other reagent red cells in a method similar to serum testing to determine the specificity.

The eluate is usually reactive with all panel cells tested when working with a warm autoantibody. This observation helps to confirm the presence of a warm autoantibody.

Eluates prepared from patients who have been recently transfused and are experiencing a possible delayed serologic or hemolytic reaction usually demonstrate the antibody causing the reaction. An eluate prepared from a newborn's red cells that have a positive DAT demonstrates an antibody that was passed to the infant by the mother during pregnancy. Identification of this antibody is important if HDFN is suspected. Testing the eluate against a panel of red cells helps determine the antibody specificity causing a positive DAT.

Nonreactive eluates may also be associated with warm autoantibodies. Antibodies to medications and nonspecific binding of proteins to red cell membranes can cause a positive DAT and a negative eluate. Evaluation of patients' medications and clinical symptoms should be considered in determining whether a warm autoantibody exists when the eluate is nonreactive. In addition, patients who show serologic evidence of warm autoimmune disease might not always demonstrate the same reactions in the serum and eluate with each transfusion request. Eluates are not useful if only complement is attached to the red cell.

Adsorption

As discussed in the section describing cold autoantibodies, adsorption procedures may be necessary to remove the autoantibody from the serum to determine whether an underlying alloantibody exists; an autologous adsorption may be performed. In a warm autoadsorption procedure, initial pretreatment of the patient's red cells with DTT is necessary to remove as many of the in vivo attached autoantibodies as possible. In addition, treating the red cells with enzymes such as papain and ficin increases the capacity of cells to attach more autoantibodies. The combination of DTT and enzymes is sometimes referred to as "ZZAP" and is commercially available as W.A.R.M. reagent (Immucor, Norcross, GA). After treatment of the red cells the patient's serum is combined with his or her red cells and incubated for 30 to 60 minutes to remove the nonspecific warm antibody (Fig. 7-7).

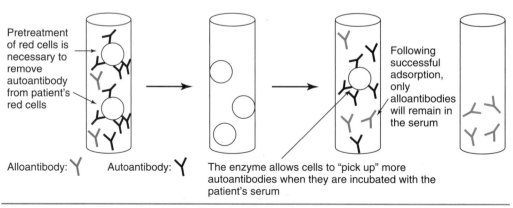

Fig. 7-7   Autologous adsorption.

The serum is removed from the red cells and retested with reagent red cells. If the patient has been transfused within the last 3 months, transfused red cells may exist in the patient's circulation. An autoadsorption is not appropriate in this circumstance because the transfused cells may adsorb the alloantibody necessary to identify.

For patients who have been transfused within the preceding 3 months, a **differential**, or allogeneic, **adsorption** technique should be performed to investigate underlying alloantibodies. An allogeneic adsorption uses known red cell types that either match the patient's phenotype or represent a combination of antigens that "selectively remove" certain known antibody specificities. Often a set of three separate adsorptions are performed, which include an R_1R_1 cell, R_2R_2 cell, and rr cell. Each tube adsorbs the autoantibody and leaves underlying alloantibodies in the serum. As in the autoadsorption procedure, enzyme pretreatment of red cells enhances autoantibody uptake. After incubation of the patient's serum with the allogeneic red cells, the serum is removed and retested against screening or panel cells to determine whether underlying alloantibodies exist. Fig. 7-8 outlines autologous adsorption and differential adsorption procedures.

Another challenge in working with warm autoantibody samples is phenotyping red cells that are coated with IgG. If a typing reagent requiring the antiglobulin phases such as anti-Fy^a is used to test red cells that are coated with IgG, a false-positive result occurs. To type the red cells, treatment with chloroquine diphosphate or an EDTA-glycine-HCL solution such as EGA (Immucor, Norcross GA) may be necessary before

Differential adsorption: adsorption or attachment of antibodies in the serum to specific known antigens, usually to different aliquots of red cells.

Autoadsorption

Differential (allogeneic) adsorption

Cells used for adsorption:
1. R_1R_1, K+, Jk(a+b−), Fy(a−b−), S−s+
2. R_2R_2, K−, Jk(a−b+), Fy(a−b−), S−s+
3. Rr, K−, Jk(a−b+) Fy(a−b−), S−s−
    (Duffy and S antigens removed by enzymes)

Fig. 7-8 Adsorption procedure outline. **A,** Autoadsorption. **B,** Differential (allogeneic) adsorption.

antigen typing. Chloroquine diphosphate and EDTA-glycine-HCL disassociate the IgG from the red cell, without damaging the antigen characteristics.[2] It is important to follow the manufacturers' directions and test controls to avoid erroneous results. It is also important to check the patient's transfusion history. If transfused cells are still circulating, the antigen typing may be misleading. Molecular methods are alternative typing techniques that can provide antigen typing results when the DAT and/or transfused cells are a problem.[3]

Warm autoantibodies represent more complicated antibody identification procedures. Patients with WAIHA may require frequent transfusions, which further complicates the serologic results. Good communication with the physician caring for the patient must be initiated early to assess alternatives to transfusion and monitor the clinical symptoms associated with immune red cell destruction.

CHAPTER SUMMARY

The process of identification of alloantibodies and resolving complex autoantibody problems becomes easier and more interesting with experience. Fig. 7-9, which incorporates an acronym for the words "BLOOD BANK," outlines some of the clues in antibody identification that are helpful in resolving the problems. The use of case studies is a good way to develop and enhance the problem-solving process necessary in becoming proficient in antibody identification. Antibody problems generally fall into the following categories:

- *Single antibody specificity* has a pattern easily identifiable with a panel following the rules of panel interpretation. Confirmation that the patient or donor is negative for the corresponding antigen helps confirm the specificity.
- *Multiple antibodies* necessitate the use of carefully selected cells and antibody techniques such as enzymes. Distinguishing multiple specificities necessitates attention to detail and a good understanding of antibody characteristics. The determination of the patient's red cell phenotype is also useful.
- *Antibodies to high-incidence antigens* should be suspected if all panel cells are positive. Identification depends on locating cells that are negative for high-incidence antigens and determining whether underlying antibodies exist.
- *Low-frequency antibodies* are usually found with other antibodies. Identification depends on the availability of additional cells for testing. Transfusions should not be delayed to determine specificity.
- *Weak IgG antibodies* often can be enhanced by using a different potentiator, increasing the serum-to-cell ratio, or increasing incubation time. The detection of newly formed alloantibodies in recently transfused patients is especially important.

B	Blood typing problem?
L	Last transfusion or pregnancy?
O	Observe reactions at each phase
O	0.05 probability (use rule of 3)
D	Dosage
B	Black or white race?
A	Autocontrol results?
N	Negatives for ruling out
K	Know your reagents

Fig. 7-9 Clues for antibody identification.

- *Cold alloantibodies* are usually clinically insignificant. Avoiding the reactions or using neutralization or prewarm techniques to eliminate agglutination is sometimes necessary.
- *Autoantibodies* are of either the cold or the warm type, and they should be suspected if the autocontrol or DAT is positive. Determining the existence of underlying alloantibodies is important to avoid additional hemolysis. Techniques such as adsorption and elution are usually performed to identify the antibody on the red cell and the alloantibody in the serum.

In each type of antibody problem, a methodical process is necessary to take into account all important clues and reach an accurate conclusion. Being comfortable with many types of antibody situations is an appreciable goal for the immunohematologist.

CRITICAL THINKING EXERCISES

EXERCISE 7-1

A donor sample from a 55-year-old white man demonstrated a positive antibody screen during routine processing testing. Results of testing with an antibody identification panel are shown. Refer to the panel to answer the following questions:

Cell	D	C	E	c	e	f	Cʷ	M	N	S	s	P₁	Leᵃ	Leᵇ	Luᵃ	Luᵇ	K	k	Fyᵃ	Fyᵇ	Jkᵃ	Jkᵇ	IS	37	IgG	CC
1 R1R1	+	+	0	0	+	0	0	+	+	+	+	+	0	+	0	+	+	+	0	+	+	0	0	0	1+	
2 R1R1	+	+	0	0	+	0	+	+	0	0	+	+	0	+	0	+	0	+	0	+	+	+	0	0	0	✓
3 R2R2	+	0	+	+	0	0	0	0	+	0	+	+	+	0	0	+	+	+	+	0	+	+	0	0	0	✓
4 r″r	0	0	+	+	+	+	0	+	0	+	0	+	0	+	0	+	0	+	+	0	+	+	0	0	2+	
5 rr	0	0	0	+	+	+	0	+	+	+	+	+	0	+	0	+	0	+	+	0	+	0	0	0	1+	
6 rr	0	0	0	+	+	+	0	+	+	+	+	+	+	0	0	+	0	+	0	0	+	+	0	0	1+	
7 R0R0	+	0	0	+	+	+	0	+	0	0	0	0	0	+	0	+	+	+	+	+	0	+	0	0	0	✓
8 rr	0	0	0	+	+	+	0	+	0	+	+	+	0	0	0	+	0	+	0	+	0	+	0	0	1+	
9 rr	0	0	0	+	+	+	0	+	+	+	0	0	+	0	0	+	0	+	+	+	+	0	0	0	2+	
10 R1R1	+	+	0	0	+	0	+	0	+	0	+	+	0	+	0	+	0	+	0	+	+	0	0	0	0	✓
Patient cells																							0	0	0	✓

Header groups: Rh (D, C, E, c, e, f, Cʷ); MNSs (M, N, S, s); P₁; Lewis (Leᵃ, Leᵇ); Lutheran (Luᵃ, Luᵇ); Kell (K, k); Duffy (Fyᵃ, Fyᵇ); Kidd (Jkᵃ, Jkᵇ); LISS (IS, 37, IgG, CC)

1. At what phase are the reactions occurring?
2. What does the phase of the reaction suggest regarding the immunoglobulin class of antibody?
3. Is this an alloantibody or an autoantibody?
4. What is the most likely antibody specificity?
5. Are there antibodies that cannot be ruled out on this panel?
6. What additional testing should be performed to verify the specificity?
7. What caused the production of this antibody in this donor?
8. Referring to the antigram, which cell or cells are homozygous for the S antigen?
9. Which cell is probably U-negative?

EXERCISE 7-2

A sample from a 25-year-old obstetric patient was referred to the hospital for antibody identification. One of the antibody screening cells was weakly positive using LISS enhancement. A panel was tested, and the results are shown:

Cell	D	C	E	c	e	f	Cw	M	N	S	s	P1	Lea	Leb	Lua	Lub	K	k	Fya	Fyb	Jka	Jkb	IS	37	AHG	CC
1 R1R1	+	+	0	0	+	0	0	+	+	+	0	+	0	+	0	+	+	+	+	0	+	0	1+	0	0	✓
2 R1R1	+	+	0	0	+	0	+	+	0	0	+	+	+	0	+	0	+	0	+	0	+	+	2+	1+	1+	
3 R2R2	+	0	+	+	0	0	0	0	+	0	+	+	+	0	0	+	+	+	0	0	+	+	0	0	0	✓
4 r'r	0	+	+	+	+	+	0	+	0	+	+	+	0	+	0	+	0	+	+	0	+	+	3+	2+	1+	
5 rr	0	0	0	+	+	+	0	+	+	0	+	+	0	+	0	+	0	+	0	0	+	0	1+	0	0	✓
6 rr	0	0	0	+	+	+	0	+	+	+	+	+	+	0	0	+	0	+	+	0	+	+	1+	0	0	✓
7 rr	0	0	0	+	+	+	0	0	+	+	0	0	0	+	0	+	+	0	+	+	0	+	0	0	0	✓
8 rr	0	0	0	+	+	+	0	+	0	+	+	+	0	0	0	+	0	+	0	+	0	+	3+	2+	1+	
9 rr	0	0	0	+	+	+	0	+	+	+	+	0	+	0	0	+	0	+	+	+	+	0	1+	0	0	✓
10 R1R1	+	+	0	0	+	0	+	0	+	+	0	+	0	+	0	+	0	+	0	+	+	0	0	0	0	✓
Patient cells																							0	0	0	✓

1. At what phase are the reactions the strongest?
2. What does the phase suggest about the immunoglobulin class of this antibody?
3. Is this an alloantibody or an autoantibody?
4. Could this antibody cross the placenta?
5. What is the most likely identity of the antibody that is demonstrated?
6. If the panel cells were treated with enzymes and retesting followed, what would be the expected reactions?
7. Is this antibody usually clinically significant? Define clinically significant.

EXERCISE 7-3

A sample from a 65-year-old white man was submitted for a 2-unit crossmatch. He is scheduled for an outpatient transfusion at the cancer clinic. A transfusion history indicated that he received 2 units of RBCs 4 months ago. Results of the ABO and D phenotypes and antibody screen follow:

Anti-A	Anti-B	Anti-D	A_1 cells	B cells	ABO/D interpretation
4+	0	3+	0	3+	A, D–positive

		LISS	
	IS	37° C	AHG
SC I	0	0	2+
SC II	0	0	2+

1. Is it possible to make an initial interpretation regarding the type of antibody present in this patient's serum?
2. What additional testing should be performed?
3. What types of medical history questions are important with this type of patient?

Additional Testing

The laboratory's policy is to perform a DAT only on samples with a positive screen unless specifically ordered. Results are as follows:

Polyspecific AHG: 3+   Anti-IgG: 3+   Anti-C3: 0

4. Based on the DAT results, what type of antibody problem should be suspected?
5. When a DAT is positive, what procedure can be performed to identify the antibody attached to the red cells?

Panel Results

An antibody panel was performed using LISS and observing reactions at all phases. All cells were positive (2+) by the IAT. The autocontrol was 3+. An elution was performed, and the eluate reacted 3+ with all panel cells (the last wash was negative).

6. What is the specificity of the antibody?
7. What additional procedures are necessary before releasing units?
8. Would different procedures be necessary if the patient had been transfused within the last 3 months?

EXERCISE 7-4

A specimen from a 70-year-old white woman was submitted for pretransfusion work-up for hip surgery in 1 week. There were 2 units of autologous RBCs reserved. Because the physician anticipated the need for additional units, routine compatibility testing procedures were performed. The patient had no recent transfusions. Results of the ABO and D phenotypes and antibody screen follow:

Anti-A	Anti-B	Anti-D	A₁ cells	B cells	ABO/D interpretation
0	0	3+	4+	4+	O, D–positive

		LISS		
	IS	37° C	IAT*	
SC I	2+	1+	+w	
SC II	2+	1+	+w	

*Anti-IgG.

1. Based on the antibody screen results, what type of antibody is demonstrated?
2. Is this an alloantibody or an autoantibody?
3. What additional testing should be performed to determine the answer to question 2?

Additional Testing

The DAT results are as follows:

Polyspecific AHG: 1+   Anti-IgG: 0 (check cells 2+)   Anti-C3: 1+

4. Do the results of the DAT confirm your suspicions?
5. What additional testing should be performed to confirm the antibody specificity?

Additional Testing

A "mini-cold panel" was tested and yielded the following results:

	SC I	SC II	Cord 1	Cord 2	Auto
4° C	3+	3+	0	0	3+

6. What is the probable specificity of the antibody?
7. What procedures could be performed to avoid the reactivity?

STUDY QUESTIONS

1. The antibody screen:
   a. detects most clinically significant antibodies
   b. detects all low-frequency antibodies
   c. helps to distinguish between an alloantibody and autoantibody
   d. can be omitted if the patient has no history of antibodies

2. HTLA antibodies:
   a. typically react at room temperature
   b. can be enhanced with PEG
   c. are usually clinically insignificant
   d. are associated with HDFN

3. Which of the following statements is associated with anti-I?
   a. It has weaker reactions with stored blood
   b. It can be neutralized with commercially prepared substance
   c. It reacts best at 37° C
   d. It does not react with cord blood cells

4. A multiple antibody problem was resolved using enzymes. One of the antibody reactions was eliminated after treatment. Which of the following antibodies was probably present?
   a. anti-c
   b. anti-I
   c. anti-Jk^a
   d. anti-Fy^a

5. An antibody demonstrating dosage would mean that:
   a. homozygous cells were stronger
   b. heterozygous cells were stronger
   c. cells reacted best with PEG
   d. cells reacted best at 4° C

6. The neutralization technique was performed on a sample containing an anti-Le^b. The control and the Lewis-neutralized sera were both negative when retested with panel cells. How should this test be interpreted?
   a. the anti-Le^b was successfully neutralized and no underlying antibodies were found
   b. the panel cells were not washed sufficiently
   c. the sample was probably diluted
   d. the antibody originally identified was probably not anti-Le^b

7. The rule of three used in antibody identification ensures which p value?
   a. 0.09
   b. 0.02
   c. 0.05
   d. 0.15

8. A DAT performed on a clotted sample stored at 4° C may demonstrate:
   a. in vivo complement attachment
   b. in vivo IgG attachment
   c. in vitro complement attachment
   d. in vitro IgM attachment

9. Which of the following antibodies may not be detected in the screen?
   a. anti-Js^b
   b. anti-V
   c. anti-k
   d. anti-s

10. The procedure that removes intact antibodies from the red cell membranes is:
    a. autoadsorption
    b. neutralization
    c. enzyme pretreatment
    d. elution

11. The removal of an antibody from serum or plasma using the individual's own red cells is:
    a. autoadsorption
    b. differential adsorption
    c. neutralization
    d. elution

12. An antibody was detected in the screen at 37° C and did not react at the AHG phase. Which of the following should be suspected?
    a. anti-s
    b. anti-e
    c. anti-N
    d. anti-Jk^a

13. Antigen typing on red cells should not be performed if the patient has been transfused within the following:
    a. 30 days
    b. 2 months
    c. 3 months
    d. 6 months

14. DTT is useful in evaluating a sample when which antibody is suspected?
    a. anti-Js^b
    b. anti-Kp^b
    c. anti-k
    d. all of the above

15. The purpose of additional procedures when working up a warm autoantibody is to:
    a. identify the warm autoantibody specificity in the serum
    b. locate RBC units that are compatible with the autoantibody
    c. identify potential underlying alloantibodies
    d. identify the antibodies coating the red cells

REFERENCES

1. Judd WJ, Barnes BA, Steiner EA, et al: The evaluation of a positive direct antiglobulin test (autocontrol) in pretransfusion testing revisited, *Transfusion* 26:220, 1986.
2. Roback JD: *Technical manual*, ed 17, Bethesda, MD, 2011, AABB.
3. Alexander L: Personalized therapy reaches transfusion medicine, *AABB News*, Nov 2011.
4. Moulds MK: Selection of procedures for problem solving weak reactions in the antiglobulin phase. In Wallace ME, Green TS, editors: *Selection of procedures for problem solving*, Arlington, VA, 1996, AABB.
5. Pierce SR: Anomalous blood bank results. In Dawson RB, editor: *Troubleshooting the crossmatch*, Washington, DC, 1997, AABB.
6. Judd WJ: Controversies in transfusion medicine. Prewarmed tests: con, *Transfusion* 35:271, 1995.
7. Mallory D: Controversies in transfusion medicine. Prewarmed tests: pro—why, when, and how—not if, *Transfusion* 35:268, 1995.
8. Leger RM, Garratty G: Weakening or loss of antibody reactivity after prewarm technique, *Transfusion* 43:1611, 2003.
9. Shan Y, et al: Immunoglobulin M red blood cell alloantibodies are frequently adsorbed by rabbit erythrocyte stroma, *Transfusion* 50, 2010.
10. Johnson SJ, Fueger JT, Gottschall JL: One center's experience: the serology and drugs associated with drug-induced immune hemolytic anemia—a new paradigm, *Transfusion* 47:697, 2007.

SUGGESTED READINGS

Judd WJ, Johnson S, Storry J: *Judd's methods in immunohematology*, ed 3, Bethesda, MD, 2008, AABB Press.

Compatibility Testing

CHAPTER OUTLINE

LEARNING OBJECTIVES

On completion of this chapter, the reader should be able to:

1. Define compatibility testing and the crossmatch.
2. List the procedures included in the routine compatibility test and explain their purpose.
3. Explain the AABB's *Standards for Blood Banks and Transfusion Services* as related to compatibility testing.
4. Select the appropriate plasma, platelets, and cryoprecipitated products for recipients with all possible ABO and D types.
5. Propose strategies for transfusion when compatible blood cannot be located.
6. Select alternative ABO and D typed donor units if ABO-identical red blood cells (RBCs) are not available in the blood bank inventory.
7. Outline the limitations of the crossmatch with regard to prevention of transfusion reactions.
8. Describe how crossmatching is handled in a massive transfusion situation.

9. Summarize the advantages and issues related to the computer crossmatch.
10. Compare and contrast the purpose and application of the immediate-spin crossmatch and antiglobulin crossmatch.
11. Explain the elements of patient identification and their importance in compatibility testing.
12. Explain the use of a type and screen protocol and a Maximum Surgical Blood Order Schedule.
13. Explain how compatibility testing is performed for an infant younger than 4 months old.
14. Discuss the principles of the crossmatch using autologous blood.
15. Evaluate laboratory results in compatibility testing.
16. Provide compatible donor RBCs for patients with multiple antibodies.

Compatibility testing: all steps in the identification and testing of a potential transfusion recipient and donor blood before transfusion in an attempt to provide a blood product that survives in vivo and provides its therapeutic effect in the recipient.

Compatibility testing is a term often considered synonymous with crossmatching.[1] In the transfusion service, a broader view of this term is taken. Compatibility testing includes recipient identification, sample collection and handling, and required pretransfusion testing. This approach ensures the greatest compatibility (no adverse reactions from transfused blood) technically possible between the donor unit and the proposed recipient. Compatibility testing encompasses all the steps highlighted in Fig. 8-1. The process begins with the transfusion request and ends with the transfusion of blood product to the patient. Because the antibody screen, ABO and D phenotyping, and donor testing are discussed elsewhere in this book, this chapter concentrates on the issues related to crossmatching, a component of compatibility testing, and provides an overview of important steps in the process of compatibility testing.

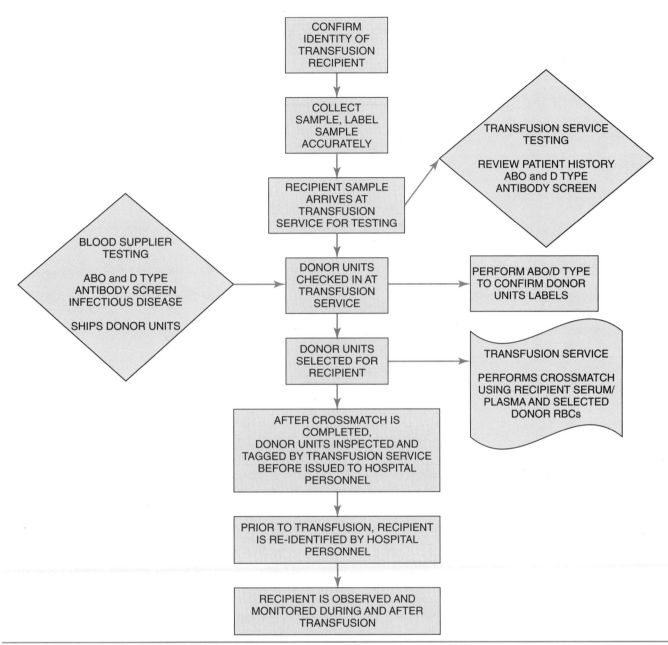

Fig. 8-1 Process of compatibility testing. The process begins at the recipient and ends with a safe transfusion into the recipient.

The history of compatibility testing and transfusion practices is an interesting progression of events that begins with the discovery of the circulation of blood in 1628 by William Harvey,[2] an event that made the first human venous transfusions possible. The first in vivo transfusion was attempted with animal blood, and later human blood, using a quill or a metal apparatus introduced into a recipient's vein. Early recipients often died because no understanding existed of ABO blood group system antibodies (elucidated by Landsteiner in 1900) or of other blood group system alloantibodies.

Direct transfusions were performed again in the first decade of the twentieth century with some success, despite the lack of compatibility testing (Fig. 8-2). A crossmatch procedure was first attempted in 1907 in New York by Weil and Ottenberg. Sera of recipient and donor were separately subjected to lengthy room temperature incubation with red cells from the opposite sources to detect hemolysins. Major and minor crossmatches were part of routine testing. Antibody screening did not become routine until the late 1950s to mid-1960s. Progress from the era of no testing to a century of rapid discoveries led to

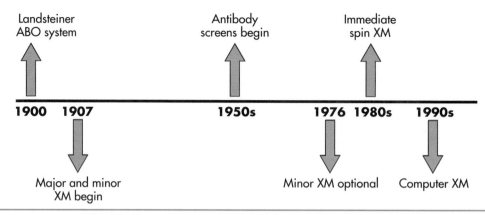

Fig. 8-2   Important events in compatibility testing. *XM,* Crossmatch.

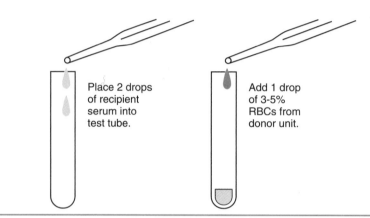

Fig. 8-3   Crossmatch. Patient serum is crossmatched with donor red cells. The minor crossmatch used donor serum crossmatched with patient red cells. Antibody screen testing on donor samples has replaced the minor crossmatch. (Modified from Immucor, Norcross, GA.)

a proliferation of testing protocols that peaked in the 1960s. A movement existed for the discovery and characterization of every possible blood group antigen and the detection of every corresponding antibody. Over the past several decades, however, the forces of cost containment, practicality, and safety abbreviated, and ultimately eliminated, many of the previous testing protocols from routine practice. The AABB made the minor crossmatch unnecessary in 1976. In the 1980s, the abbreviated, or immediate-spin, crossmatch was implemented in the absence of antibodies in the current antibody screen or the patient's past record. In the 1990s, the blood banking community proposed the elimination of the in vitro crossmatch under certain defined circumstances and the adoption of the computer crossmatch.

SECTION 1
PRINCIPLES OF THE CROSSMATCH

WHAT IS A CROSSMATCH?

Crossmatching is routinely performed only with donor products containing red cells. A crossmatch must be performed for red cell transfusions; the exception is situations requiring an urgent need for blood. The term crossmatch implies a crossway mixing of donor and recipient blood components.[3]

The crossmatch procedure involves the mixing of serum or plasma from the recipient with red cells from the donor (Fig. 8-3). Hemolysis or agglutination at any phase or step of the process indicates the presence of recipient antibodies interacting with donor red cell antigens and a mismatch between donor and recipient (Table 8-1). A crossmatch is

TABLE 8-1 Compatible versus Incompatible Crossmatch

CROSSMATCH INTERPRETATION	APPEARANCE
Compatible	No agglutination and no hemolysis
Incompatible	Agglutination or hemolysis

interpreted as compatible when no agglutination and no hemolysis are present in testing. The donor unit is acceptable for transfusion purposes. A crossmatch is interpreted as incompatible when agglutination or hemolysis is present in testing. The donor unit is unacceptable for transfusion purposes.

PURPOSES OF CROSSMATCH TESTING

The purposes of crossmatching are to:
- Prevent life-threatening or uncomfortable transfusion reactions
- Maximize in vivo survival of transfused red cells.

The crossmatch procedure attempts to fulfill these goals in the following ways:
- The crossmatch serves as a double check of ABO errors caused by patient misidentification or donor unit mislabeling.
- If the recipient possesses a clinically significant antibody or a history of one, the crossmatch provides a second means of antibody detection and checks the results of the antibody screen.

The crossmatch, designed to detect donor units unlikely to survive normally once transfused, must be rapid and simple enough to be practical. Actual measurement of the survival rates of transfused red cells may be considered to constitute the best crossmatch. This technique can be performed directly through the use of radioisotope labeling, but this is impractical for regular use. Posttransfusion hematocrit or hemoglobin values are often determined to provide a working measure of successful transfusion. One unit of transfused red blood cells (RBCs) should increase the hematocrit by 3% and the hemoglobin by 1 g/dL.

> One unit of RBCs should increase the hematocrit by 3% and the hemoglobin by 1 g/dL.

STANDARDS AND REGULATIONS GOVERNING THE CROSSMATCH

The AABB and the U.S. Food and Drug Administration (FDA) are the two principal organizations applying standards to the blood banking and transfusion service communities in the United States. The College of American Pathologists and The Joint Commission also inspect blood establishments.

The AABB *Standards* provides the most inclusive summary of crossmatch standards. It requires that a crossmatch procedure always be performed using the recipient's serum or plasma and a sample of donor cells taken from a segment originally attached to the blood product bag. The exception is an emergency situation in which blood may be released for transfusion before crossmatch. The crossmatch defined by the AABB *Standards*[4] is a technique that "shall use methods that demonstrate ABO incompatibility and clinically significant antibodies to red cell antigens and shall include an antiglobulin test." Again, an exception is provided. If no clinically significant antibodies were detected in the current sample or in the patient's past records, an immediate-spin crossmatch is permitted to fulfill the requirement of detecting ABO incompatibility. The AABB provision for a computer crossmatch as an alternative to these requirements is presented later in this chapter.

CROSSMATCH PROCEDURES

There are two classifications of the crossmatch procedure: serologic crossmatch and computer crossmatch (Fig. 8-4).

Fig. 8-4 Comparison of immediate-spin, computer, and antiglobulin crossmatch requirements. *XM,* Crossmatch.

Serologic Crossmatch

The serologic crossmatch procedure tests the recipient's serum or plasma with the RBCs from the donor unit in an immediate-spin crossmatch or an antiglobulin crossmatch. A crossmatch can be performed using multiple methods, including the tube test, solid phase red cell adherence test, and gel test. This discussion illustrates the principles relative to tube testing.

Immediate-spin Crossmatch

The immediate-spin crossmatch may be used for recipients with no evidence of clinically significant antibody or antibodies in the current sample and in the historical record. In this procedure, recipient serum or plasma and donor red cell suspensions are added to a tube, and the tube is immediately centrifuged. This procedure meets the AABB standard for detecting ABO incompatibility.

Antiglobulin Crossmatch

In the event the patient demonstrates a clinically significant antibody in the current antibody screen or has done so in the past, antigen-negative units should be crossmatched by the antiglobulin crossmatch procedure. Commercial high-titered antiserum is necessary when selecting these antigen-negative donor units. For the antiglobulin crossmatch, a reading is required only at the antiglobulin phase. However, the antiglobulin crossmatch procedure usually includes an immediate-spin phase, a 37° C incubation period, and an antiglobulin phase. Enhancement media used in the antibody screen are usually added to the crossmatch tubes to mirror the conditions in which the antibody was detected. Antiglobulin crossmatches performed in the gel test or solid phase red cell adherence test have only antiglobulin phase results.

When a crossmatch is performed on a patient with a warm autoantibody, some laboratories use patient's serum or plasma that is not adsorbed. The crossmatch is reported as incompatible. Other laboratories use the adsorbed serum to screen and select nonreactive units for transfusion for patients with underlying clinically significant alloantibodies. These units would be issued as "serologically compatible with adsorbed serum." However, this practice can also be misinterpreted as false sense of security for transfusion.[6]

Computer Crossmatch

A computer crossmatch uses a computer to make the final check of ABO compatibility in the selection of appropriate units for transfusion. The same prerequisite pertains to the computer crossmatch and the immediate-spin method: The recipient does not possess clinically significant antibody or antibodies in the current or any previous sample. The computer program should provide a flag indicating the recipient's eligibility or ineligibility for computer crossmatch. The AABB *Standards*[4] contains the required provisions for an acceptable computer crossmatch. Table 8-2 summarizes criteria for the computer crossmatch.

Keystroke errors are easy to make when using a computer. The system must alert the user to nonsense entries or mismatches with hard-coded ABO logic tables and require

There should be no delays in the centrifugation step of the immediate-spin crossmatch or reading the reaction. If the immediate-spin crossmatch is not properly performed, false-negative results may occur with failure to detect ABO incompatibility.

Refer to the *Laboratory Manual* that accompanies this textbook for details of the immediate-spin and antiglobulin crossmatch procedure.

TABLE 8-2	Computer Crossmatch Requirements

- Computer-system validation onsite and assurance that ABO incompatibilities are detected; incompatible blood products not released
- ABO phenotype determination has been performed on a current sample
- Second ABO phenotyping interpretation may be a retype of the same current sample, a second current sample, or a comparison with previous records
- Individual facility determines whether ABO phenotyping is performed by two technologists or whether two samples must be collected at different times
- Computer system includes donor unit information: product name, ABO and D phenotype, unique number, and interpretation of ABO confirmation test
- Computer system includes recipient ABO and D phenotyping, antibody screen results, and interpretation of compatibility
- Logic to alert user to ABO incompatibility between donor unit and recipient and between donor unit label and ABO confirmation test
- Method to verify correct entry of all data before release of blood or blood components

From Carson TH, editor: *Standards for blood banks and transfusion services,* ed 27, Bethesda, MD, 2011, AABB.

confirmation points along the way, which forces the user to verify or accept crucial conclusions with an additional entry. The bar coding of blood components and recipient specimens adds another measure of safety.

The first large-scale implementation of a computer crossmatch protocol occurred in 1992 at the blood bank at the University of Michigan Hospital, under an AABB exemption that met the FDA requirements for alternative compatibility procedures.[5] The FDA *Code of Federal Regulations* (640.120) requires that transfusion services seek approval in writing for its use.

The computer crossmatch has numerous advantages, including the following:
- Increased time efficiency
- Reduced volume of sample needed on large crossmatch orders
- Greater flexibility in staffing
- Better management of blood bank inventory
- Potential for a centralized transfusion service

LIMITATIONS OF CROSSMATCH TESTING

The performance of acceptable crossmatch testing does not guarantee a successful transfusion outcome. Adverse transfusion reactions may still occur. The risks of viral transmission, allergic reactions, and white blood cell reactions are complications that can be consequences of transfusions. These adverse complications of transfusions are discussed further in Chapter 10.

The antibody screen and the crossmatch have inherent limitations as separate tests and should be used in tandem. A recipient could have a negative antibody screen result and an incompatible crossmatch. A negative antibody screen does not guarantee that the recipient's serum does not have clinically significant red cell antibodies. The negative antibody screen means that the recipient's serum contains no antibodies that react with the screening cells by the method used. In this example, a recipient might possess an antibody directed against a low-incidence antigen not contained in the commercial screening cells, and a crossmatch might detect this situation. An antibody detected with screening cells might not react with a weak expression of the antigen on donor cells in a crossmatch, leading to the situation of a positive antibody screen with compatible crossmatch.

A compatible crossmatch also does not guarantee the optimal survival of red cells. Aspects of the patient's clinical course (e.g., bleeding, red cell sequestration) may limit the benefit of the transfusion. A delayed transfusion reaction could occur if a preexisting, undetectable recipient antibody is boosted in strength by the infusion of the corresponding antigen in the donor unit and rapidly destroys the donor red cells.

TABLE 8-3	Unexpected Incompatibilities in Immediate-Spin Crossmatch		
PROBLEM	**CAUSES**	**RESOLUTIONS**	
ABO phenotyping errors	Patient identification error	Repeat ABO testing	
	Sample labeling error	Redraw patient	
Unexpected antibodies	Cold alloantibody (M, P1)	Test panel cells	
	Anti-A_1 in A_2 patient	Test A_2 cells	
	Cold autoantibody (I, IH)	Determine clinical significance	

TABLE 8-4 Steps in Compatibility Testing

- Accurate patient (recipient) identification
- Proper sample collection, labeling, and handling
- Review of recipient's past blood bank records
- ABO and D phenotyping, antibody screening, and infectious disease testing on donor units
- ABO and D phenotyping and antibody screening of recipient; crossmatch of recipient's sample with donor units
- If recipient is determined to possess a clinically significant antibody, donor units are screened and found negative for the corresponding antigen and crossmatched
- Tagging, inspecting, and issuing blood products
- Reidentification of recipient before transfusion
- Careful observation of recipient's vital signs after transfusion and monitoring of posttransfusion hematocrit and hemoglobin levels for efficacy of transfusion

---

Even if red cell destruction does not occur, a recipient may become alloimmunized to the donor antigens, rendering subsequent compatibility work-ups more time-consuming and complicated. Non–life-threatening transfusion reactions may also occur, making the transfusion uncomfortable for the recipient (e.g., hives, low-grade fever, chills, itching).

PROBLEM SOLVING INCOMPATIBLE CROSSMATCHES

Because pretransfusion testing encompasses antibody screening and identification and crossmatching, interpreting incompatibilities in conjunction with the results of these tests is important. Table 8-3 summarizes the causes of incompatible crossmatches in the immediate-spin crossmatch and presents suggestions for resolutions. The antiglobulin crossmatch is more commonly performed in the presence of a clinically significant antibody or previous history of one. Problem solving has revolved around identification of the antibody's specificity and the location of antigen-negative donor units. An incompatible antiglobulin crossmatch occasionally may be detected. Often the primary reason for this incompatibility is the presence of a preexisting positive direct antiglobulin test (DAT) in the donor unit.

SECTION 2
PRINCIPLES OF COMPATIBILITY TESTING

OVERVIEW OF STEPS IN COMPATIBILITY TESTING

As discussed in the introduction of this chapter, compatibility testing is a process that begins and ends with the recipient. The process involves many steps and requirements designed to ensure the safety of both the donor and the recipient of the transfusion. The steps are outlined in Table 8-4 and are discussed individually.

Recipient Blood Sample

Safe and accurate pretransfusion testing begins with the recipient's blood sample, properly collected and labeled with accurate patient identification procedures.

Antibodies can be missed in compatibility testing if:
- The corresponding antigen is absent from screening cells
- The antibody is so weak that it detects only homozygous expressions of the antigen (dosage effect)
- The antibody is detectable only by a method not routinely employed (e.g., in the presence of a particular enhancement medium)
- Antibody history is unknown

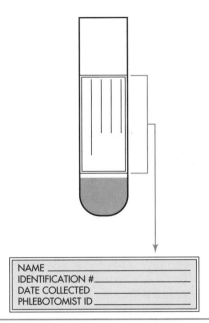

NAME _____
IDENTIFICATION #_____
DATE COLLECTED _____
PHLEBOTOMIST ID _____

Fig. 8-5   Recipient sample labeling.

Patient Identification and Sample Labeling Requirements

Minimum labeling requirements are defined in the AABB *Standards*[4]: "The identifying information for the patient and the blood sample shall correspond and be confirmed using two independent identifiers." The two independent identifiers should include the patient's first and last name and an identification number unique to the recipient.

The patient must be positively identified by comparing the requisition and sample label to the identification band attached to the patient (not to the wall or the bed). The patient should also state his or her name without prompting from the phlebotomist. A caregiver may identify the patient if the patient is incoherent or a language barrier exists. Commercial banding systems are available whereby a number on the patient's band is also attached to the specimen, request form, and eventual blood product to be transfused. Bar-coding technology has been applied to patient identification systems and has been implemented in many laboratories. The sample must be labeled at the bedside. To prevent a possible sample mix-up, prelabeled tubes should never be used. The label must include first and last name of recipient; unique identification number; date of collection; and signature, initials, or a method to identify the phlebotomist. The label must also be legible and indelible (Fig. 8-5).

Information on the label must match the request form. This request form must also include the types of blood product being ordered and the requesting physician's name. The request form is in effect a prescription. Other useful information on the request form includes the location of the patient, sex, diagnosis, date of the proposed transfusion, and priority indicator (e.g., routine, stat, transfuse on date, preoperative, standby).

Sample Collection Tubes

Patient samples for compatibility testing may be serum or plasma.[6] Plasma samples are preferred. Plain tubes with a red top (no anticoagulant) and purple or pink top (ethylenediaminetetraacetic acid [EDTA]) tubes are most commonly used. Many laboratories have adopted the pink-stoppered blood collection tubes for blood bank samples. The collection tubes are spray-coated with K_2EDTA and provide anticoagulated blood with plasma and red cells for testing. Historically, any form of anticoagulated blood sample was discouraged for compatibility testing because of the anticomplementary properties of anticoagulants and the possible presence of fibrin in plasma. Most clinically significant antibodies are now recognized not to depend solely on the presence of complement for their detection. Considerable time can be saved in emergencies in not waiting for a blood

Accurate patient identification is a fundamental practice for patient safety.

Good laboratory practice recommends labeling blood sample tubes in the presence of the patient.

specimen to clot, especially when most crossmatches are performed at immediate-spin, where fibrin is less likely to interfere.

Age of Sample

Patient samples and a segment from the donor unit used for crossmatching must be stored for at least 7 days following transfusion in the event that a transfusion reaction investigation is necessary.[4]

Samples should be collected no more than 3 days (with the date of draw being day 0) of the scheduled transfusion, if the patient has been transfused or was pregnant in the previous 3 months or the history is unclear or unknown.[4] This practice ensures that the sample used in testing reflects the recipient's current immunologic status. The 3-day requirement applies only to recently transfused patients or women with pregnancy in the last 3 months. Many laboratories prefer to standardize their operations by setting a 3-day limit for all pretransfusion testing samples.

If a reliable history exists of no recent pregnancy or transfusion and no current or past unexpected antibodies, the sample may be kept and reused. This practice allows preoperative testing before a patient's surgical procedure and crossmatching at the time of need. In some settings where patients are being repeatedly transfused, new samples may be required for these patients (e.g., every other day). This decision must be made after considering the volume of extra work and expense entailed compared with the number of new transfusion-induced antibodies detected.

Considerations in Sample Collection and Appearance

Hemolyzed or lipemic samples create difficulty in the interpretation of crossmatch results.

Serum or plasma hemolyzed during the collection process is an unacceptable specimen, and the sample should be collected again. Mechanical hemolysis may be caused by the use of small-gauge needles, trauma to a small vein, the forcing of blood into the tube through a small needle, or the further addition of blood to a partially clotted sample. Mechanical hemolysis can mask the detection of antibody-induced hemolysis (a positive reaction in some examples of ABO, P1, Lewis, Kidd, or Vel system antibodies).

Samples potentially diluted with intravenous fluids (e.g., Ringer's lactate) are also unacceptable because of the chance of missing a weak antibody or the inducement of false-positive reactions caused by the molecules in the intravenous fluid. Blood samples for the blood bank and all other laboratory testing should always be collected from below an intravenous site, preferably from a different vein and ideally from the other arm. If the intravenous site is the only site for drawing blood, the intravenous catheter should be turned off and flushed with saline, and the first 5 to 10 mL of blood should be discarded.

Comparison with Previous Records

The AABB *Standards*[4] requires comparison of results of current blood typing with ABO and D typing performed over the past 12 months. It also mandates that all previous records be consulted for typing anomalies, presence of clinically significant antibodies, significant transfusion reactions, and special transfusion requirements. Inconsistencies or problems must be investigated and resolved before proceeding with transfusion.

Repeat Testing of Donor Blood

Segment: sealed piece of integral tubing from the donor unit bag that contains a small aliquot of donor blood; used in the preparation of red cell suspensions for crossmatching.

The transfusing facility is responsible for confirming the correct ABO labeling of all donor blood (whole blood or red blood cells) received from the donor center if the units were not previously confirmed. The AABB *Standards*[4] dictates that the ABO phenotype must be retested on all units and that the D typing must be retested on all units labeled "negative." For instance, if a D-negative unit was mislabeled D-positive, the unit would be transfused to a D-positive person, and no clinical harm would result. However, if a D-positive unit was mislabeled D-negative, the unit would be selected for a D-negative recipient and could effect an immunization to the D antigen in this individual. Testing for the weak D antigen is not required in repeat testing of donor blood. Retyping is performed by making a red cell suspension of the donor blood from a **segment** attached to the donor bag. Records of these repeat tests must be kept for 5 years. Any discrepancy with the typing on the label must result in rejection of the unit and notification to the collecting facility. Plasma and platelet products do not require retyping. Fig. 8-6 shows RBC donor units with attached segments.

Fig. 8-6 Labeled donor RBC units with attached segments. The segments are attached to each donor unit and are used as a sample of the donor unit RBCs for crossmatch and retyping.

Pretransfusion Testing on Recipient Sample

Pretransfusion testing on the recipient's sample includes the determination of the patient's ABO and D phenotype, an antibody screen, and a crossmatch.

ABO and D Phenotype of Recipient

The recipient's ABO and D phenotype is established to transfuse ABO-compatible and D-compatible blood components. For ABO group determination, the recipient's red cells are tested with commercial anti-A and anti-B reagents. The recipient's serum or plasma is also tested with reagent red cells, group A_1 and group B. See Chapters 2 and 4 for a review of this testing. Any ABO discrepancy should be resolved before any blood is transfused. If transfusion is required before resolution of the ABO discrepancy, group O RBCs should be administered.

For D antigen typing, the recipient's red cells must be tested with commercial anti-D reagent with appropriate observations or controls to avoid a false-positive interpretation. See Chapters 2 and 5 for a review of this testing. In D phenotyping discrepancies, the recipient should be transfused with D-negative RBCs until the D phenotype has been established. Weak D testing on a recipient is not necessary.[6] The transfusion of D-negative RBCs to recipients of the weak D phenotype causes no deleterious effects. Some transfusion services perform weak D testing on recipient samples to identify patients who can be transfused with D-positive blood components and to conserve the D-negative blood components. Routine testing for other Rh antigens is not necessary.

Antibody Detection Test

The recipient is also tested for expected and unexpected antibodies before components containing red cells are issued for transfusion. Antibody screening methods should detect as many clinically significant antibodies as possible and as few clinically insignificant antibodies as possible. The antibody screening procedure should be completed in a timely manner to prevent delays of transfusion. The AABB *Standards*[4] requires the use of unpooled reagent red cells in antibody screen methods used for the detection of clinically significant antibodies in recipients' samples. See Chapters 2 and 7 for a review of this testing.

> ABO phenotype, ABO type, and ABO group are terms used to describe the detectable ABO red cell antigens. These terms are used interchangeably in the blood bank literature.

TABLE 8-5	ABO Compatibility for Whole Blood, Red Blood Cells, and Plasma Transfusions		
RECIPIENT		DONOR	
ABO PHENOTYPE	WHOLE BLOOD	RED BLOOD CELLS	PLASMA
A	A	A, O	A, AB
B	B	B, O	B, AB
AB	AB	AB, A, B, O	AB
O	O	O	O, A, B, AB

Crossmatch Test

As stated earlier, a crossmatch must be performed for RBC transfusions, with the exception of circumstances requiring an urgent need for blood. The crossmatch uses procedures to demonstrate ABO incompatibility and clinically significant antibodies to red cell antigens.

Selection of ABO Donor Units

Whenever possible, recipients should receive ABO-identical blood. If the component for transfusion contains 2 mL or more of red cells, the donor's red cells must be ABO compatible with the recipient's plasma.[6] In the transfusion of plasma products, the ABO antibodies in the transfused plasma should be compatible with the recipient's red cells. Table 8-5 reviews compatibility of ABO grouping for whole blood, red blood cells, and plasma.

Selection of D Antigen Donor Units

D-positive blood components should be selected for D-positive recipients. D-negative recipients should receive RBCs that are D-negative to avoid immunization to the D antigen, especially women of childbearing age. If the recipient has a clinically unexpected antibody, the recipient should receive antigen-negative blood. If there is difficulty obtaining crossmatch-compatible donor units, the medical director should be involved in the decision to pursue transfusion.

Selection of Antigen-Negative Donor Units for Recipients with Antibodies

See Chapter 3 for the calculations of the number of donors required to find antigen-negative compatible units for a patient with multiple antibodies.

The provision of antigen-negative donor units for transfusion to recipients with blood group antibodies may be difficult, expensive, and unnecessary. Poole and Daniels[7] proposed a policy for the selection of suitable donor units for recipients with blood group antibodies using information about the antibody's history of clinical significance and availability of compatible blood. Antigen-negative RBC donor units were recommended for ABO, Rh, Kell, Duffy, and Kidd blood group system antibodies; anti-Co[a]; and anti-Vel. Donor units compatible by indirect antiglobulin test (IAT) at 37° C were recommended for anti-A$_1$, anti-P1, anti-Lu[a], anti-Do[a], anti-Do[b], and anti-Co[b]. The transfusion of donor units that are crossmatch compatible with anti-M and anti-N is a generally accepted practice, provided that the antibodies are not reactive at 37° C. Antigen-negative donor units are not required.

Tagging, Inspecting, Issuing, and Transfusing Blood Products

When the appropriate compatibility testing has been completed and the unit or units are suitable for transfusion, a tag is produced and attached to each donor unit. The donor unit tag must clearly state the patient's full name and identification number, name of the product, donor number, expiration date, ABO and D phenotype of the unit, interpretation of the crossmatching test (if performed), and identity of the person doing the testing or selection of the unit (Table 8-6). If compatibility testing is incomplete or shows incompatibility, this information must be indicated in bold on the tag.

A physician's order for blood or a blood product must be on file for the transfusion to occur. Ideally, the person requesting the donor unit presents a transfusion request

TABLE 8-6	Requirements for the Tag on the Crossmatched Donor Unit

- Patient's full name and second independent identifier
- Name of blood product
- Unique donor unit number or pool number
- Unit expiration date and ABO and D phenotype
- Interpretation of crossmatch
- Technologist's identification

TABLE 8-7	Requirements for the Issue of Donor Units

- Physician's order
- Intended recipient's two independent identifiers, ABO group, and D phenotype
- Requisition form: patient name and blood product
- Compare requisition form with donor unit tag
- Compare donor unit tag with blood product label
- Blood product expiration date
- Visual check of unit: Discoloration? Clot? Abnormal appearance?
- Documentation of person issuing and person receiving donor unit
- Special transfusion requirements
- Date and time of issue, unit destination

form to the blood bank staff indicating the desired product and the intended recipient. This form is checked carefully and independently by both persons against the unit tag. The unit tag information is also checked against the unit label. The expiration date is carefully checked to ensure that outdated units are not issued. The unit is visually checked for discoloration, clots, or other abnormal appearance. These checks are documented with the name of the person issuing the unit and the person picking it up. The date and time of issue and the unit's ultimate destination are also documented (Table 8-7). After the transfusion is complete, a copy of the tag is attached to the patient's chart.

The visual check of the donor unit before issue is an important step. Bacteria-contaminated or traumatized donor units can be detected.

Patient identification is crucial for safe transfusion and is the ultimate responsibility of the nursing or medical personnel who hang the unit. A wristband with the patient's full name and identification number must be on the patient and must exactly match the information on the unit tag. Commercial transfusion identification tagging systems use a separate wristband with special numbers to be attached to the patient specimen and any units prepared on the basis of that specimen. This system can be useful to ensure correct patient identification, and bar-code features and handheld scanners provide even greater accuracy.

Once issued for transfusion, blood products may be returned to the transfusion service for storage if they are not going to be used immediately. Unmonitored refrigerators in patient care areas should never be used for storage of blood products. Reissuing of blood products from the transfusion service is permitted, if the closure has not been entered and the unit has not exceeded the upper or lower temperature conditions for that product (1° C to 10° C for RBCs). RBCs, if not stored in a monitored refrigerator, should be returned to the transfusion service within 30 minutes to allow reissue.

SECTION 3
SPECIAL TOPICS

URGENT REQUIREMENT FOR BLOOD AND BLOOD COMPONENTS

Provision must be made by the transfusion service to expedite the release of blood in cases of life-threatening hemorrhage before completion of the usual compatibility tests. If possible, a pretransfusion sample and recent transfusion history are highly desirable.

However, obtaining such a sample is complicated if the patient received donor units that were ABO compatible, (e.g., group O, D-negative) but not identical at another facility. Because the chaotic atmosphere of an emergency situation increases the likelihood of making errors such as mislabeling or obtaining suboptimal specimens, personnel responsible for obtaining the blood bank sample must remain focused on the task of proper identification of the patient and acquisition of an adequate specimen.

After the specimen is in the blood bank, the most important test to complete is ABO and D phenotyping so that blood can be issued. The recipient's past records should also be consulted at the outset to provide a check on the ABO and D phenotype and to acquaint personnel with knowledge of any antibodies. Records alone (without current typing) may not be used as a basis for issuing blood. While these procedures are being performed, only group O, D-negative RBCs or group AB plasma should be issued. If group O, D-negative RBCs are in short supply, they should be reserved preferentially for emergency release to women younger than or of childbearing age. Group O, D-positive RBCs may be substituted for emergency release to men and to women older than childbearing age. When the phenotype is determined and confirmed, ABO-identical blood products should be issued. If an antibody is noted in the record and if time permits, the RBC products should be screened for the corresponding antigen before being issued.

The second most important test to complete is the antibody screen. Crossmatching may be initiated simultaneously. If a positive reaction is noted at any step of the antibody screen, antibody identification procedures and antiglobulin crossmatches (on the issued units and additional ones) should be initiated at once. The patient's physician must be advised of the problem. Further transfusion should be delayed, if possible, until the problem is identified and safe units can be provided, but the patient's physician must make this decision. The AABB *Technical Manual*[8] states: "The risk that the transfused unit might be incompatible may be judged to be less than the risk of depriving the patient of oxygen-carrying capacity."

The AABB *Standards*[4] stipulates that detailed records be kept of the emergency release of blood products. These records must include the patient's full name, unique identifiers, ABO and D phenotype, list of all issued units, name of the person who issued them, and name of the physician who requested emergency release of blood (Table 8-8). The AABB *Standards* and the FDA *Code of Federal Regulations* (606.151) require that the physician sign a release. Although this step can wait until after the emergency, the physician should understand that it is his or her ultimate responsibility. In addition, the tag or label on each unit that was issued uncrossmatched must include a conspicuous indication that the unit was issued that way. Segments must be pulled from the donor bags as soon as possible before they are issued and must be placed in tubes labeled with the donor unit number for subsequent crossmatching.

During the acute emergency, the blood bank personnel should "stay ahead" by crossmatching additional RBC units, preparing platelets, and thawing cryoprecipitate and frozen plasma in anticipation of need by (and in consultation with) the team caring for the patient. If the patient dies as a result of the emergency, remaining compatibility testing may be waived or abbreviated at the discretion of the transfusion service physician. Testing should be complete enough to show that the death was unrelated to the transfusion of uncrossmatched blood.

> In emergency situations, group O RBCs are issued uncrossmatched if the patient's ABO group is unknown. D-negative blood is also provided if the D type is unknown, especially if the patient is a woman of childbearing potential.

TABLE 8-8	**Urgent Requirement for Blood and Blood Components**

- Release signed by physician
- Tag on donor unit indicating emergency release: compatibility or infectious disease testing was not completed at the time of issue
- Patient name and identifiers
- Donor unit number(s), ABO and D phenotype, expiration date
- Retain segments from units for crossmatching
- Name of person issuing units

MASSIVE TRANSFUSION

A massive transfusion is defined as a total volume exchange of blood through transfusion within a 24-hour period, whether in an infant or in an adult patient. The blood products transfused in 24 hours approximate or exceed the recipient's original blood volume (approximately 10 to 12 units of whole blood in an average man). At that point, the recipient's circulation contains almost entirely transfused blood and essentially no autologous blood. The original patient's sample no longer represents the circulating blood of the patient. The transfusion service physician should have a policy clearly in place dictating what is done under these circumstances and at what point a new "recipient" sample is required. Some policies indicate that the serologic immediate-spin crossmatch is eliminated for a time, and ABO-identical donor units are simply tagged and issued. If a computer crossmatch protocol was in place, this step would be unnecessary. When clinically significant antibodies are involved, all units issued must be negative for antigens, but an immediate-spin crossmatch still could be used.

The other consideration in massive transfusion is the availability first of group O, D-negative blood and then of ABO-identical blood. When the blood group is established, group-specific blood should be transfused to protect the supply of group O, D-negative blood. However, if ABO-identical blood begins to run out, ABO-compatible blood may be used. In the case of group AB, A, or B recipients, group O RBCs may always be substituted. Group AB recipients could receive group A or group B but not both; group A typically would be used because of greater availability. See Table 8-5 for a review of these concepts. In the selection of the D-antigen type, women negative for the D antigen with childbearing potential should receive only D-negative blood. Other D-negative recipients may receive D-positive blood. However, approximately 50% to 70% of D-negative individuals subsequently develop anti-D, which sharply diminishes flexibility in a subsequent bleeding episode.[9]

Only one way exists to determine the safe point of switching the patient back to the original ABO phenotype. A new "recipient" sample must be obtained and used to determine whether the level of passively transfused anti-A, anti-B, or anti-A,B is sufficient to cause incompatibility with group A, B, or AB donors.

MAXIMUM SURGICAL BLOOD ORDER SCHEDULE

Many transfusion services have a philosophy for preparing blood for scheduled surgery that is based on statistical measures of average blood use for certain surgical procedures in their own facility. A list of all surgical procedures performed in the facility is first drawn up, and then actual usage figures for each procedure are compiled. The average number of blood units used is then determined. The surgeons, anesthesiologists, and blood transfusion physician agree on this number as the standard blood order for the stated procedure. For example, a procedure for a total hip replacement is determined to require a preoperative order of 5 units of RBCs. Such a list is called the Maximum Surgical Blood Order Schedule (MSBOS). The MSBOS may also be used as a guide for the number of autologous units the patient may donate before surgery.

TYPE AND SCREEN PROTOCOLS

If the average use for a particular surgical procedure is less than 1 unit of RBCs, many transfusion services decide that these are the cases where only a type and screen (T/S) is performed (unless clinically significant antibodies are found). If blood is subsequently needed, the T/S specimen is retrieved. Donor units are crossmatched by the immediate-spin or computer crossmatch technique. Some institutions initially perform only a T/S on all preoperative patients and crossmatch (immediate-spin or computer) only when the blood is ordered. This policy allows greater inventory availability. The physician must be able to trust that blood is always issued quickly if the T/S protocol is used. If clinically significant antibodies are or were ever present, antigen-negative units should be identified and reserved or crossmatched.

Passively transfused: when an antibody is transferred to the recipient from the plasma portion of a blood product during transfusion.

Fig. 8-7 Type and screen request flow chart for appropriate testing requirements of samples and the selection of the crossmatch procedure.

These approaches are intended to conserve blood inventory by not "tying up" excess numbers of units unlikely to be transfused. Sufficient blood supply to cover unexpected needs must be readily available, although units may not be crossmatched until the time of issue. A flow chart for T/S testing decision making is outlined in Fig. 8-7.

CROSSMATCHING AUTOLOGOUS BLOOD

Autologous blood is blood donated by the prospective recipient for later use, usually in the context of elective surgery. Special procedures must exist (whether manual or computerized) to ensure that these units are located and transfused to the intended recipient. The extent of pretransfusion testing for autologous units varies in individual facilities.

A system must exist to ensure that the autologous units are transfused before any directed or allogeneic donor units. Computerized tracking makes this step easier, but it can be done manually when necessary. If autologous units are donated, many issues of liability arise if these units are not made available, and allogeneic units are transfused instead, particularly if subsequent antibody production is stimulated or a disease is transmitted.

> Directed donations are crossmatched using the same methods as an allogeneic transfusion.

CROSSMATCHING OF INFANTS YOUNGER THAN 4 MONTHS OLD

Infants younger than 4 months old are unable to produce their own antibodies. Antibodies detected in the circulation of a newborn are maternal in origin. At 4 to 6 months of age, infants begin producing their own ABO antibodies and become capable of producing antibodies, if immunologically challenged through transfusion.

Initial compatibility testing in an infant must include a pretransfusion ABO and D phenotype on a sample obtained from the neonate. Because ABO antibodies are not present in an infant, performance of ABO reverse grouping is not required. ABO and D typing does not need to be repeated for the duration of the current admission or until the neonate reaches the age of 4 months, whichever is sooner. An initial antibody screen needs to be performed on either the infant's or mother's sample. If clinically significant antibodies are found, the blood for transfusion needs to be antigen-negative or compatible in an antiglobulin crossmatch. Crossmatching continues until maternal antibody is no longer detectable in the infant's serum. If the antibody screen is negative, however, no crossmatches or repeat screens are needed during the current admission as long as group O RBCs are used.[6]

Donor centers customarily prepare pediatric units for infants by dividing a full unit of RBCs into sterile portions. The transfusing facility may subdivide these pediatric units further if necessary. The use of syringes for transfusions to infants is also a common practice. This method transfuses the same donor blood repeatedly to the infant if multiple transfusions are needed, limiting the exposures to undetected diseases and immunologic stimuli from donor blood.

PRETRANSFUSION TESTING FOR NON–RED BLOOD CELL PRODUCTS

Plasma, platelet concentrates, and **cryoprecipitate** contain almost no red cells and do not need to be crossmatched. **Apheresis platelets** and especially **granulocyte concentrates** may contain red cells, but they need to be crossmatched only if the unit contains more than 2 mL of red cells.[4]

It is assumed that the serum or plasma of the donors of non–red cell products has been thoroughly screened for antibodies. Therefore, a repeat antibody screening and ABO and D phenotype for these products by the transfusing facility are not required. Products containing a large volume of plasma must be selected on the basis of ABO serum compatibility with the recipient. Cryoprecipitate and platelet concentrates may be transfused with combinations of ABO compatible units and units that are not ABO compatible if the cumulative volume is not large. For example, a group A recipient may receive a mixture of group A and group O platelets for transfusion. The transfusion of platelets with the same ABO phenotype as the patient may increase platelet survival rates in vivo.

Plasma: blood component prepared from whole blood that contains only the plasma portion of whole blood and is frozen after separation.

Platelet concentrates: platelets obtained from a whole blood donation; contain a minimum of 5.5×1010 platelets.

Cryoprecipitate: blood component recovered from a controlled thaw of fresh frozen plasma; the cold-insoluble precipitate is rich in coagulation factor VIII, von Willebrand's factor, factor XIII, and fibrinogen.

Apheresis platelets: apheresis procedure in which the platelets are removed from a donor, and the remaining red cells and plasma are returned.

Granulocyte concentrates: blood component collected by cytapheresis; contain a minimum of 1.0×1010 granulocytes.

In the transfusion of plasma, the D antigen is not important for compatibility because Rh antigens are found only on the red cells and are absent from plasma products. ABO antibodies are more important in the transfusion of plasma. Unlike the ABO antibodies, anti-D is not a non–immune stimulated red cell antibody.

CHAPTER SUMMARY

This chapter emphasizes that the process of compatibility testing extends beyond the boundaries of the transfusion service. The procedure begins and ends with the most important individual in the process: the recipient of the transfusion. Responsibilities of blood bank personnel include evaluating, monitoring, and following transfusion procedures and policies to meet the needs of these patients.

Process of Compatibility Testing

Patient:	✓	Accurate identification
Patient:	✓	Proper sample collection and handling
Patient:	✓	Review of past blood bank records
Patient:	✓	ABO and D type, antibody screen, crossmatch
Donor:	✓	ABO and D type, antibody screen, and infectious disease testing
Donor:	✓	Double check of unit's ABO and D typing label
Patient:	✓	Tagging, inspecting, and issuing blood products
Patient:	✓	Accurate reidentification and monitoring of transfusion

Crossmatch Procedure

The crossmatch procedure combines serum or plasma from the recipient with red cells from the donor.

- **Compatible crossmatch:** No agglutination and no hemolysis at any phase of testing. Donor unit can be transfused.
- **Incompatible crossmatch:** Hemolysis or agglutination at any phase of testing. Donor unit is not acceptable for transfusion.

Crossmatch Types

- **Serologic crossmatch:** Uses procedures to demonstrate ABO incompatibility and clinically significant antibodies to red cell antigens. There are two types of serologic crossmatches: immediate-spin for ABO compatibility and antiglobulin for clinically significant antibodies.

- **Computer crossmatch:** Uses computer to make the final check of ABO compatibility in the selection of appropriate donor units. Recipient cannot possess clinically significant antibodies in the current or any previous sample.

Urgent Requirement for Blood and Blood Components

In emergency situations, group O RBCs are issued uncrossmatched if the patient's ABO group is unknown. D-negative blood is also provided if the D type is unknown, especially if the patient is a woman of childbearing age.

Massive Transfusion

Massive transfusion refers to total volume exchange of blood through transfusion within a 24-hour period, whether in an infant or in an adult patient. The blood products transfused in 24 hours approximate or exceed the recipient's original blood volume (approximately 10 to 12 units of whole blood in an average man). The recipient's circulation contains almost entirely transfused blood and essentially no autologous blood.

Maximum Surgical Blood Order Schedule

The MSBOS is a list of blood component requirements for scheduled surgery that is based on statistical measures of average blood use for certain surgical procedures in a facility.

Type and Screen Protocols

If the average use for a particular surgical procedure is less than 1 unit of RBCs, the pretransfusion order is a T/S unless clinically significant antibodies are found. If blood is subsequently needed, the T/S specimen is used to crossmatch units by the immediate-spin or computer crossmatch technique.

Crossmatching Autologous Blood

Autologous blood is blood donated by the prospective recipient for later use, usually in the context of elective surgery. The extent of pretransfusion testing for autologous units varies in individual facilities.

Crossmatching of Infants Younger than 4 Months Old

- Initial compatibility testing in an infant must include pretransfusion ABO and D typing with no serum testing. ABO and D type does not need to be repeated for the duration of the current admission or until the neonate reaches the age of 4 months, whichever is sooner.
- An initial antibody screen needs to be performed on either the infant's or the mother's sample.
- If clinically significant antibodies are found, the blood for transfusion needs to be antigen-negative or compatible in an antiglobulin crossmatch.
- Crossmatching continues until maternal antibody is no longer detectable in the infant's serum.
- If the antibody screen is negative, no crossmatches or repeat screens are needed during the current admission as long as RBCs are used that are ABO compatible with the infant and specific for the infant's D-antigen typing (or D-negative).

Pretransfusion Testing for Non–Red Blood Cell Products

- Frozen plasma, platelet concentrates, and cryoprecipitate contain almost no red cells and do not need to be crossmatched.
- Apheresis platelets and especially granulocyte concentrates may contain red cells, but they need to be crossmatched only if the unit contains more than 2 mL of red cells.

CRITICAL THINKING EXERCISES

EXERCISE 8-1

A 60-year-old woman with anemia is admitted to the hospital. Her hematocrit is 17%, and she has been experiencing subtle gastrointestinal bleeding over many weeks. Her physician requests 4 units of RBCs for transfusion. The patient's RBCs are phenotyped as group AB, D-positive. Her antibody screen is negative on the sample drawn in the emergency department, but her records indicate a previously detected anti-E. Only 3 group AB, D-positive RBC units are available in the blood bank's inventory. The blood bank's inventory contains RBC donor units of all ABO and D types.

1. What ABO phenotype should be selected for the fourth donor unit? State your reasons for this choice.
2. What type of crossmatches should be performed?
3. Is any additional screening required on the donor units before crossmatching?

Additional Testing

After antigen screening of the 4 units of RBCs for the E antigen, one of the group AB, D-positive units is E-positive.

4. How many donor units should be screened to find the 4 units ordered, plus 2 more units to hold in reserve for the patient?

Additional Testing

Having located 6 E-negative donor units, you perform crossmatching on the units. One of the units is incompatible in the antiglobulin phase (2+ reactivity). The physician is becoming insistent on beginning the transfusion because the patient is having some shortness of breath.

5. How do you respond to the physician's request?
6. List several reasons to explain the incompatible donor unit.
7. What additional testing do you perform?

Additional Testing

Antibody-identification testing reveals no detectable antibodies, and the autologous control is negative. Additional testing revealed a positive DAT on the donor unit.

8. What is the usual transfusion service policy on donor units with a positive DAT?

STUDY QUESTIONS

1. Detection of serologic incompatibility between donor RBCs and recipient serum is performed in the:
   a. antibody screen
   b. crossmatch
   c. DAT
   d. autologous control

2. What incompatibilities are detected in the antiglobulin phase of a crossmatch?
   a. IgM alloantibodies in recipient's serum
   b. ABO incompatibilities
   c. IgG alloantibodies in recipient's serum
   d. room temperature incompatibilities

3. Which of the following statements is true regarding compatibility testing for infants younger than 4 months of age?
   a. A DAT is required
   b. A crossmatch is needed when the antibody screen is negative
   c. Maternal serum can be used for the crossmatch
   d. Testing for ABO antibodies is required for the infant

4. What tests are included in compatibility testing?
   a. blood typing of recipient
   b. antibody screening of recipient
   c. crossmatch
   d. all of the above

5. One group B, D-positive unit of RBCs is received in the transfusion service. What repeat testing is required on this donor unit?
   a. ABO typing only
   b. ABO and D typing
   c. ABO, D, and weak D typing
   d. ABO and D typing; antibody screen

6. What ABO and D types are selected for RBC units issued to a patient in emergency release?
   a. group O, D-positive
   b. group O, D-negative
   c. group A, D-positive
   d. group AB, D-negative

7. What antibodies are detected in the immediate-spin crossmatch?
   a. Rh antibodies
   b. high-titer, low-avidity antibodies
   c. ABO antibodies
   d. Kell antibodies

For questions 8 and 9, use the following information. Current pretransfusion testing on John Smith reveals a negative antibody screen with a previous history of anti-K. He is group A, D-positive.

8. Which of the following crossmatch procedures is performed to identify compatible units?
   a. immediate-spin crossmatch
   b. electronic crossmatch
   c. antiglobulin crossmatch
   d. none of the above

9. Given the following inventory, which donor unit should be selected to use for crossmatching?
   a. group A, D-positive, K+k+
   b. group A, D-negative, K–k+
   c. group O, D-positive, K+k–
   d. group O, D-negative, K+k–

10. What information is sufficient for a properly labeled blood sample for the blood bank?
    a. name, unique identification number
    b. name, unique identification number, date of collection
    c. name, unique identification number, date of collection, physician name
    d. none of the above

11. Which of the following products is crossmatched with the recipient before transfusion if the unit contains greater than 2 mL of RBCs?
    a. granulocyte concentrates
    b. plasma
    c. platelet concentrates
    d. cryoprecipitate

12. A patient who has a phenotype group AB, D-negative requires 1 unit of plasma. Which of the following units of plasma would be best for transfusion?
    a. group A, D-negative
    b. group B, D-positive
    c. group AB, D-positive
    d. group O, D-negative

13. The type of a donor unit of RBCs was tested with the following results:

Red Blood Cells Tested with:		
Anti-A	Anti-B	Anti-D
4+	0	3+

The donor unit was labeled group A, D-negative. What is the next step?
    a. transfuse as a group A, D-negative
    b. transfuse as a group A, D-positive
    c. discard the unit
    d. notify the collection facility

14. An antiglobulin crossmatch is performed with a donor red blood cell unit. The antiglobulin crossmatch result is a 2+ agglutination reaction. What is the most likely explanation for this result?
    a. recipient's RBCs are demonstrating polyagglutination
    b. recipient's RBCs have a low-frequency antigen
    c. recipient possesses an IgG alloantibody
    d. recipient possesses a cold autoantibody

15. A recipient's antibody screen is negative; however, the recipient is incompatible with the selected donor unit. Select a possible explanation for these results.
   a. recipient RBCs possess a high-frequency antigen
   b. recipient has a warm autoantibody
   c. recipient possesses an antibody to a low-frequency antigen
   d. recipient RBCs possess a cold autoantibody

True or False

_____ 16. The computer crossmatch is easily implemented in the blood bank and does not require validation.

_____ 17. A crossmatch detects most errors in the identification of antigens on patient's red cells.

_____ 18. A crossmatch demonstrating a 2+ agglutination is interpreted as compatible.

_____ 19. An immediate-spin crossmatch of a D-positive recipient with a D-negative donor unit is usually incompatible.

_____ 20. The computer crossmatch requires two ABO and D phenotypes on the recipient.

_____ 21. A crossmatch prevents the immunization of the recipient to blood group antigens.

_____ 22. A type and screen protocol provides a mechanism to increase the number of uncrossmatched donor units in inventory.

_____ 23. The only component that requires crossmatching is a unit of RBCs.

_____ 24. Group O plasma is considered the universal donor of plasma products.

_____ 25. The recipient sample must be labeled with full name, a second unique identifier, date collected, and some means of identifying the phlebotomist.

REFERENCES

1. Guy LR, Huestis DW, Wilson LR: *Technical methods and procedures*, ed 4, Chicago, 1966, AABB.
2. Oberman HA: The crossmatch, a brief historical perspective, *Transfusion* 21:645, 1981.
3. Spraycar M, editor: *Stedman's medical dictionary*, ed 26, Baltimore, 1995, Williams & Wilkins.
4. Carson TH, editor: *Standards for blood banks and transfusion services*, ed 27, Bethesda, MD, 2011, AABB.
5. Butch SH, Oberman HA: The computer or electronic crossmatch, *Transfus Med Rev* 11:256, 1997.
6. Roback JH, editor: *Technical manual*, ed 17, Bethesda, MD, 2011, AABB.
7. Poole J, Daniels G: Blood group antibodies and their significance in transfusion medicine. *Transfus Med Rev* 21:58, 2007.
8. Vengelen-Tyler V, editor: *Technical manual*, ed 12, Bethesda, MD, 1996, AABB.
9. Issitt PD, Anstee DJ: *Applied blood group serology*, ed 4, Durham, NC, 1998, Montgomery Scientific.

Blood Bank Automation for Transfusion Services

CHAPTER OUTLINE

LEARNING OBJECTIVES

On completion of this chapter, the reader should be able to:

1. Compare and contrast the forces driving the move to automation in the transfusion service.
2. Identify the potential benefits and challenges associated with change to automation.
3. Define the characteristics of an ideal instrument for blood bank testing.
4. Evaluate a vendor, base technology, and instrument for desired features.
5. Compare and contrast gel technology and solid phase red cell adherence assays (SPRCA).
6. Compare and contrast the automated platforms available for the transfusion service.
7. Select an automated platform for a transfusion service.

SECTION 1

INTRODUCTION TO AUTOMATION IN IMMUNOHEMATOLOGY

Automation in immunohematology is not a new concept. In larger blood donor centers, automated blood bank systems have performed donor unit testing for many years. Until more recently, automation was practical only for these donor centers because no technology was available to address the needs of the hospital transfusion services. Advances in test technologies and robotics are opening new opportunities for automation to meet the requirements of hospital transfusion services and medium-sized blood banks. Instruments are available for handling lower sample volumes and more individualized testing requests. Gel technology and solid phase red cell adherence assays (SPRCAs) can be performed on automated platforms. Consequently, automation is becoming more feasible for immunohematology testing performed in multiple settings. Facilities have a selection of instruments to meet their needs. In context with other coincidental driving forces, the time is optimal for medium-sized blood centers and hospital transfusion services to move forward toward automation. As automated platforms are investigated as a potential tool for the improvement of laboratory services, the selection of the appropriate automation platform becomes key in achieving this goal. Targeting the appropriate automated blood bank platform has become a major pursuit for these laboratories.

A component of the process in the selection of an automated system is an understanding of the answers to the following questions highlighted in this chapter:

- What are the forces driving the trend toward automation in the blood bank?
- What are the benefits and barriers in the adoption of an automated system?
- What are the characteristics of an "ideal" instrument for the blood bank?
- What are the major differences between fully automated and semiautomated blood bank systems?
- What automated technology is available to meet the laboratory's needs?

FORCES DRIVING THE CHANGE TO AUTOMATION

Although other disciplines within the clinical laboratory have been operating in an automated mode for many years, incentives to change to automated testing in the blood bank have received significant attention only more recently. Besides the availability of technology for automated systems, many other factors have been cited as stimulants in the movement toward automation of the blood bank. The movement toward an automated immunohematology laboratory has been attributed to the following contributing external forces[1]:

- Financial environment encouraging new economies
- Pressures to operate more efficiently; trend toward consolidation of hospitals and blood banks
- Higher testing volumes as a result of consolidation
- Compliance with increased regulations
- Standardization of testing and technology within the blood bank
- Shortage of skilled technologists attributed to the presence of fewer training programs in operation and the increase of opportunities in other professional careers
- Reduction in staff positions
- Spectrum of automated systems with technology capable of automating the reading of reactions

The combined effect of all of the above-listed factors has propelled blood banks, plasma centers, and hospital transfusion services of all sizes to pursue the evaluation of blood bank automation.

BENEFITS AND BARRIERS OF AUTOMATED INSTRUMENTS

In the investigation of any new process, both the positive and the negative aspects of automation need to be taken into consideration. An awareness of the potential benefits and challenges can assist in the planning and implementation of the automated platform.[2]

Potential Benefits

Many potential benefits accompany the switch to automation. These benefits include but are not limited to the following items.

Opportunity for Reduction in Operating Costs

With the prevalent pressures of cost containment, a major goal in the adoption of an automated system is to save operating funds. These savings may originate from laboratory expenses in labor, reagents and supplies, and biohazardous waste disposal. Labor costs represent a significant portion of laboratory expenses. Laboratory managers are concerned with controlling this cost. The implementation of automation allows a review of staffing pictures with the potential to decrease the number of full-time equivalent positions for optimal operations. Automation also provides the opportunity to cross-train technologists more readily between the blood bank and other areas of the clinical laboratory potentially generating economies in labor. The same testing platform in all laboratories in a health care network allows a standardization of inventory and more efficient usage of supplies. Avoidance of needless waste of reagents and potential savings in this area are achieved with the more efficient usage. Generally, less biohazardous waste is generated, which decreases the volume of disposal waste and its accompanying costs.

Opportunity to Redesign Work Processes and Support Systems

As automated technology is considered, the laboratory is provided an opportunity to question and examine work processes and identify areas for improvement. With an automated system, workflow may be conducive to reengineering with the potential for batch testing. Batch processing of samples saves time, materials, and reagents. More efficient workplace configurations for the workload may also be possible with automated technology. Current staffing configurations may be reviewed and reconfigured in a manner that optimizes use of staff members. Automation reduces hands-on time for the technologist freeing staff to perform other functions such as the preparation of customized blood products and compliance activities. The concept of work process redesign provides the tools for the successful implementation of these changes.[3]

Opportunity for Increased Productivity

An obvious benefit of automation is the increase in productivity. Testing capacity is increased. Turnaround times for testing are consistent and reliable. Technologists are free to perform other tasks. Automation technology can also be used in the laboratory as a mechanism to generate new revenue growth by adding new business.

Opportunity to Enhance Total Quality

Although saving and generating money are positive motivations for automated technology, the opportunity to improve total quality of testing is a top priority for any laboratory. Tube agglutination tests are associated with limitations related to sample identification, manual reagent and sample dispensing, subjective interpretation, and manual recording of results. Human errors and variations in technique are uncontrollable factors in the overall quality. Automated technology systems containing positive identification with bar coding, automated reagent and sample dispensers, automated readers, and computer interfaces for data generation and documentation eliminate these unpredictable sources of errors. Consequently, through the elimination of variability in the testing process, the end product possesses better precision and accuracy. In addition, the standardization of the automated systems enhances the laboratory's compliance with regulatory bodies.

Potential Challenges

The utopian viewpoint previously discussed is not free of its negative points. Several challenges may be encountered during the transition period.

Concerns among Staff Members

Any change to an existing system generates apprehension for the individuals who operate within the system. Although managers may tout the efficiencies of the automated technology, the staff members may view the new instrument as a job replacement. The apprehension of possible position elimination among staff members is an item to be addressed. Involving staff members in the decision-making process and discussing their concerns are keys to the acceptance of the automated technology within the laboratory. Implementation of the automation requires thorough staff training for confidence and competence with the new technology, the operation of the selected instrument, and the computer software and interface.

Cost Justification Issues

The investment in the automated technology requires an initial capital investment for equipment purchases. Because laboratories must make a valid business case before committing to the significant capital investment, management should develop a capital investment plan for presentation to the administration. The plan sets a realistic budget and outlines ways to justify the investment with labor savings, improved efficiency, increased capacity, and improvement in the quality of operations. If the purchase of equipment is undesirable, the laboratory may consider other contractual configurations with the automation suppliers that preclude an initial capital investment.

Automation Implementation Issues

In any work process redesign, the startup of the operation requires an investment of time to accomplish validation protocols, conduct training, and get procedures in order. This step requires good planning because status quo testing is ongoing in a parallel manner. The transition time requires extra staffing coverage to allow the completion of training and validation.

CHARACTERISTICS OF AN IDEAL INSTRUMENT FOR THE BLOOD BANK

If available technology had no limitations, the "ideal" instrument would possess a proven track record with the ability to automate testing, sample, and data handling. Plapp and Rachel[4] presented some characteristics of the ideal blood grouping analyzer that meet these handling criteria. The automation ideals suggested by Plapp and Rachel[4] plus other important criteria are outlined as follows:

1. Criteria important in the automation of testing include:
   - **Random-access** operating mode to accommodate STAT testing
   - Simultaneous multiple analyses to increase **throughput**
   - Extensive testing menu
   - Automated reader for reactions
   - Automatic reagent dispensing and reagent recognition
   - Precision pipetting
   - No excessive maintenance
2. Criteria important in the automation of sample handling include:
   - Clot detection
   - Liquid detection
   - Positive identification link between sample tube and test results—bar-code reading of specimen labels
   - Direct closed tube sampling of whole blood to reduce infectious disease risks
   - Automated sampling of red cells and plasma with precision and negligible carryover
   - Multiple sample tube acceptance
3. Criteria important in the automation of data handling include:
   - Flexible software for blood banks
   - Automatic comparison of current and previous test results to flag discrepancies
   - **Laboratory information system (LIS) interface** capabilities
   - Automatic update of patient files in the LIS

Random-access: system devices or workstations are used for multiple occurrences of a given laboratory operation within the automated procedure.

Throughput: productivity of a machine, procedure, process, or system over a unit period.

Laboratory information system (LIS) interface: laboratory information system interface for reporting results from the computer.

SECTION 2

SELECTION OF AUTOMATION TO MEET LABORATORY NEEDS

When considering the switch from manual to automated testing, it is important first to identify what is the appropriate automation for the facility and how much is needed. The philosophy of "one size fits all" is incorrect. After an evaluation of the automation goals of the facility and the completion of a needs assessment, the laboratory's needs should be compared with the characteristics of the analyzers on the market. In the evaluation of the available systems, several items should be considered, as discussed next.[5]

VENDOR ASSESSMENT

A thorough investigation of the automation vendors is vital to learn what they can do. In considering an automation partner, the laboratory should determine the level of the vendor's automation experience and the vendor's proven record for implementation and customer support. A list of reputable users can be very informative. These laboratories can be consulted for information on their experiences with the instrumentation and the vendor.

When selecting an automation partner, a laboratory should also ascertain its requirements in terms of customer support, training, and service. The amount and availability

TABLE 9-1	Checklist for Vendor Assessment

- Automation experience
- Record of installations
- Customer service
- Training programs
- Technical support—rapid response time
- Preventive maintenance programs
- Instrument validation and performance verification guides

TABLE 9-2	Checklist for Base Technology

- Sensitivity and specificity
- Technology lends itself to automation
- Test turnaround time
- Workload capacity
- Direct costs for reagents and equipment
- Ease of performance
- Ability to cross-train technologists

of customer service and technical support are important factors. Is there a guaranteed response time for technical consultation? Is there an adequate training program for the new instrument? Is there customer service available to diagnose instrument problems and a guaranteed on-site supply of essential replacement parts? Important considerations in the selection of an automation vendor are summarized in Table 9-1.

BASE TECHNOLOGY ASSESSMENT

The foundation of any automated platform begins with a proven technology. The reliability and accuracy of the base technology require investigation. Is the technology proven in terms of desired sensitivity and specificity? Is the technology easy to use with stable reactions? Does the technology lend itself to automation? Does the technology possess the appropriate test repertoire to meet desired needs? Other considerations in the selection of the appropriate base technology are outlined in Table 9-2.

INSTRUMENT ASSESSMENT

Automation should make it easier to do things the right way and more difficult to do the wrong things.[5] In the assessment of an instrument's performance, the adaptability, availability, and cost-effectiveness of the automated platform are important factors to evaluate.

Clinical laboratories must operate in terms of efficiency and economy of effort. Rapid turnaround times for selected samples and the ability to accommodate large volume batch testing contribute to overall operational efficiency. Instrument maintenance requirements should have a minimal impact on instrument operation. The amount of hands-on time required by the user and the workload flexibility contribute to economy of effort. The user should be able to load a STAT sample efficiently. The instrument should also be able to meet the testing profiles requirements of the clinical facility. The instrument's ability to interface with the existing LIS and the level of difficulty and required time and effort to link the two should be thoroughly investigated before purchase. The amount of training required for employees to gain confidence with the new system and the physical plant requirements to accommodate the new analyzer should also be considered.

In addition to demonstrating efficiency and economy of effort, clinical laboratories must operate in a cost-effective manner. Before the purchase of the automated platform, all of the associated immediate and long-term expenses require accounting. Beyond the capital cost of the analyzer itself lies the annual price tag for the operation of the instrument. Items that require attention include the following:

TABLE 9-3 Checklist for Assessment of Instrument

Item 1. Installation	Item 3. Test Repertoire
• Power requirements • Space and drainage requirements • Waste disposal • Heat output • Delivery • Installation assistance	• ABO/Rh phenotyping • Antibody screening/identification • Crossmatch • Direct antiglobulin test • User-defined testing profiles • Accuracy/reproducibility of test results • Errors in ABO/Rh typing • Rate of no type determined • Operator interpretation of unresolved tests
Item 2. Operation and Specifications	**Item 4. Maintenance and Reliability**
• 24-hour continuous availability • Password level access controls • Startup/shutdown and maintenance • Instrument throughput • Sample tube capacity • STAT capability • Supported bar-code types • Range of sample types • Range of sample tube sizes • Pediatric sample capability • Minimum sample volume • Liquid level detection of samples and reagents • Clot detection • Hemolyzed, icteric, and lipemic samples • Carryover • Reagent capacity • Reagent volumes monitored • Reagent waste • Reagent preparation	• Daily and weekly maintenance • Typical downtime • Maintenance contract • Ambient temperature requirements • Service representative response time • Diagnostic online service
	Item 5. Data Management
	• Windows-based software • Password access to instrument software • Bidirectional interface • Ability to configure screen and reports • Relevant information stored with results • Remote access to database

- Costs associated with reagents and disposable items
- Costs for the linkage of the analyzer to the LIS
- Costs for replacement parts
- Costs to keep equipment in working condition
- Costs for training personnel
- Costs for physical plant modifications to accommodate the analyzer

Table 9-3 provides a checklist for the assessment of blood bank instruments. With so many choices of analyzers, laboratory professionals need to call on their collective management and technical expertise to make the right choice for the future of their institutions. Evaluating the vendor and base technology in conjunction with the instrument provide valuable tools for targeting blood bank automation.

SECTION 3

AUTOMATED TESTING SYSTEMS

Automated testing systems have been developed for SPRCAs, gel technology, and microtiter plates. These systems can perform ABO and Rh phenotyping, antibody detection and identification, and crossmatching. For the purposes of an introduction to automation, SPRCA and gel technology instrumentation are discussed.

> See Chapter 2 for a review of solid phase red cell adherence assays, gel technology, and microtiter plate testing.

AUTOMATED SYSTEMS FOR SOLID PHASE RED CELL ADHERENCE ASSAYS

SPRCAs are manufactured by Immucor (Norcross, GA) under the trade name Capture-R Ready-Screen and Capture-R Ready ID.[6] Capture technology is also referred to as SPRCA. The automated instruments that support this technology include Galileo, Galileo ECHO (Fig. 9-1), and NEO (Fig. 9-2). In addition, the Capture Workstation provides a means

Fig. 9-1   ECHO. ECHO is an automated microplate-based solid phase technology, a bench-top instrument. (Courtesy Immucor, Norcross, Ga.)

Fig. 9-2   NEO. NEO is an automated microplate-based solid phase technology for high-volume testing. (Courtesy Immucor, Norcross, Ga.)

to perform a manual version of the Capture-R procedure (Fig. 9-3). The automated instruments use microplates and microwell strips to perform various predefined assays including hemagglutination assays and SPRCAs, which are described subsequently.

Hemagglutination Assays

Hemagglutination assays are used for testing the following:
- ABO and D antigen phenotype
- Antigen screen
- Immediate-spin crossmatch

Hemagglutination assays performed in microplates use the same principle as tube agglutination but in a smaller medium. Bar-coded patient samples, reagents, and

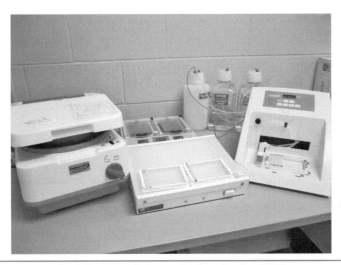

Fig. 9-3 Manual Capture Workstation for SPRCA.

Results - Group

Sample ID	Interp.	Flags	Mono Ctrl	Anti-A	Anti-B	Anti-D1	Anti-D2	A1 Cells	B Cells
R28786	0 Pos		0	0	0	3+	3+	4+	3+
			◯	◯	◯	◉	◉	◉	◉

Fig. 9-4 Results and interpretation of an ABO/Rh phenotype. In the hemagglutination test, agglutination is a positive result, and no agglutination is a negative result. (Courtesy Immucor, Norcross, Ga.)

microtiter plates provide a means of ensuring positive identification and system verification. After sample and reagent pipetting, the plate is automatically centrifuged and then read by the instrument's camera-reader. Grading and interpretations are made by the instrument, which appear on the computer monitor (Fig. 9-4). The reactions and interpretations must be verified by the operator before releasing results. ABO forward and reversed discrepancies are flagged, and a weak D test can be automatically ordered for D-negative sample results.

The immediate-spin crossmatch can also be performed by automated solid phase hemagglutination methods and has the advantage of bar-code technology to enhance patient and donor sample identification and verification. If online with the hospital information system, historical test results can also be checked for ABO/Rh and antibody history results. This technology is especially helpful when performing the computer (electronic) crossmatch.

Solid Phase Red Cell Adherence Assays

SPRCAs are performed for the following tests:
- Antibody screen
- Antibody identification
- Direct antiglobulin test
- Weak D test
- IgG crossmatch

SPRCAs can be used for both indirect and direct antiglobulin tests. For antibody screen and identification procedures, pretreated wells are purchased that have red cell membranes bound to the surface of the polystyrene microtiter wells (Fig. 9-5).

The antigen configurations vary with the lot, similar to standard reagent red cells. The first step in testing is the addition of the specially formulated low-ionic-strength saline (LISS) reagent, followed by the patient serum. The plate is automatically moved in to the 37° C incubator for a predetermined time. If antibodies are present, they attach to the

Capture microstrips:

Fig. 9-5 Capture Ready-Screen and Ready-ID. Capture Ready-Screen and Ready-ID precoated test wells for antibody screen **(A)** and panel Capture microstrips **(B)** are purchased with red cell membranes preattached to the wells. Pooled and two-cell, three-cell, and four-cell screens are available. Several panel options are also available that provide different antigen configurations, such as D-positive and D-negative panels. (Courtesy Immucor, Norcross, Ga.)

corresponding antigen on the well surface. Unbound serum proteins are washed away. To detect bound antibody, an IgG-coated indicator red cell is added, and the strip is centrifuged, which allows the cells to adhere to the antibody that may be attached to the membrane. Adherence is a positive result. If the cells pellet to the bottom of the well in a tightly packed button, antibodies either were not present or were not specific for the antigen on the well and interpreted as negative. Fig. 9-6 illustrates the principle of this test and the reaction interpretations.[7-9]

The Capture-R Select provides microwells for the immobilization of red cells other than the screen cells or panel cells. Red cells used may be patient cells for a direct antiglobulin test, patient or donor cells for a weak-D test, or donor cells for IgG crossmatch. An example of antibody screen and antibody detection using the Capture assay system is provided in Fig. 9-7.

Solidscreen[R] II Technology

The TANGO™ optimo System is a platform combining Erytype[R] S and Solidscreen[R] II technologies with state-of-the-art instrumentation to provide laboratories of all sizes with outstanding productivity, reliability, and true hands-off convenience. The automated platform is offered by Bio-Rad Laboratories, Inc. (Hercules, CA). The TANGO™ optimo is a fully automated, random access system for blood group serology assays (antibody screen, antibody identification, direct antiglobulin test, IgG crossmatch, Weak D, and ABD/Kell red cell phenotype). Similar to the Immucor Capture system, microtiter wells are designed to accommodate either antiglobulin tests or hemagglutination tests (Fig. 9-8).

Solidscreen[R] II is a solid phase assay for antiglobulin testing. The wells in this assay are precoated with Protein A, a component of the cell wall of *Staphylococcus aureus*, which has a high affinity for the Fc portion of most immunoglobulin classes.[10] The instrument pipettes LISS (MLB2), plasma (or serum), and test erythrocytes into wells coated with Protein A. The wells are incubated at 37° C and then washed with PBS to remove

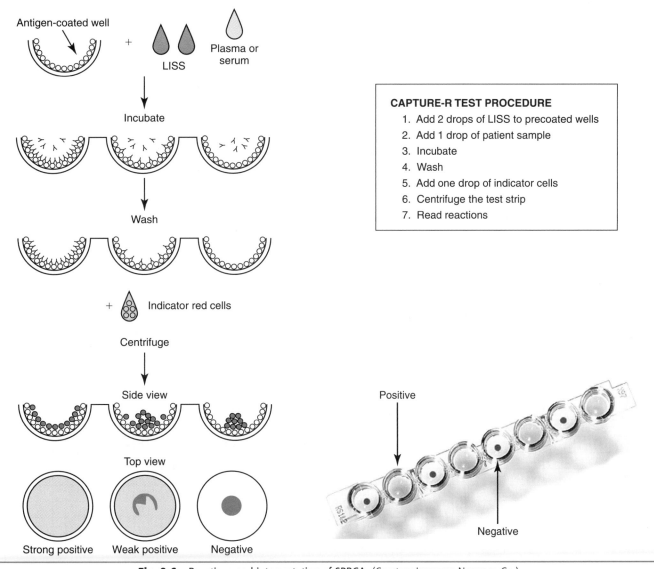

CAPTURE-R TEST PROCEDURE

1. Add 2 drops of LISS to precoated wells
2. Add 1 drop of patient sample
3. Incubate
4. Wash
5. Add one drop of indicator cells
6. Centrifuge the test strip
7. Read reactions

Fig. 9-6 Reactions and interpretation of SPRCA. (Courtesy Immucor, Norcross, Ga.)

any unbound immunoglobulin. After washing, the instrument adds IgG AHG and centrifuges the strip. If antibody was bound to its corresponding antigen during incubation, the IgG AHG Fab portion will bind to the antibody on the red cell. When spun, the Fc portion of the IgG AHG will attach to the Protein A layer at the bottom of the well, yielding a smooth monolayer of red cells, a positive reaction. If no antibody has been bound to red cells during incubation, no IgG AHG is attached and, after centrifugation, a compact cell button will indicate a negative reaction. The instrument reads and interprets the results. Fig. 9-9 illustrates this procedure.

Erytype^R S Technology

The TANGO™ optimo System uses Erytype^R S microplate wells/strips for hemagglutination assays. ABD (forward and reverse) typing, plus C, c, E, e, and Kell red cell antigen typings may be performed on these strips. Wells are precoated with dried, monoclonal antisera.[11] The instrument pipettes the sample, centrifuges, reads, and interprets the results. The Erytype^R S ABD + A$_1$, B procedure is outlined in Fig. 9-10.

Results - Screen

Sample ID	Interp.	Flags	Screen 1	Screen 2	Screen 3	Pos Ctrl
R28786	Positive		4+	4+	0	4+

Results - Ready ID

Sample ID	Interp.	Flags	R-ID 1	R-ID 2	R-ID 3	R-ID 4	R-ID 5	R-ID 6	R-ID 7	R-ID 8
R28786	Complete	*	4+	4+	4+	4+	0	0	0	0

Sample ID	Interp.	Flags	R-ID 9	R-ID 10	R-ID 11	R-ID 12	R-ID 13	R-ID 14	Pos Ctrl	Neg Ctrl
R28786	Complete	*	0	0	0	0	0	4+	4+	0

CAPTURE-R READY-ID
Master List

ID144

IMMUCOR, INC. Norcross, GA 30071 USA
US LICENSE NO: 886
LOT NO: ID 144
EXPIRES 2011/08/30

NAME _____
NO. R28786
INSTITUTION _____
BLOOD GROUP _____
ANTIBODY IDENTITY _____
TECH _____ DATE _____

CELL	Special Type	Donor	D	C	c	E	e	V	Cᵂ	K	k	Kpᵃ	Kpᵇ	Jsᵃ	Jsᵇ	Fyᵃ	Fyᵇ	Jkᵃ	Jkᵇ	Leᵃ	Leᵇ	P₁	M	N	S	s	Luᵃ	Luᵇ	Xgᵃ	CELL	PATIENT'S TEST RESULTS
1		RzR1 A3481	+	+	0	+	+	0	0	0	+	0	+	0	+	+	+	+	+	0	0	+	0	+	0	+	+	+	1	4+
2		R1wR1 B3785	+	+	0	0	+	0	+	+	+	0	+	0	+	0	+	+	+	0	+	+	0	+	0	+	0	+	+	2	4+
3		R2R2 C3723	+	0	+	+	0	0	0	0	+	0	+	0	+	0	+	+	+	0	+	+	+	0	0	0	0	+	+	3	4+
4		Ror D691	+	0	+	0	+	+	0	0	+	0	+	0	+	0	+	+	+	0	+	+	+	0	+	0	0	+	+	4	4+
5		r'r E766	0	+	+	0	+	0	0	0	+	0	+	0	+	+	+	0	+	0	+	0	+	+	+	0	0	+	0	5	0
6		r"r F792	0	0	+	+	+	0	0	+	+	0	+	0	+	+	+	+	+	0	0	+	+	+	+	0	+	+	6	0
7		r'r E831	0	+	+	0	+	0	0	0	+	0	+	0	+	0	+	+	0	+	0	+	0	+	0	+	0	+	+	7	0
8		rr G483	0	0	+	0	+	0	0	0	+	0	+	0	+	0	+	0	+	0	+	+	0	+	0	+	0	+	+	8	0
9		rr H1281	0	0	+	0	+	0	0	0	+	0	+	0	+	0	+	0	+	0	+	+	0	+	0	+	0	+	+	9	0
10	Yt(bᵀ)	rr H347	0	0	+	0	+	0	0	0	+	0	+	0	+	0	0	+	0	+	+	+	+	0	+	0	0	10	0
11		rr V163	0	0	+	0	+	+	0	0	+	0	+	0	+	0	+	0	W	+	+	+	+	0	+	0	+	+	11	0
12		rr N3073	0	0	+	0	+	0	0	0	+	+	0	+	0	+	+	+	+	0	+	+	0	+	0	0	0	+	0	12	0
13		rr G964	0	0	+	0	+	0	0	+	+	0	+	0	+	+	0	0	+	+	0	+	+	0	+	+	+	+	13	0
14	Di(aᵀ)	R1R1 B7587	+	+	0	0	+	0	0	0	+	0	+	0	+	0	+	+	0	0	+	+	0	0	+	0	+	+	14	4+
15		POSITIVE CONTROL	/	/	/	/	/	/	/	/	/	/	/	/	/	/	/	/	/	/	/	/	/	/	/	/	/	/	/	PC	4+
16		NEGATIVE CONTROL	/	/	/	/	/	/	/	/	/	/	/	/	/	/	/	/	/	/	/	/	/	/	/	/	/	/	/	NC	0

* Indicates those antigens whose presence or absence may have been determined using only a single example of a specific antibody.

NOTES:
An antigen designated with a 'w' represents a weakened expression of the antigen that may or may not react with all examples of the corresponding antibody.

426-17

I	4+
II	4+
III	0
IV	

Fig. 9-7 Capture Ready-Screen and Ready-ID test results and interpretation. Panel results show wells 1 to 4 and 14 as positive. These results are transferred to the panel below, which can be interpreted by ruling out with the negative reactions. As with tube testing methods, it is important that the correct panel lot number is chosen. Interpretation by ruling out demonstrates an anti-D. (Courtesy Immucor, Norcross, Ga.)

Fig. 9-8   TANGO™ optimo automated blood bank system. (Courtesy Bio-Rad Laboratories, Inc., © 2012.)

Solidscreen® II Test Principle

Test Menu for Solidscreen® II Assays

- Antibody screening
- Antibody Identification
- Direct Antiglobulin test
- Crossmatch – Anti-IgG
- Weak D

Solidscreen II is suitable for the following applications:

✓   Antibody screen with pooled cells, two, three, or four combinations

✓   Antibody identification with 8 or 11 panel cells

✓   IgG crossmatch

✓   Enzyme-treated red cells for antibody screen and identification

✓   Auto control

✓   Antibody titration

✓   Direct antiglobulin test

✓   Anti-D (RH1) blend for weak D and partial D tests

Fig. 9-9   Solidscreen II technology. (Courtesy Bio-Rad Laboratories, Inc., © 2012.)

Erytype® S Test Principle

Wells Pre-coated with Antisera

Red Cells Diluted in Bromelin

Incubation at RT

Centrifugation

Strong Positive

Weak Positive

Negative

Ready-to-use microplate wells pre-coated with monoclonal blood grouping antisera

Red cells suspended in Bromelin are pipetted into wells

Antisera dissolves and antigen-antibody reaction occurs – Incubation at RT

Centrifugation and resuspension of agglutination

TANGO™ optimo System interprets agglutination patterns

Anti-A	Anti-B	Anti-AB	Anti-D	Anti-D	Neg.con.	A1-cell	B-cell
--	--	--	++++	++++	--	+	+++

Test Menu for Erytype® S Assays

- ABO/Rh
- Rh and Kell Phenotype
- ABO donor confirmation
- Rh donor confirmation

Fig. 9-10 Example of Erytype S assay. (Courtesy Bio-Rad Laboratories, Inc., © 2012.)

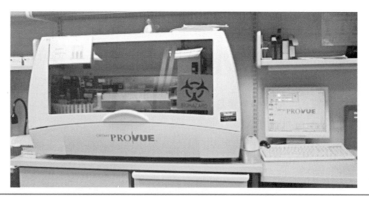

Fig. 9-11 ORTHO ProVue instrument.

AUTOMATED SYSTEM FOR GEL TECHNOLOGY ASSAYS

Gel technology assays are manufactured by Ortho Clinical Diagnostics (Raritan, NJ) under the trade name ID-MTS Gel Test. The automated instrument that supports this technology is the ORTHO ProVue (Fig. 9-11). The instrument is a modular and microprocessor-controlled unit, which was designed to automate in vitro immunohematologic testing of human blood using the ID-MTS Gel Test.[12] As a standalone instrument or interfaced to the customer's LIS, ORTHO ProVue automates test processing functions and data management requirements using gel cards and digital image processing.

The ORTHO ProVue consists of the following primary components:

- ProVue computer (or computer)
- ProVue software
- ProVue (or instrument)
- Handheld bar-code scanner
- Printer
- Uninterruptible power supply (UPS)

ORTHO ProVue has been qualified for use with ID-MTS Gel Test gel cards and diluents and Ortho 0.8% Reagent Red Blood Cells.[13] The following test types are supported by the ORTHO ProVue:

- Direct agglutination tests: ABO forward and reverse grouping, D antigen typing, Rh phenotyping, immediate-spin crossmatch
- Direct antiglobulin tests (DAT): Anti-IgG DAT, anti-IgG, -C3d DAT
- Indirect antiglobulin tests (IAT): Antibody screen, antibody identification, IAT crossmatch

This analyzer helps to eliminate labor-intensive, time-consuming processes. The instrument increases productivity through random access, discrete testing, and continuous throughput. It also possesses a STAT interrupt capability. The unit enhances process control with dispense verification, bar-code tracking from start to finish, and multilevel password protection. Its quality control features monitor reagent expiration and gel card integrity and can reduce transcription errors owing to a bidirectional interface.

The unit has a sample carousel that holds 48 sample tubes up to 16 × 100 mm in diameter and height. The reagent carousel holds 16 reagents and 2 diluents. The dilution station prepares sample red cell suspensions. The system has three cameras for sample, reagent, and card identification and image analysis. There is also a 24-position capacity card block with the option of 16 gel cards at 25° C and 8 cards at 37° C or all gel cards at one temperature. A robotic handler probe pierces the foil and performs sample dilutions. The gel card gripper transports cards to a 12-position centrifuge and a 12-position service rack for cards that need review (Fig. 9-12).

The ORTHO ProVue computer handles the software for the operation of the instrument. Using the software, the operator orders a specified test, such as ABO and Rh phenotyping (Fig. 9-13). Bar-coded patient samples are loaded into the sample carousel. The instrument determines the gel card type, number, and position of gel cards placed in the incubator block. For phenotyping A, B, and D antigens, MTS Monoclonal A/B/D Grouping Cards are required to be placed in the 25° C incubator block. MTS Diluent 2 PLUS is loaded in the assigned position in the reagent carousel. The diluent is required to dilute red cells to 4 ± 1% for the gel test. Once reagents and samples are loaded on the instrument, the operator gives the start command for the operation of the

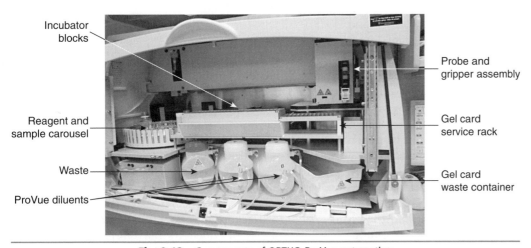

Fig. 9-12 Components of ORTHO ProVue automation.

Fig. 9-13   Software image of the ORTHO ProVue.

ID-MTS GEL TEST PROCEDURE

ABD Phenotyping

1. Prepare 4% red cell suspensions in MTS Diluent 2 PLUS.
2. Pipet 10 μL of 4% red cell suspension into gel card.
3. Place gel cards into gel card centrifuge.
4. Centrifuge for 10 minutes.
5. Read and grade gel card reactions.

Fig. 9-14   ID-MTS Gel Test procedure for the detection of A, B, and D antigens. (Courtesy ID-MTS Interpretation Guide, Ortho Clinical Diagnostics, Raritan, NJ.)

Results by sample

Date: 4/28/2011 12:30:28 PM
Batches: 666-702
Template: TX pin

Samples	A	B	D	Ctl	A1Cel	B Cell	Group	Rh	Cell 1	Cell 2	XIAT	XIS
1111802053A	4+	-	4+	-	-	4+	A	Pos	-	-		

Fig. 9-15   Example of sample results for ABO and D typing and antibody screen on the ORTHO ProVue.

ORTHO ProVue. The ABO and Rh phenotyping program begins operation of the test procedure.

The ID-MTS Gel Test procedure for the phenotyping of A, B, and D antigens is outlined in Fig. 9-14.[14] These operations are performed by the ORTHO ProVue. The gel card is read by a camera, and the results are graded according to the reading algorithms built into the software. A printout of the results is provided by the ORTHO ProVue. An example of a printout screen is provided in Fig. 9-15.

The ORTHO ProVue is equivalent to the standard manual method for both direct agglutination test and DAT and IAT using the ID-MTS Gel Test.[13] More recent studies showed that, on average, one ORTHO ProVue operator did the serologic testing previously performed by two technical staff members and reduced the total processing time by 40%. The research also showed an 81.6% overall hands-on time reduction compared with manual tube testing and a 75.9% reduction compared with manual gel testing.[15]

CHAPTER SUMMARY

- Advances in test technologies and robotics are opening new opportunities for automation to meet the requirements of hospital transfusion services and medium-sized blood banks.
- Automated testing systems have been developed for the detection of antigen-antibody reactions in immunohematologic testing.
- The test system's computer may be interfaced with a laboratory's information system for reporting results.
- The benefits of automation in the transfusion service include opportunities for reduction in operating costs, redesign of work processes and support systems, increased productivity, and increased quality.
- The challenges of automation implementation include staff concerns, justification of investment costs, and issues associated with implementation.
- A thorough investigation of automation vendors is vital to learn what they can do for the transfusion service.
- The foundation of any automated platform begins with a proven technology. The reliability and accuracy of the base technology requires investigation.
- In the assessment of performance of an instrument, the adaptability, availability, and cost-effectiveness of the automated platform are important factors to evaluate.
- Automated testing systems have been developed for SPRCA, gel technology, and microtiter plates. These systems can perform ABO and Rh phenotyping, antibody detection, and identification and crossmatching.

CRITICAL THINKING EXERCISES

EXERCISE 9-1

The transfusion service at JHM Hospital has been asked to implement the electronic crossmatch to reduce turnaround time. The lead technologist has been assigned the task of investigating the various automated technology currently available to accomplish this task. What important criteria should be considered when deciding which automated testing system to bring on board to accommodate the electronic crossmatch procedure?

EXERCISE 9-2

A small remote hospital is having difficulty in staffing the transfusion service section due to the lack of experience and hesitancy of many of the staff techs who work in other sections of the laboratory. An automated platform for the blood bank area is being considered to work around this issue. How could an automated system help in this circumstance?

EXERCISE 9-3

A blood bank using the ECHO found a discrepant result on a donor sample that was tested for weak D. Prior donor records showed the result as weak D positive, while current testing was weak D negative. A review of the records indicated that previous testing was performed in the tube, prior to implementing the automated system. What items should be considered when investigating this discrepancy? What are possible causes of these differing results and how should it be resolved?

STUDY QUESTIONS

1. Which of the following statements is true regarding interpretation of SPRCA results?
   a. Grading reactions is based on a 1-to-4 grading scale where 4+ is a strong positive.
   b. A tight button of cells on the bottom of the well would be interpreted as a positive reaction.
   c. Hemagglutination assay results are interpreted the same as SPRCA results.
   d. An evenly distributed layer of cells on the well surface is a negative reaction.

2. Indicator cells used in SPRCA are:
   a. IgM-coated red cells useful in determining the presence of ABO antibodies
   b. cells used to agglutinate IgG antibodies to form a pellet in the well after centrifugation
   c. IgG-coated red cells that cross-link with IgG antibodies attached to the well
   d. check cells that are added to negative reactions to validate the washing step

3. In the gel test, a button of cells at the bottom of the well is a:
   a. 4+ positive reaction
   b. 1+ positive reaction
   c. negative reaction
   d. invalid reaction

4. The gel test and SPRCA share which of the following advantages over the antiglobulin tube testing method?
   a. both use prediluted cells, saving reagent expense
   b. endpoints are stable and reviewable for at least 2 days
   c. centrifugation is not required for either system
   d. a washing step is not required for either system

5. Which method is used in the automated Immucor system for ABO and D phenotype?
   a. solid phase red cell adherence assay (SPRCA)
   b. enzyme-linked immunosorbent assay (ELISA)
   c. reverse-passive hemagglutination (RPHA)
   d. hemagglutination in a microwell

6. False-negative reactions can occur in both gel test and SPRCA for which of the following errors?
   a. failing to centrifuge
   b. not mixing reagent red cells sufficiently
   c. incubation time was too short
   d. all of the above

7. Mixed-field reactions were observed in the ID-MTS Gel Test for ABO and D phenotype using the ORTHO ProVue. What is the most likely cause of this observation?
   a. improper pipetting technique
   b. the use of contaminated reagents
   c. transfusion of group O cells to an A or B patient
   d. centrifugation error

8. After centrifugation using the ID-MTS anti-IgG gel cards, a layer of agglutinated cells was observed at the top of two of the three screening cell microtubes. What should be done next?
   a. repeat the test
   b. proceed to an antibody identification panel
   c. perform a DAT to determine if the patient has an autoantibody
   d. verify the negative reaction with check cells

9. The MTS Monoclonal A/B/D Grouping Gel Card is used for:
   a. typing A, B, and D antigen
   b. antiglobulin crossmatches
   c. typing Rh system antigens
   d. direct antiglobulin tests

10. The Capture-R select microwell strips are used for:
    a. direct antiglobulin test
    b. antiglobulin testing of selected panel cells
    c. weak D test
    d. all of the above

True or False

____ 11. Bar-code technology is used in automated instruments to ensure positive sample identity.

____ 12. LIS interfaces link the automated test system with a laboratory information system for reporting results.

____ 13. Automation should make it easier to do things the right way and more difficult to do the wrong things.

____ 14. When selecting an automation partner, a laboratory does not need to determine its requirements in terms of customer support, training, and service.

____ 15. Rapid turnaround times for selected samples and the ability to accommodate large volume batch testing contribute to overall operational efficiency.

____ 16. Vendors of automation for the transfusion service require prior approval from the FDA.

____ 17. Vendor assessment, base technology, and instrument assessment are important considerations in the selection of an automated system.

____ 18. Automation can be purchased for gel technology and SPRCAs.

____ 19. Because of the sensitivity of the SPRCAs and gel assays, the immediate-spin crossmatch for detecting ABO compatibility is no longer necessary.

REFERENCES

1. Paxton A: Blood banks step up move to automation, *CAP Today* 13(10):1, 28-32, 34, 1999.
2. Wilde M: Automation a simple solution to do more with less, *Adv Med Lab Prof* 9:6, 1997.
3. South SF: *Automation and work process redesign*, Raritan, NJ, Ortho-Clinical Diagnostics, 1999, Inc.
4. Plapp FV, Rachel JM: Automation in blood banking, *AJCP* 98(Suppl 1):17, 1992.
5. Johnson SM, Aller RD: Weeding out the wrong coagulation analyzer, *CAP Today* 14:46, 2000.
6. Harmening D: *Modern blood banking and transfusion practices*, ed 5, Philadelphia, 2005, FA Davis.
7. Capture-R Select, Solid Phase System for the Immobilization of Human Erythrocytes (package insert), Immucor, Norcross, GA.
8. Capture-R Ready Screen and Capture-R Ready ID (package insert), Immucor, Norcross, GA.
9. Sinor L: Advances in solid phase red cell adherence methods and transfusion serology, *Transfus Med Rev* 6:26, 1992.
10. Erytype ABD+Rev.A₁, B (package insert). *Bio-Rad*. www.bio-rad.com. Accessed December, 2011.
11. Solidscreen II (package insert). *Bio-Rad*. www.bio-rad.com. Accessed December, 2011.
12. Micro Typing Systems, Inc. Ortho ProVue 510K Summary. *Food and Drug Administration*. www.fda.gov. Accessed December, 2011.
13. Casina TS, Weiland D, Howard P, et al: AP108: evaluation of a fully automated system for gel testing. *Transfusion* 43(Suppl):166A, 2003.
14. MTS Monoclonal A/B/D Grouping Card (package insert), *Ortho Clinical Diagnostics*. www.orthoclinical.com. Accessed December, 2011.
15. Sorenson EA, Pless D, Yu MG: AP109 continuous throughput, discrete testing and random access: a new reality in blood bank automation, *Transfusion* 43(Suppl):166A, 2003.

10 Adverse Complications of Transfusions

CHAPTER OUTLINE

LEARNING OBJECTIVES

On completion of this chapter, the reader should be able to:

1. Describe the hemovigilance model and its role in improving transfusion safety.
2. List common signs and symptoms of adverse transfusion reactions.
3. Distinguish between acute and delayed transfusion reactions and provide examples.
4. Compare and contrast immune-mediated and non–immune-mediated red cell destruction.
5. Describe the distinguishing features of the following transfusion reactions: febrile, urticarial, anaphylactic, transfusion-related acute lung injury, and transfusion-associated graft-versus-host disease.
6. Discuss the causes and clinical features of bacterial contamination of blood products.
7. Describe the clinical features of transfusion reactions caused by circulatory overload and patients at risk of this transfusion reaction.
8. Describe the mechanisms and prevention of transfusion hemosiderosis, citrate toxicity, and posttransfusion purpura.
9. Provide direction to medical personnel performing the transfusion in the event of a reported adverse reaction.
10. List initial tests performed in the transfusion service on receipt of a patient sample following a reaction.
11. Identify additional testing that might be required in the investigation of transfusion reactions and the rationale for selecting these tests.
12. Describe the required documentation and reporting in the investigation of a transfusion reaction.

Transfusion safety measures are incorporated at all steps of the blood collection, donor unit processing, and transfusion protocols. Despite careful pretransfusion testing and patient monitoring, noninfectious complications of transfusions occur and are not always preventable. Many systems and procedures have been designed to reduce the risk of adverse complications of blood transfusions. This chapter provides an overview of the proposed mechanisms, risks, and preventive measures associated with complications of blood transfusion.

SECTION 1
OVERVIEW OF ADVERSE REACTIONS TO TRANSFUSION

HEMOVIGILANCE MODEL

An **adverse transfusion reaction** is "an undesirable response or effect in a patient temporarily associated with the administration of blood or blood component."[1] Statistically, noninfectious complications of transfusions pose a greater risk to patients than infectious diseases.[2] Table 10-1 summarizes the U.S. Food and Drug Administration (FDA) reportable transfusion fatalities for 2010. The "Hemovigilance Model" under the National Healthcare Safety Network (NHSN) was developed with the cooperation of the AABB and the Centers of Disease Control and Prevention (CDC) to track, to analyze, and ultimately to improve transfusion outcomes. This confidential, voluntary reporting system collects data from participating hospitals that report to the CDC on a monthly basis. The CDC publishes these results to assist facilities in quality improvement activities, collaborative research, and recognition of trends. The contents of this chapter follow the case definition criteria for adverse reactions of blood transfusion used in the hemovigilance model, which is based on International Society of Blood Transfusion (ISBT) definitions.[3]

Adverse transfusion reaction: undesirable response by a patient to the infusion of blood or blood products.

RECOGNITION OF A TRANSFUSION REACTION

Clinical signs and symptoms of a complication of transfusion may be associated with more than one type of reaction, and early recognition and evaluation is important for the best outcome. Transfusion reactions may occur as an **acute reaction** (immediately or within 24 hours) or a **delayed reaction** (>24 hours). In patients who are anesthetized or medicated, clinical symptoms may not be as obvious. Signs of a transfusion reaction may include the following:

Acute reaction: reaction occurring within 24 hours of transfusion.

Delayed reaction: reaction occurring more than 24 hours following transfusion.

- Fever ≥1° C increase or >38° C
- Chills/rigors
- Respiratory distress—wheezing, coughing, dyspnea, cyanosis
- Hypertension or hypotension
- Pain—abdominal, chest, flank or back, infusion site
- Skin manifestations—urticaria, rash, flushing, edema
- Jaundice, hemoglobinuria
- Nausea/vomiting
- Abnormal bleeding
- Oliguria/anuria

TABLE 10-1	Fatal Transfusion Reactions Reported to the Food and Drug Administration in 2010	
COMPLICATION	**NUMBER**	**%**
TRALI	145	47
Non-ABO hemolytic transfusion reaction	47	15
TACO	37	12
Microbial infection	35	11
ABO hemolytic transfusion reaction	28	9
Anaphylactic	11	4
Other	4	1
Total	*307*	*100*

Data from *Fatalities reported to FDA following blood collection and transfusion: annual summary for fiscal year 2010.* http://www.fda.gov/downloads/BiologicsBloodVaccines/SafetyAvailability/ReportaProblem/TransfusionDonationFatalities/UCM254860.pdf.
TRALI, Transfusion-related acute lung injury; *TACO,* transfusion-associated circulatory overload.

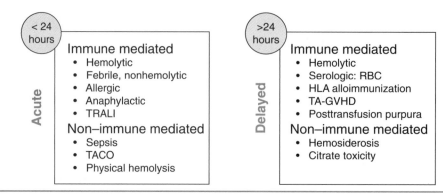

Fig. 10-1 Categories of transfusion reactions. *TACO,* Transfusion-associated circulatory overload; *TRALI,* transfusion-related acute lung injury; *RBC,* red blood cell; *HLA,* human leukocyte antigen; *TA-GVHD,* transfusion-associated graft-versus-host disease.

Immune-mediated reactions: reactions involving antigen-antibody complexes, cytokine release, or complement activation.

Non–immune-mediated reactions: reactions that may be due to the component transfused, the patient's underlying condition, or the method of infusion.

Reactions are further classified as either **immune-mediated reactions** or **non–immune-mediated reactions,** meaning that the recognition of foreign proteins and cells by the immune system may or may not be involved. In a nonimmune reaction, the component given, the method of transfusion, or the patient's underlying condition may be the cause of the reaction. Fig. 10-1 presents the categories of reactions to be discussed further in this chapter.

SECTION 2
CATEGORIES OF TRANSFUSION REACTIONS

HEMOLYTIC TRANSFUSION REACTION

A hemolytic transfusion reaction is the destruction of transfused red cells that results in intravascular or extravascular hemolysis or a combination of both. Hemolytic reactions are classified as acute or delayed, and both types may stem from immune or nonimmune causes.

Acute Hemolytic Transfusion Reaction

An acute hemolytic transfusion reaction (AHTR) is the rapid destruction of red cells during, immediately after, or within 24 hours following a transfusion of red cells. The clinical presentation of an AHTR ranges in severity from fever to death. Signs and symptoms associated with an acute hemolytic reaction include fever, chills, pain or oozing at the infusion site, back or flank pain, hypotension, epistaxis (nosebleed) hemoglobinuria, disseminated intravascular coagulation (DIC), oliguria, anuria, and renal failure.[1]

Multiple simultaneous clinical events contribute to the degree of severity resulting from the destruction of red cells. The interaction of preformed antibodies with red cell antigens, usually an ABO incompatibility, is the immunologic basis for AHTR. Events in an immune-mediated AHTR include the following:

Severe symptoms of an AHTR can occur after the infusion of as little as 10 mL of incompatible blood.[4]

- Antibody binding to red cells
- Activation of complement
- Activation of mononuclear phagocytes and release of cytokines
- Activation of the coagulation system
- Shock and renal failure

Pathophysiology of Acute Hemolytic Reactions

The first event in an immune-mediated AHTR is the interaction of red cell antibodies with respective red cell antigens. This antigen-antibody complex formation initiates the clinical sequence of events associated with hemolysis. Characteristics of both the red cell alloantibody and the corresponding antigen are major determinants for the course and severity of a hemolytic transfusion reaction. Preformed antibodies in the recipient interact with the transfused red cells to create the most severe hemolytic reactions.

The concentration or titer of the red cell alloantibody also influences the extent and severity of an AHTR. Higher concentrations of circulating antibody in a transfusion recipient are more likely to produce severe clinical manifestations. The density (number of antigens per red cell) and distribution of the targeted red cell antigens also influence the severity of an AHTR. Scattered surface antigens bind fewer antibody molecules per red cell and are less likely to initiate severe hemolytic episodes. In contrast, antigens that are clustered together on the red cell surface increase the chances for the activation of the classical pathway of complement.

ABO antibodies of the IgM class readily activate the classical pathway of complement, leading to the potential for intravascular hemolysis (destruction of the transfused red cells within the vascular component). Intravascular hemolysis releases free hemoglobin and **red cell stroma** into the plasma. ABO antibodies of the IgG class less commonly activate the complement pathway but can interact with Fc receptors of mononuclear phagocytes, effecting phagocytosis and cellular activation. In an AHTR, complement functions in three capacities: opsonization, anaphylatoxin generation, and red cell lysis.

- *Opsonization* occurs because the membrane-bound complement products are cleared by mononuclear phagocytic cells.
- *Anaphylatoxins,* potent inducers of inflammation, are liberated into the plasma. These products act on mast cells, smooth muscle, and neutrophils. C5a acts on smooth muscle to effect contraction with an overall net effect of vascular dilation and bronchospasm. C3a and C5a also cause vasoactive amine (**serotonin** and **histamine**) release by mast cells and basophils and effect degranulation of neutrophils. The net effect of the systemic release of serotonin and histamine is increased vascular permeability. **Bradykinin,** a potent vasodilator and one of the plasma **kinins**, is generated to increase vasodilation and hypotension. In addition, antigen-antibody complex deposition and thrombus formation contribute to the vascular compromise observed in the kidneys.[4]
- *Red cell lysis* is the final outcome in complement activation following the assembly of the membrane attack complex. Liberated hemoglobin is bound by plasma haptoglobin. When the hemoglobin-binding capacity of plasma **haptoglobin** is exceeded, hemoglobinemia and hemoglobinuria are detectable.

Antigen-antibody-complement complexes may initiate the coagulation and fibrinolytic systems. DIC is often associated with an AHTR. The cardinal signs of DIC include the consumption of clotting factors (particularly fibrinogen, factor V, and factor VIII) and platelets with resulting diffuse, uncontrolled microvascular bleeding. The microvascular thrombi promote tissue **ischemia** and release of tissue factor, encouraging the activation of more thrombin. Hemostatic profiles of patients in DIC demonstrate low platelet counts and decreased fibrinogen levels with the presence of fibrin degradation products.

With the release of anaphylatoxins, vasoactive amines, kinins, and cytokines into the circulation as consequences of intravascular red cell destruction, the patient may present with shock. Shock is an abnormal condition of inadequate blood flow to the body's peripheral tissues, with life-threatening cellular dysfunction.

Renal failure caused by a severe AHTR is a multifactorial event and is most prominent in an untreated AHTR.[4] Contributing factors to renal failure include systemic hypotension, reactive renal vasoconstriction, and deposition of intravascular thrombi whose cumulative effects compromise the renal cortical blood supply. The release of norepinephrine in a physiologic reaction to the hypotension and shock produces vasoconstriction observed in the kidneys and lungs. The developing renal ischemia may be transient or advance to acute tubular necrosis and renal loss. Fig. 10-2 illustrates the clinical consequences of an AHTR.

Prevention of Acute Hemolytic Transfusion Reactions

Clerical and misidentification errors that lead to the transfusion of ABO incompatible red blood cell (RBC) units continue to be the most common cause of AHTRs.[4] Misidentification of the patient, incorrect sample collection, and incorrect or missed entry of test results occur because of failure to follow standard operating procedures when collecting, testing, and transfusing units of blood. Results of an analysis of contributing factors to

Red cell stroma: red cell membrane that remains after hemolysis.

Serotonin: potent vasoconstrictor liberated by platelets.

Histamine: compound that causes constriction of bronchial smooth muscle, dilation of capillaries, and decrease in blood pressure.

Bradykinin: potent vasodilator of the kinin family.

Kinins: group of proteins associated with contraction of smooth muscle, vascular permeability, and vasodilation.

Haptoglobin: plasma protein that binds free hemoglobin and carries the molecule to the hepatocytes for further catabolism.

Ischemia: decreased supply of oxygenated blood to an organ or body part.

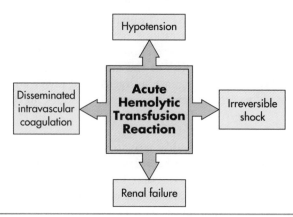

Fig. 10-2 Clinical consequences of an acute hemolytic transfusion reaction.

TABLE 10-2 Errors Contributing to Acute Hemolytic Transfusion Reactions	
ERRORS KNOWN TO CAUSE AHTR	**CONTRIBUTING FACTORS CAUSING ERRORS**
• Collection of blood from the incorrect patient • Incorrect labeling of blood samples • Misidentification of sample at blood bank • Issuance of wrong unit from blood bank • Transfusion of blood to incorrect patient • Alloquoting a patient sample to improperly labeled test tube	• Insufficient segregation of units • Preprinted sample labels • Patients with similar or identical names • Sequential patient identifiers • Verbal and STAT orders • Manual issuance of blood • Simultaneous processing of specimens from multiple patients • Tested the correct sample but recorded results on the wrong patient record • Overriding computer error messages

Data from Sazama K: Reports of 355 transfusion-associated deaths: 1976 through 1985, *Transfusion* 30:583-590, 1990.
AHTR, Acute hemolytic transfusion reaction.

AHTRs are shown in Table 10-2. Awareness of potential errors is important in preventing the serious consequences of AHTRs.

Delayed Hemolytic Reaction

As outlined in the previous section, an AHTR in a transfusion recipient may produce serious clinical consequences. These reactions are usually associated with the transfusion of ABO incompatible red cells. In contrast, delayed hemolytic transfusion reactions (DHTRs), with symptoms appearing after 24 hours, are usually less severe and require no treatment.[5]

The cause of a DHTR is an IgG antibody that the patient made from red cell exposure from prior transfusion or pregnancy. Normally, pretransfusion testing detects clinically significant antibodies. However, the antibody may have been below detectable levels when pretransfusion testing was performed. In some cases, the antibody may have been missed in error or not detected because of the sensitivity of the test method. In rare cases, an antibody to a low-frequency antigen may not have been detected because the antigen may not have been demonstrating on the screening cells.

The first detectable sign of a delayed hemolytic reaction may be an inadequate increase of posttransfusion hemoglobin levels, a rapid decrease back to pretransfusion levels, or an unexplained appearance of spherocytes. Newly identified red cell alloantibodies demonstrating between 24 hours and 28 days after transfusion provide definitive criteria for an immune-mediated DHTR.[1] Blood group antibodies associated with delayed hemolytic reactions include, in order of decreasing frequency, antibodies in the Kidd, Duffy, Kell, and MNS systems.[6]

Pathophysiology of Delayed Hemolytic Reaction

Red cells, sensitized with either immunoglobulin or complement, are removed from the circulation by the mononuclear phagocyte system. The macrophages, located in the spleen, are probably most active in this mechanism, although Kupffer cells of the liver also participate.

These mononuclear phagocytes also generate cytokines that mediate the systemic effects often associated with AHTRs. Cytokines are protein hormones involved in cell-to-cell communication. The combined effects of these cytokines include fever, hypotension, activation of T cells and B cells, and activation of endothelial cells to express procoagulant activity. A delayed hemolytic reaction may be asymptomatic or similar but milder than an AHTR.[1] AHTRs and DHTRs are compared in Table 10-3.

Non–Immune-Mediated Mechanisms of Red Cell Destruction

For a transfusion reaction in a patient experiencing hemoglobinemia and hemoglobinuria, the initial focus is to investigate the possibility of an immune-related response. When alloantibodies are not implicated, an investigation into the nonimmunologic mechanisms of red cell destruction should be initiated. This process necessitates examination of the segments or remaining blood from the unit in question with careful questioning of personnel regarding the transfusion process itself. If a hemolyzed donor unit is accidentally transfused, the recipient receives free hemoglobin and red cell stroma. The red cell stroma may stimulate complement activation and a procoagulant state.

TABLE 10-3   Acute versus Delayed Hemolytic Transfusion Reactions

	ACUTE	DELAYED
Clinical signs and symptoms	Fever, chills, flushing, pain at site of infusion, tachycardia, tachypnea, lower back pain, hemoglobinemia, hemoglobinuria, hypotension; dramatic and severe; rapid onset	>24 hours posttransfusion; fever—temperature increase ≥1° C (or 2° F) with or without chills; unexplainable decrease in hemoglobin and hematocrit; occasional mild jaundice
Major complications	DIC, renal failure, irreversible shock, death	No major complications; less severe reaction
Causes	Complement activation; ABO incompatibility	Anamnestic response to red cell antigen; alloantibody not demonstrating or missed
Clinical laboratory tests	Clerical check; visual inspection of posttransfusion sample; DAT—positive or negative; repeat ABO testing; tests for hemolysis; ↑ plasma free hemoglobin; ↑ serum bilirubin; ↓ haptoglobin; hemoglobinuria	DAT—positive; posttransfusion antibody screen—positive; ↓ hemoglobin/hematocrit; tests for hemolysis
Management	Treat hypotension and DIC; maintain renal blood flow	Provide antigen-negative donor units; no additional treatment necessary
Prevention	Avoid errors of mislabeled samples and patient identification; design systems to decrease chances of technical error	Check patient records

DIC, Disseminated intravascular coagulation; *DAT,* direct antiglobulin test; ↑, increased levels; ↓, decreased levels.

Fig. 10-3   0.9% saline. No medications or solutions other than 0.9% sodium chloride injection (USP) should be administered with blood components through the same tubing.

Examples of the causes from non–immune-mediated red cell hemolysis include the following:

• Exposure of red cells to extreme temperatures (>50° C or <0° C)

Exposure to extreme temperatures may produce hemolysis of red cells. The use of malfunctioning or unregulated blood warming devices or warming during refrigerated storage may lead to hemolyzed units. RBC units stored frozen without additive cryoprotectants induce the hemolysis of the units.

• Improper deglycerolization of an RBC unit on thawing

A simple test to prevent this complication of transfusion is to observe the supernatant of a red cell suspension for evidence of hemolysis after the deglycerolization has been completed.

• Mechanical destruction of red cells

Small-bore needles, mechanical valves, excessive pressure, and blood salvage equipment have been linked with nonimmune hemolysis of red cells.

• Incompatible solutions

The only solution that may be added to a donor unit is physiologic saline (Fig. 10-3). Blood mixed with nonphysiologic solutions such as half-strength saline, 5% dextrose in 0.18% saline, Ringer's lactate, and medications may cause osmotic rupture of the red cells. Exceptions to normal saline can be made if they have been approved by the FDA or documentation is available to show that the addition is safe and does not adversely affect the blood and blood component.[4]

• Transfusion of bacterially contaminated blood products
• Intrinsic red cell defect attributable to a clinical condition

Certain clinical disease states may be responsible for hemolysis unrelated to the transfusion, including sickle cell disease, thermal burns, glucose-6-phosphate dehydrogenase deficiency, and paroxysmal nocturnal hemoglobinuria.

> Thermal damage, mechanical damage, osmotic destruction, and bacterial contamination are nonimmune mechanisms that can generate a hemolytic episode in a transfusion recipient.

DELAYED SEROLOGIC TRANSFUSION REACTIONS

In addition to immune-mediated acute or delayed hemolytic transfusion reaction, a delayed serologic reaction should be considered if an antibody develops between 24 hours and 28 days after transfusion, even though there is an adequate, maintained hemoglobin response.[1] A newly identified antibody or a positive direct antiglobulin test (DAT) would confirm the diagnosis of this type of reaction. Blood group antibodies associated with delayed serologic reactions may go unrecognized because most patients do not undergo red cell antibody screening after transfusion unless additional units are requested.[7]

FEBRILE NONHEMOLYTIC TRANSFUSION REACTIONS

The febrile nonhemolytic transfusion reaction is a commonly observed adverse effect of transfusion. Because the presenting clinical features are similar to an AHTR, a careful investigation is necessary to rule out hemolysis. A febrile nonhemolytic reaction is typically manifested by a temperature elevation of more than 1° C (or 2° F) occurring during or shortly after transfusion. The most common cause is transfused cytokines or the action of cytokines generated by the recipient in response to transfused leukocytes.[1] Prestorage leukocyte reduction of platelets and RBC units decreases the frequency of febrile reactions (Fig. 10-4).[8] It also has been suggested that premedication with acetaminophen may be beneficial in avoiding febrile nonhemolytic reactions.[9] A summary of febrile nonhemolytic transfusion reactions appears in Table 10-4.

Fig. 10-4 Leukocyte removal filter. Removing leukocytes before storage reduces the cytokines and leukocytes in blood components, which can cause febrile transfusion reactions.

TABLE 10-4	Febrile Nonhemolytic Transfusion Reactions
Clinical signs and symptoms	Fever—temperature increase ≥1° C (or 2° F); chills; nausea; vomiting; headache; and back pain
Major complications	Usually not life-threatening for recipient
Causes	Recipient HLA antibodies to HLA antigens on donor lymphocytes Cytokines released by WBCs during blood product storage
Clinical laboratory tests	DAT—negative No visible hemolysis
Management	Antipyretics—acetaminophen
Prevention	Prestorage leukocyte reduction of blood products

HLA, Human leukocyte antigen; *WBC,* white blood cell; *DAT,* direct antiglobulin test.

ALLERGIC AND ANAPHYLACTIC TRANSFUSION REACTIONS

Allergic reactions to transfusion range in clinical severity from minor urticarial effects to fulminant anaphylactic shock and death. The cause of these reactions derives from soluble allergens present in donor plasma. These reactions are more commonly associated with the transfusion of blood products containing a plasma component, and symptoms usually occur within seconds or minutes of the start of the transfusion.[1] In the classic type I hypersensitivity response, preformed IgE antibodies in the recipient react with the allergen (plasma protein), which activates mast cells. Mast cell activation results in degranulation and the release of histamine, proteases, and chemotactic factors.

More severe anaphylactic reactions sometimes have life-threatening outcomes. Mast cell degranulation has been triggered by non-IgE mechanisms. IgA antibody–deficient patients may demonstrate severe anaphylactic reactions if they have made an antibody to the IgA immunoglobulin and receive plasma components. It may be necessary for IgA antibody–deficient patients with antibodies to IgA to receive IgA-deficient plasma from the rare donor registry or washed red cell and platelet components to avoid reactions. Severe reactions may require treatment with methylprednisolone, prednisone, or epinephrine.[1]

Two or more of the following signs or symptoms, observed within 4 hours of transfusion, are definitive characteristics of an allergic reaction:

- Urticaria (hives)
- Pruritus (itching)
- Maculopapular rash
- Generalized flushing
- Localized angioedema
- Edema of the lips, tongue, and uvula
- Erythema and edema of the periorbital area
- Conjunctival edema
- Respiratory distress; bronchospasm
- Hypotension

Treatment of allergic transfusion reactions with antihistamines is usually adequate, and transfusions can be resumed once symptoms have dissipated. This is the only type of transfusion reaction where the component may continue to be administered following prompt treatment.[10] In patients with prior allergic reactions to transfusions, premedication with antihistamines 30 minutes before transfusion may be beneficial. Table 10-5 summarizes and compares allergic transfusion reactions.

TRANSFUSION-RELATED ACUTE LUNG INJURY

Transfusion-related acute lung injury (TRALI) can be a life-threatening or fatal transfusion reaction; this reaction has many overlapping symptoms with transfusion-related sepsis, circulatory overload, and anaphylactic reactions. Respiratory distress and pulmonary edema occur within 1 to 2 hours after transfusion. Symptoms include severe hypoxemia, tachycardia, cyanosis, hypotension, and fever. Specific criteria for diagnosing acute hypoxia associated with acute lung injury following transfusion are defined by respiratory measurements along with a chest x-ray showing bilateral infiltrates.[1]

The exact mechanism of lung injury in TRALI has not been determined.[3] The mechanism is associated with the infusion of antibodies to leukocyte antigens, which activates neutrophils in the pulmonary microvasculature. The activated neutrophils cause pulmonary epithelial damage, capillary leakage, and pulmonary edema. Transfused donor antibodies to class I and class II human leukocyte antigen (HLA) antigens and neutrophil antigens have been implicated as the most probable cause of TRALI. Because multiparous women are more likely to have antibodies associated with TRALI, an effort to reduce the risk by using male donors for plasma products has decreased the fatalities reported to the FDA.[11] Table 10-6 provides a summary of TRALI.

TABLE 10-5	Allergic Transfusion Reactions	
	URTICARIAL	**ANAPHYLACTIC**
Clinical signs and symptoms	Hives, erythema, itching within 15-20 minutes of transfusion	Rapid onset and severe, after small volume is transfused; wheezing, coughing, dyspnea, bronchospasm, respiratory distress, vascular instability; no fever
Major complications	None	Shock, loss of consciousness; death
Causes	Recipient antibodies to foreign plasma proteins or other substances such as drugs or food consumed by blood donor	Associated with genetic IgA deficiency in recipient; possesses IgG, complement-binding anti-IgA antibodies
Clinical laboratory tests	DAT—negative No visible hemolysis	DAT—negative No visible hemolysis
Management	Transfusion interrupted and antihistamine administered	Transfusion terminated; epinephrine administered Oxygen administered and open airways maintained
Prevention	Premedication with antihistamine if patient history reveals repetitive allergic reactions May necessitate washed cellular products	Plasma-containing products from IgA-deficient donors Washed red cell and platelet products

DAT, Direct antiglobulin test.

TABLE 10-6	Transfusion-Related Acute Lung Injury
Clinical signs and symptoms	Marked respiratory distress; fever, hypotension, chills, cyanosis; rapid onset—occurs during transfusion or within 6 hours of completion
Major complications	Severe and dramatic presentation, can be fatal
Causes	Interaction of granulocytes and HLA-specific donor antibodies, complement activation, aggregation of granulocytes that leads to blockage of pulmonary microvasculature; capillary damage, vascular leakage, pulmonary edema
Clinical laboratory tests	DAT—negative; no visible hemolysis; WBC antibody screen in donor and recipient
Management	Respiratory support
Prevention	Defer implicated donor for plasma containing components Avoid use of plasma components from multiparous women

HLA, Human leukocyte antigen; *DAT,* direct antiglobulin test; *WBC,* white blood cell.

TRANSFUSION-ASSOCIATED GRAFT-VERSUS-HOST DISEASE

Transfusion-associated graft-versus-host disease (TA-GVHD) is a rare but highly lethal complication of transfusion; it is associated with a 90% mortality rate.[4] This immune reaction is mediated by immunocompetent donor lymphocytes in cellular blood components. Symptoms can occur 3 days to 6 weeks after transfusion and include maculopapular rash, fever, diarrhea, and elevated liver function tests.[1] Following the transfusion of donor lymphocytes to a recipient who is immunologically incompetent, or closely HLA

TABLE 10-7 Indications for Irradiated Components

INDICATED	NOT INDICATED
Intrauterine transfusions	Patients with HIV
Premature, low-birth-weight infants	Full-term infants
Congenital immunodeficiencies	Nonimmunosuppressed patients
Hematologic malignancies	
HLA-matched components	
Directed donations from related donors	
Granulocyte components	
Newborns with erythroblastosis fetalis	

Data from Hemovigilance module: adverse reaction case definition exercises, July 2009. http://www.cdc.gov/nhsn/wc_BioVig_AdverseReaction.html.
HIV, Human immunodeficiency virus.

TABLE 10-8 Transfusion-Associated Graft-versus-Host Disease

Clinical signs and symptoms	Onset 3-30 days posttransfusion; fever, erythematous maculopapular rash, abnormal liver function; nausea, vomiting, jaundice, abdominal pain, diarrhea
Major complications	Sepsis and hemorrhage; 90% mortality rate
Cause	Transfused immunocompetent T lymphocytes mount immunologic response against recipient
Clinical laboratory tests	Confirmation by HLA typing to demonstrate a disparity between donor lymphocytes and recipient tissues
Management	Unresponsive to medical intervention
Prevention	Irradiation of blood products before transfusion in at-risk recipients; gamma irradiation (25 Gy) to prevent blast transformation of donor lymphocytes[10]

HLA, Human leukocyte antigen.

similar, the donor lymphocytes engraft and mount an immune response against the host tissues. Because the host is unable to destroy the transfused cells, the donor lymphocytes proliferate and respond to unshared histocompatibility antigens in the host. TA-GVHD is only rarely successfully treated; therefore, identifying patients at risk and providing irradiated blood products is essential. Table 10-7 lists indications for irradiated components.

Immunocompromised patients and recipients who are receiving blood products from donors that share similar HLA phenotypes are at high risk of developing TA-GVHD and should receive blood products that have been irradiated at specific doses required by AABB standards.[10] Irradiation eliminates the ability of leukocytes to replicate and mount an immune response. Leukocyte reduction of the blood component is *not* sufficient to avoid TA-GVHD. Table 10-8 summarizes the important concepts regarding TA-GVHD.

BACTERIAL CONTAMINATION OF BLOOD PRODUCTS

A serious and potentially fatal adverse complication of transfusion is secondary to bacterial proliferation in donor units during storage. The major sources of the bacterial contamination include a transient bacteremia in an asymptomatic donor or improper cleansing of the donor's skin during blood collection. Bacterial endotoxins, generated during the storage period, result in a dramatic clinical picture on transfusion of the contaminated blood product. Transfusion recipients may experience shock rapidly. Fatalities attributed to transfusion of contaminated blood are more common following platelet transfusions.[2]

The introduction of plastic collection bags and closed systems has considerably decreased the probability of bacterial contamination. Care during the donor phlebotomy process is necessary to prevent entry of bacteria from the donor's skin into the collection system. To reduce this type of contamination, the AABB has required since 2008 that diversion pouches be used for all platelet collections (described in Chapter 12).[9] Any contaminating bacteria in the donor unit that are unable to survive at 4° C die after several days of storage. However, organisms capable of growth at 4° C find an ideal environment for their perpetuation. Gram-negative bacteria such as *Yersinia enterocolitica, Serratia liquefaciens,* and *Pseudomonas fluorescens* can thrive under these conditions and promote transfusion reactions. Gram-positive organisms are more often observed in platelets stored at 20° C to 24° C and include bacteria such as *Staphylococcus* species and *Bacillus cereus.*[4] The AABB requirement for bacteria detection testing in apheresis platelets before transfusion has also reduced the incidence of sepsis transmitted by transfusion.[10]

The clinical symptoms of bacterial contamination mimic acute hemolytic transfusion reactions. The number of infused organisms influences the symptomatic presentation and the clinical outcome. Treatment of the reaction must be initiated before confirmation of the cause to prevent a fatal outcome. Broad-spectrum antibiotic therapy is provided to the recipient.[1] Blood cultures from the patient and the blood bag are obtained. Transfusion service personnel perform visual checks of all donor units at the time of issue. The individual inspecting the donor unit should be alert for any visible discoloration, clots, cloudiness, or hemolysis.

TRANSFUSION-ASSOCIATED CIRCULATORY OVERLOAD

Transfusion-associated circulatory overload (TACO), as a category of adverse complications of transfusion, occurs when a patient's cardiopulmonary system exceeds its volume capacity. Patients older than 70 years old and infants are at greatest risk.[4] This complication of transfusion is considered if dyspnea, severe headache, peripheral edema, or other signs of congestive heart failure occur during or shortly after transfusion. Patients with compromised cardiac and pulmonary status poorly tolerate rapid elevations in total blood volume and are more susceptible to TACO. Because this type of reaction can lead to fatality, prompt aggressive treatment with oxygen therapy and diuretic medications is imperative to prevent further complications.

Transfusion candidates susceptible to TACO should receive RBC units, not whole blood. The units should be administered at a slow rate in small-volume aliquots. The transfusion period should proceed over 4 to 6 hours. Infusions of large volumes of plasma should be avoided.

TRANSFUSION HEMOSIDEROSIS

Hemosiderosis is a condition that results from the accumulation of excess iron in macrophages in various tissues. Iron overload is a potential complication in patients undergoing long-term transfusions, such as patients with **thalassemia** and sickle cell disease with persistent hemolysis. In transfusion hemosiderosis, iron intake (250 mg/unit) exceeds the daily iron excretion (1 mg/day) with the subsequent deposition of excess iron in the liver, heart, and kidney. When patients have received more than 100 transfusions, iron deposition may interfere with the function of the liver, heart, or endocrine glands. Prevention of iron toxicity through the use of iron chelators such as deferiprone or deferoxamine allows the body to bind and excrete excess iron through the urine and feces.[4]

Thalassemia: inherited disorder causing anemia because of a defective production rate of either α or β hemoglobin polypeptide.

CITRATE TOXICITY

The transfusion of large quantities of citrated blood in a relatively short time frame introduces the risk of citrate toxicity for the transfusion recipient. Citrate, which is present in the formulation of the anticoagulants used in the blood collection process, binds ionized calcium. Excess citrate may be toxic to patients receiving large volumes in massive transfusion situations or in patients with impaired liver function for the metabolism of the citrate. Citrate toxicity is a possible adverse event in the transfusion of preterm infants with severe hepatic or renal insufficiency. Removing the additive-containing plasma may be beneficial in these patients. Injections of calcium chloride or calcium gluconate negate the toxic effects.[4]

POSTTRANSFUSION PURPURA

In posttransfusion purpura (PTP), the patient's platelet count plummets 5 to 12 days after the transfusion of blood or blood products containing platelets. Generalized purpura and an increased probability of bleeding episodes follow. This complication is an anamnestic response to a previous sensitization with the high-incidence platelet antigen, HPA-1a, which has a 98% frequency in the population. Antigen-negative individuals are at risk of developing PTP. HPA-1a-negative women are sensitized through multiple pregnancies and respond with the immune production of anti-HPA-1a. This platelet-specific alloantibody destroys not only the transfused HPA-1a platelets but also the patient's HPA-1a negative platelets. The mechanism for the concomitant destruction of the autologous platelets with transfused platelets has not been determined. Treatment of PTP includes plasmapheresis, exchange transfusion, and use of intravenous immunoglobulin (IVIG).[4]

SECTION 3
EVALUATION AND REPORTING A TRANSFUSION REACTION

INITIATING A TRANSFUSION REACTION INVESTIGATION

Protocols for the initiation of a transfusion necessitate that the transfusionist carefully check all the identifying information and document informed patient consent before the infusion of the blood product. This information is documented in the transfusion record with the date and time of the start of the transfusion.[9] In addition to verifying identification, the transfusionist records the patient's pretransfusion vital signs, including temperature, blood pressure, pulse, and respiration rate. The transfusionist should remain with the patient for the first few minutes of the infusion to detect any indications of acute hemolysis, anaphylaxis, or bacterial contamination. After the first 15-minute period, the patient should be observed, and the vital signs should be recorded. Clinical personnel should continue to observe the patient periodically throughout the transfusion and up to 1 hour after completion.[4]

If an adverse reaction is suspected, the following procedure is performed:
- The transfusion should be stopped; reidentification of the patient and the transfused component is initiated.
- The transfusion service and the patient's physician are notified immediately of the suspected reaction.
- An intravenous line is maintained (for administration with blood) with normal saline or a solution approved by the FDA.
- The physician evaluates the patient to determine any clinical intervention and potential medical management.
- If signs and symptoms of possible AHTR, anaphylaxis, TRALI, transfusion-induced sepsis, or other serious complications are seen, a postreaction blood sample is sent to the transfusion service for evaluation. This specimen must be properly labeled and forwarded to the transfusion service with the blood bag, the administration set, the attached intravenous solutions, and all related forms and labels. In some cases, the first voided postreaction urine is collected for possible evaluation.
- If the presenting clinical signs and symptoms are indicative of urticarial or circulatory overload, the transfusion service does not need to evaluate any postreaction blood and urine samples.[4]

An outline of transfusion reaction instructions to medical personnel is provided in Fig. 10-5.

Fig. 10-5 Instructions to medical staff when a transfusion reaction is suspected.

Fig. 10-6 Postreaction work-up. Initial investigation to determine if a hemolytic transfusion reaction is occurring.

Any suspected transfusion reaction becomes a high priority in the transfusion service. On receipt of the postreaction clinical materials, the transfusion service personnel perform the following four steps (Fig. 10-6):

1. *Clerical check* for any errors in identification

   The patient sample and blood component are checked for any errors relating to identification. If such an error is discovered, notification is provided to the medical personnel handling the transfusion reaction. All records are double-checked to determine whether another potential transfusion recipient is at risk because of this error. The source of the error is evaluated in light of the overall transfusion process to determine where the system failed.

2. *Visual check* for hemolysis or icterus

   Because red cells immediately release free hemoglobin into the plasma during intravascular hemolysis, the postreaction sample is evaluated for any evidence of hemolysis or **icterus** and is compared with the pretransfusion sample, if available in the laboratory. Any pinkish or reddish discoloration suggests the presence of free hemoglobin. If a transfusion has occurred over a 3- to 4-hour period, icterus may be noted as the degradation of free hemoglobin to bilirubin progresses. Bilirubin levels usually peak at 5 to 7 hours after a hemolytic event.

   Icterus: pertaining to or resembling jaundice.

3. *DAT*

   To check for a serologic incompatibility, a DAT is performed on a postreaction (preferably anticoagulated) sample. A microscopic DAT is recommended because the ratio of donor to recipient cells is small. If the postreaction sample is positive, a recipient alloantibody may have sensitized the transfused red cells. A positive DAT from a transfusion reaction appears as mixed field with the transfused red cells demonstrating agglutination and the autologous red cells remaining unagglutinated. If the transfused red cells have experienced a rapid clearance, the DAT may be negative at the time of sample collection. Comparison of the postreaction sample with the DAT performed on the pretransfusion sample is helpful in evaluating the transfusion reaction.

4. *Other serologic tests performed as needed*

TABLE 10-9	Additional Testing in a Transfusion Reaction Investigation
TEST	**REASON**
ABO/D phenotyping	Errors in patient or sample identification
Antibody screen	Newly detected antibodies
Crossmatch	Serologic compatibility
Hemoglobin/hematocrit	Therapeutic effectiveness
Haptoglobin	Hemolytic process
Bilirubin	Hemolytic process
Urine hemoglobin	Hemolytic process
Inspection of donor unit	Nonimmune hemolysis or bacterial contamination
Gram stain and blood culture	Bacterial contamination

Additional Laboratory Testing in a Transfusion Reaction

Depending on the results of the aforementioned testing, further laboratory testing may be performed (Table 10-9). The extent of the additional testing is in part at the discretion of the physician in charge of the transfusion service and preestablished policies for the investigation of a transfusion reaction.[10] According to AABB *Standards,* "there must be a process for evaluation for suspected non-hemolytic transfusion reactions including, but not limited to febrile reactions, possible bacterial contamination and TRALI."[10] A review and interpretation by the medical director is also required. Additional laboratory testing that may follow the initial investigation includes any combination of the following analyses:

* ABO typing of pretransfusion and posttransfusion patient samples along with a reconfirmation of the ABO of the donor unit
  Any discrepancies of typing confirm an error in sample or patient identification; if an error in the patient's sample has occurred, an investigation of another potential clerical error affecting another patient should be initiated.
* Parallel testing of pretransfusion and posttransfusion patient samples for antibody detection
  The use of additional enhancement techniques in the antibody screen may be helpful in the detection of a weakly reactive antibody. Polyethylene glycol or enzyme techniques may provide additional information in the work-up. If a new antibody is detected, antibody identification procedures are performed. A previously undetected antibody, now evident in the posttransfusion sample, is indicative of a possible anamnestic immune response following the recent transfusion exposure. The donor unit transfused to the recipient is checked for the presence of the antigen.
* Repetition of crossmatch using pretransfusion and posttransfusion patient samples
  The recommended crossmatch procedure includes both the immediate-spin and the antiglobulin crossmatch phases.
* Frequent checks of hematologic status
  Hemoglobin and hematocrit values are evaluated after transfusion for expected therapeutic elevations of 1 g/dL hemoglobin and 3% hematocrit for each RBC unit transfused.[4]
* Analysis of haptoglobin levels on both the pretransfusion and the posttransfusion patient samples
  Haptoglobin is a plasma protein with the sole function of binding free hemoglobin and carrying the molecule to hepatocytes for further catabolism. During a hemolytic process, haptoglobin levels decrease in plasma because haptoglobin-hemoglobin complexes are formed. Free hemoglobin, released during intravascular red cell destruction, is excreted into the urine after exceeding the plasma haptoglobin-binding capacity.

TABLE 10-10	Case Definition Criteria for Hemovigilance Reporting
CRITERIA	**DEFINITIONS**
Signs and symptoms	*Definitive:* Conclusive *Probable:* Evidence in favor *Possible:* Evidence indeterminate
Laboratory/radiology	*Definitive:* Conclusive *Probable:* Evidence in favor *Possible:* Evidence indeterminate
Severity (graded)	*Grade 1:* Nonsevere *Grade 2:* Severe—requires medical intervention or prolongation of hospitalization or both *Grade 3:* Life-threatening; major intervention needed to prevent death *Grade 4:* Death as a result of adverse transfusion reaction
Relationship to transfusion (imputability)	*Definitive:* Conclusive *Probable:* Evidence in favor *Possible:* Evidence indeterminate

Data from NHSN manual: biovigilance component protocol hemovigilance module, June 2011. *Guidelines and procedures for monitoring hemovigilance.* http://www.cdc.gov/nhsn/bio.html.

- Examination of returned donor unit and administration tubing for abnormal appearance or hemolysis
  If bacterial sepsis is suspected, Gram stain and culture of the donor unit may be performed.
- Other postreaction testing
  Other postreaction testing may include bilirubin, IgA levels, and HLA and granulocyte antibody detection.

RECORDS AND REPORTING OF TRANSFUSION REACTIONS AND FATALITIES

Hemovigilance Component

Facilities that elect to participate in the hemovigilance component of the NHSN are required to use case definition criteria in reporting reactions.[3] The reactions are also assessed as definitive, probable, or possible on whether they meet the defined criteria. The severity of the reactions is graded on a scale of 1 to 4 where 1 is least severe and 4 is death. The relationship of the reaction to the transfusion is also assessed as definitive, probable, or possible. These reporting guidelines allow for consistency and thus more accurate evaluation and assessment of data collected by the participating facilities. Case definition criteria are outlined in Table 10-10.

Records

Records of patients who experience an adverse reaction to a transfusion remain indefinitely in the transfusion service.[10] Cases of transfusion-transmitted disease and bacterial contamination must also be reported to the blood collection facility. These records serve as a determining factor in the prevention of future reactions. For example, a patient with a history of a previous clinically relevant alloantibody, currently not demonstrable in the antibody screen test, would require a transfusion with antigen-negative donor units.

FDA Reportable Fatalities

Fatalities attributable to transfusion must be reported as soon as possible by telephone, express mail, or electronic means to the director of the FDA Office of Compliance, Center for Biologics Evaluation and Research,[11] followed by a written report within 7 days. The formal report includes medical and laboratory documentation and an autopsy report.

CHAPTER SUMMARY

The major immune-mediated and non–immune-mediated adverse complications of transfusion are summarized in the following table:

Adverse Complications of Transfusion			
	Cause	Signs and Symptoms	Clinical Tests
Immune-mediated			
Hemolytic	Acute: ABO incompatibility	Fever, chills, pain, hypotension	Positive DAT, eluate, serum antibody, elevated plasma hemoglobin or bilirubin
	Delayed: Primary or secondary alloimmunization	Unexplained decrease in hemoglobin	
Febrile nonhemolytic	Recipient leukocyte antibodies, transfused cytokines	Fever, chills, rigors	Rule out hemolysis, test for HLA antibodies
Urticarial	Plasma allergen	Rash, hives, flushing	None, responds to symptomatic treatment
Anaphylactic	Anti-IgA in IgA-deficient recipient	Respiratory distress, hypotension	IgA antibody
TRALI	Donor WBC antibodies	Hypoxemia	Bilateral infiltrates in chest x-ray
Posttransfusion purpura	Anti-HPA-1a or other platelet antibody	Thrombocytopenia (↓ 20% of pretransfusion)	Anti-HPA-1a antibody
TA-GVHD	Immunocompetent donor lymphocytes to susceptible host	Fever, rash, diarrhea	Abnormal liver dysfunction test, WBC chimerism
Non–immune-mediated			
Hemolytic	Mechanical or chemical trauma to unit	Fever, chills, pain, hypotension	Check blood administration—needles, fluid, blood warmers
TACO	Volume overload secondary to rapid, high volume	Respiratory distress, pulmonary edema, cardiac failure	Underlying cardiac or pulmonary pathology
Bacterial infection	Donor septicemia or contamination during phlebotomy	Fever, chills	Gram stain, culture of unit

CRITICAL THINKING EXERCISES

EXERCISE 10-1

An inexperienced nurse from an outpatient facility calls the transfusion service to report a transfusion reaction. The transfusion recipient is complaining of shortness of breath and chills. The nurse is seeking advice on the appropriate procedure.
1. What instructions should be provided to the nurse?
2. What documentation should be returned to the transfusion service?
3. What immediate procedures should be performed in the laboratory to initiate the transfusion reaction investigation?

EXERCISE 10-2

Seven days after the transfusion of 5 RBC units, a patient demonstrates a 5 g/dL decrease in hemoglobin and is mildly jaundiced. No evidence of bleeding is identified.
1. What tests would provide evidence for a delayed transfusion reaction?
2. What is the rationale for the test selection?

EXERCISE 10-3
A 55-year-old man was admitted to the emergency department after a motor vehicle accident. The patient is hemorrhaging from a lacerated spleen and requires emergency surgery. Pretransfusion testing determined that the patient's phenotype is group A, D-negative with a negative antibody screen. Crossmatches with RBC units were compatible by the immediate-spin crossmatch. During surgery, the patient receives 6 units of group A, D-negative RBCs and 4 units of group A frozen plasma. Three days later, during the first 15 minutes of a subsequent RBC transfusion using a blood-warming device, the patient developed fever and chills.
1. Based on the information provided, propose three possible explanations of the cause of the transfusion reaction.
2. Determine a strategy for the evaluation of the transfusion reaction to rule in or rule out any possible mechanism.

EXERCISE 10-4
Refer to the table in the Chapter Summary.
1. Outline possible preventive measures for each of the reactions listed.
2. Describe the category of patients most likely to experience each reaction.

STUDY QUESTIONS

1. A patient experiences chills and fever, nausea, flushing, and lower back pain after infusion of 150 mL of blood. To rule out an acute hemolytic transfusion reaction, one should immediately:
   a. perform a DAT and visually compare pretransfusion and posttransfusion serum samples
   b. measure serum haptoglobin on prereaction and postreaction samples
   c. repeat crossmatches on prereaction and postreaction samples
   d. perform Gram stain and culture of the unit

2. Dyspnea, severe headache, and peripheral edema occurring soon after transfusion are indicative of which type of transfusion reaction?
   a. hemolytic
   b. TRALI
   c. TACO
   d. anaphylactic

3. What is a common cause of a febrile nonhemolytic transfusion reaction?
   a. recipient is allergic to the donor's plasma proteins
   b. donor unit is cold
   c. donor unit has a positive DAT
   d. recipient has antibodies to the donor's HLA antigens

4. What plasma protein functions to bind hemoglobin following intravascular hemolysis?
   a. albumin
   b. haptoglobin
   c. transferrin
   d. C-reactive protein

5. Which of the following adverse complications of transfusion is prevented by the irradiation of blood components?
   a. TRALI
   b. hyperkalemia
   c. febrile
   d. TA-GVHD

6. Which of the following characteristics is associated with a delayed serologic transfusion reaction?
   a. hives and wheals
   b. hemosiderosis
   c. positive antibody screen in posttransfusion sample
   d. ABO incompatibility between donor unit and recipient

7. What blood group system antibodies are commonly associated with delayed hemolytic transfusion reactions?
   a. Rh
   b. ABO
   c. MNS
   d. Kidd

8. A patient has experienced two febrile nonhemolytic reactions after RBC transfusion. What is the preferred blood component if future transfusions are necessary?
   a. leukocyte-reduced RBCs
   b. irradiated RBCs
   c. cytomegalovirus-negative RBCs
   d. group O, D-negative RBCs

9. Which of the following patient histories might suggest future transfusions with saline-washed RBCs?
   a. history of multiple red cell alloantibodies
   b. history of congestive heart failure
   c. IgA-negative recipient with anti-IgA antibodies
   d. history of transfusion-associated sepsis

10. What is the cause of transfusion-induced hemosiderosis?
    a. excess citrate
    b. HPA-1a antigen
    c. iron overload
    d. circulatory overload

11. What laboratory test is useful to detect clerical errors of sample identification in an acute transfusion reaction investigation?
    a. ABO typing
    b. antibody screen
    c. crossmatch
    d. DAT

12. What microorganism grows well at 4° C and may result in a transfusion-transmitted sepsis?
    a. *Staphylococcus aureus*
    b. *Yersinia enterocolitica*
    c. *Staphylococcus epidermidis*
    d. *Bacillus cereus*

13. What is the expected therapeutic effect in the recipient's hematocrit after the transfusion of 1 unit of RBCs?
    a. increase of 0.5%
    b. increase of 1%
    c. increase of 2%
    d. increase of 3%

14. Anaphylactic reactions to transfusion are usually caused by:
    a. anti-IgA in an IgA-deficient recipient
    b. anti-IgG in an IgA-deficient recipient
    c. IgA deficiency
    d. IgG deficiency

15. A precipitous decrease in a recipient's platelet count after a transfusion is associated with:
    a. circulatory overload
    b. posttransfusion purpura
    c. citrate toxicity
    d. factor VIII deficiency

16. When evaluating a possible delayed hemolytic reaction, what is the best sample to use for bilirubin determination?
    a. 6 hours posttransfusion
    b. 12 hours posttransfusion
    c. 24 hours posttransfusion
    d. 48 hours posttransfusion

17. In a delayed serologic or hemolytic transfusion reaction, the DAT is typically:
    a. negative
    b. weak positive, mixed field
    c. positive with C3 only
    d. negative if serum antibody screen is negative

18. The use of plasma from only male donors for transfusion is a preventive method for which type of transfusion reaction:
    a. febrile
    b. TRALI
    c. allergic
    d. TACO

19. Premedication with diphenhydramine (Benadryl) is a common procedure when administrating platelets to patients undergoing frequent transfusions. Which type of transfusion reaction does this medication prevent?
    a. allergic
    b. TRALI
    c. febrile nonhemolytic reactions
    d. TACO

20. Posttransfusion purpura following transfusion of a platelet or RBC unit is usually caused by:
    a. HLA antibodies in the donor unit
    b. HLA antibodies made by the recipient
    c. anti-HPA-1a made by the recipient
    d. febrile reactions secondary to cytokines in the unit

21. Five days after a transfusion, a patient returned to his physician for postsurgical blood tests. It was noted that the hemoglobin value decreased from 11 mg/dL to 9 mg/dL during that time. The patient had not experienced any symptoms. To rule out a delayed hemolytic transfusion reaction, what test should be performed?
    a. DAT on current sample, elution if positive
    b. antibody screen on the current sample
    c. blood smear to check for spherocytes
    d. all of the above

22. According to AABB *Standards,* continuing a transfusion after treatment with medication is allowed when which type of reaction has occurred?
    a. febrile
    b. TACO
    c. TRALI
    d. allergic

REFERENCES

1. NHSN manual: biovigilance component protocol hemovigilance module, June 2011. *Guidelines and procedures for monitoring hemovigilance.* http://www.cdc.gov/nhsn/bio.html.
2. *Fatalities reported to FDA following blood collection and transfusion: annual summary for fiscal year 2010.* http://www.fda.gov/downloads/BiologicsBloodVaccines/SafetyAvailability/ReportaProblem/TransfusionDonationFatalities/UCM254860.pdf.
3. Hemovigilance module: adverse reaction case definition exercises, July 2009. http://www.cdc.gov/nhsn/wc_BioVig_AdverseReaction.html.
4. Roback JD, editor: *Technical manual,* ed 17, Bethesda, MD, 2011, AABB.
5. AABB/America's Blood Centers/American Red Cross: *Circular of information for the use of human blood and blood components,* May 2011.
6. Mollison PL, Engelfriet CP, Contreras M: *Blood transfusion in clinical medicine,* ed 9, Oxford, UK, 1993, Blackwell Scientific.
7. Schonewille H, van de Watering LMG, Brand A: Additional red cell alloantibodies after blood cell transfusion in a nonhematological alloimmunized patient cohort: is it time to take precautionary measures? *Transfusion* 46:630, 2006.
8. Pagliano JC, Pomper GJ, Fisch GS, et al: Reduction of febrile but not allergic reactions to RBCs and platelets after conversion to universal prestorage leukoreduction, *Transfusion* 44:16, 2004.
9. Ezidiegwu CN, Lauenstein KJ, Rosales LG, et al: Febrile non-hemolytic transfusion reactions: management by premedication and cost implications in adult patients, *Arch Pathol Lab Med* 128:991, 2004.
10. Carson TH: *Standards for blood banks and transfusion services,* ed 27, Bethesda, MD, 2011, AABB.
11. Food and Drug Administration: Code of federal regulations, 21 CFR 606.170, Washington, DC, 2011, US Government Printing Office (revised annually).

Hemolytic Disease of the Fetus and Newborn

CHAPTER OUTLINE

LEARNING OBJECTIVES

On completion of this chapter, the reader should be able to:

1. Discuss the etiology of hemolytic disease of the fetus and newborn (HDFN).
2. Contrast the metabolism of bilirubin in the fetus versus bilirubin in the newborn.
3. Correlate the tests included in an initial prenatal work-up with their significance in predicting HDFN.
4. Distinguish clinically significant and insignificant antibodies in terms of causing HDFN.
5. Explain the primary value of performing antibody titration, and state what results are considered significant.
6. Outline the intervention procedures used in the diagnosis and management of HDFN.
7. List the tests routinely performed on cord blood cells when HDFN is suspected, and discuss possible sources of error when performing each test.
8. Compare and contrast the clinical and laboratory findings in ABO HDFN versus HDFN caused by anti-D.

9. Discuss the composition, eligibility criteria, and principle of Rh immune globulin (RhIG).
10. Explain the principle, interpretation, and significance of a positive rosette test for fetomaternal hemorrhage.
11. Outline the principle, interpretation, and significance of the Kleihauer-Betke acid elution.
12. Evaluate laboratory test results on postpartum samples, and determine if RhIG should be administered.
13. Given the fetomaternal hemorrhage results, calculate the dose of RhIG.
14. Explain the selection of blood for an intrauterine transfusion exchange transfusion with regard to ABO and D phenotype.
15. List the special considerations that must be met when selecting blood for exchange transfusion, and explain the purpose of each requirement.

Hemolytic disease of the fetus and newborn (HDFN), also known as **erythroblastosis fetalis,** is a disorder of the fetus or newborn in which fetal red cells are destroyed by maternal IgG antibodies. These antibodies, directed against fetal antigens, cross the placenta, sensitize fetal red cells, and shorten red cell survival. This premature red cell destruction results in disease varying from mild anemia to death in utero. The transfusion service plays a critical role in the prediction, diagnosis, treatment, and prevention of this potentially life-threatening disease. The terms **prenatal, antenatal,** and **antepartum** refer to the time before delivery when testing is done to prevent or predict HDFN. **Neonatal** testing involves testing the newborn up to 28 days after delivery. The **perinatal** period extends from 28 weeks of gestation to 28 days after delivery.

SECTION 1

ETIOLOGY OF HEMOLYTIC DISEASE OF THE FETUS AND NEWBORN

During pregnancy, the placenta functions as the site of oxygen, nutrient, and waste exchange. In addition, the placenta serves as a barrier between maternal and fetal circulations. This barrier limits the number of fetal red cells entering the maternal circulation during pregnancy and reduces the chances of antibody production during pregnancy. ABO incompatibility between mother and child can also provide additional protection against immunization. Intravascular hemolysis of ABO-incompatible fetal red cells by maternal anti-A or anti-B reduces exposure to fetal cells carrying foreign antigens. At the time of delivery, when the placenta is separated from the uterus, a significant number of fetal red cells escape into the maternal circulation (known as **fetomaternal hemorrhage [FMH]**). In addition to delivery, immunization can result from fetal red cell exposure after amniocentesis, spontaneous or induced abortion, cordocentesis, ectopic pregnancy, or abdominal trauma. Fetal red cells carrying antigens that are different from the mother (paternal antigens) can stimulate an active immune response in the mother, which results in the production of IgG antibodies.

In a subsequent pregnancy, the IgG antibodies cross the placental barrier by an active transport mechanism. The antibodies bind to the fetal antigens, which ends in red cell destruction by macrophages in the fetal liver and spleen. Hemoglobin liberated from the damaged red cells is metabolized to indirect bilirubin. The indirect bilirubin is transported across the placenta, conjugated by the maternal liver, and harmlessly excreted by the mother (Fig. 11-1, *A*). As red cell destruction continues, the fetus becomes increasingly anemic. The fetal liver and spleen enlarge as erythropoiesis increases in an effort to compensate for the red cell destruction. Immature red cells (erythroblasts) are released into the fetal circulation (which explains the term erythroblastosis fetalis). If this condition is left untreated, cardiac failure can occur, accompanied by **hydrops fetalis**, or edema and fluid accumulation in fetal peritoneal and pleural cavities. The greatest threat to the fetus is cardiac failure resulting from uncompensated anemia.

After delivery, the infant faces a different challenge. Red cell destruction continues with the release of indirect bilirubin. In utero, indirect bilirubin is conjugated in the maternal liver and excreted. However, the newborn liver is deficient in glucuronyl transferase (the liver enzyme needed to conjugate indirect bilirubin). As indirect bilirubin is released, it binds to albumin and circulates harmlessly. When the binding capacity of the albumin is exceeded, indirect bilirubin binds to tissues, which results in jaundice. In particular, it may bind with tissues of the central nervous system (CNS) and cause permanent brain damage (kernicterus), resulting in deafness, mental retardation, or death (Fig. 11-1, *B*).

SECTION 2

OVERVIEW OF HEMOLYTIC DISEASE OF THE FETUS AND NEWBORN

Three important factors must be present for HDFN to occur:
1. *The red cell antibody produced by the mother must be of the IgG class.* IgG is the only immunoglobulin capable of crossing the placental barrier. This active transport across the placenta is determined by the fragment, crystallizable, or Fc, portion of the immunoglobulin molecule. IgM antibodies such as anti-Le^a, anti-Le^b, anti-M, anti-N, and anti-P1 have not been implicated in HDFN.[1]
2. *The fetus must possess an antigen that is lacking in the mother.* The gene for the antigen is inherited from the father. If the father is known to be homozygous for the

---

Prenatal: time period before birth.

Antenatal: time period before birth.

Antepartum: period of time between conception and onset of labor, used with reference to the mother.

Neonatal: time period within the first 28 days after birth.

Perinatal: period extends from 28 weeks of gestation to 28 days after delivery.

Fetomaternal hemorrhage: escape of fetal cells into the maternal circulation, usually occurring at the time of delivery.

Hydrops fetalis: edema in the fetus.

Erythroblastosis fetalis: also called hemolytic disease of the fetus and newborn.

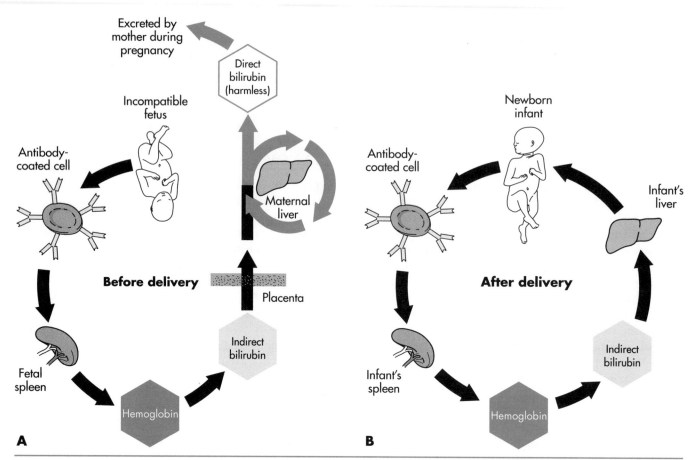

Fig. 11-1   Metabolism of bilirubin. **A,** Before delivery, fetal bilirubin produced by the breakdown of sensitized red cells in the fetal spleen is safely metabolized by the maternal liver. **B,** After delivery, the newborn's liver does not produce glucuronyl transferase and cannot convert bilirubin to an excretable form. As a result, it collects in tissues and causes brain damage. (From Ortho Diagnostics: *Blood group antigens and antibodies as applied to hemolytic disease of the fetus and newborn,* Raritan, NJ, 1968, Ortho Diagnostics.)

gene, 100% of the children inherit the gene and are at risk for HDFN. If the father is known to be heterozygous, only 50% of the children may inherit the gene and are at risk.

3. *The antigen must be well developed at birth.* Blood group antigens such as Lewis, P1, and I are not well developed at birth. Antibodies to these antigens are not expected to cause HDFN because the antigen is not available to bind with the maternal antibody.

HDFN is often classified into three categories based on antibody specificity: D, ABO, and other antibodies. These categories are described in the following section.

Rh HEMOLYTIC DISEASE OF THE FETUS AND NEWBORN

Anti-D is responsible for the most severe cases of HDFN. In most cases, D-negative women become alloimmunized or sensitized at delivery in the first pregnancy with a D-positive baby. The first pregnancy rarely demonstrates clinical signs of HDFN. Following production of anti-D, subsequent D-positive fetuses are affected to varying degrees. In some cases, the maternal anti-D binds to fetal D-positive red cells and causes a positive direct antiglobulin test (DAT) and minimal, if any, signs of red cell destruction. Moderately affected infants develop signs of jaundice and corresponding elevations in bilirubin levels during the first few days of life. Severely affected D-positive infants, in whom rapid red cell destruction occurs, experience anemia in utero and develop jaundice within hours of delivery. Exchange transfusion may be necessary to reduce bilirubin levels to prevent kernicterus after delivery.

The introduction of **Rh immune globulin (RhIG)** in 1968 dramatically reduced the incidence of Rh HDFN. However, a 1991 study estimated the incidence of Rh HDFN at 10.6 per 10,000 total births.[2] HDFN caused by anti-D continues to be the most common cause of death from HDFN.

Rh immune globulin (RhIG): commercially available human source gamma globulin consisting of high-titered anti-D that is used in preventing alloimmunization to the D antigen.

ABO HEMOLYTIC DISEASE OF THE FETUS AND NEWBORN

ABO antibodies are more commonly involved in newborn red cell destruction than anti-D. Most cases are subclinical and do not necessitate treatment. Some infants may experience mildly elevated bilirubin levels and some degree of jaundice within the first few days of life. Based on the number of infants who develop jaundice, Mollison et al[3] estimated that HDFN caused by ABO incompatibility occurs in 1 in 150 births. These cases can usually be treated with **phototherapy.** Possible explanations for the mild red cell destruction despite high levels of maternal antibody include the following:

Phototherapy: treatment of elevated bilirubin or other conditions with ultraviolet light rays.

- Presence of A or B substances in the fetal tissues and secretions that bind or neutralize ABO antibodies, which reduces the amount of ABO antibody available to destroy fetal red cells
- Poor development of ABO antigens on fetal or infant red cells
- Reduced number of A and B antigen sites on fetal or infant red cells

ABO HDFN occurs most frequently in group A or B babies born to group O mothers. Group O individuals are more likely to have higher titers of IgG ABO antibodies compared with other ABO groups. In contrast to HDFN caused by anti-D, ABO incompatibility often affects the first pregnancy because of the presence of naturally occurring ABO antibodies. In Table 11-1, the clinical and laboratory findings in HDFN caused by ABO incompatibilities and anti-D are compared.[4]

ABO HDFN is most common in type A or B babies born to type O mothers.

ALLOANTIBODIES CAUSING HEMOLYTIC DISEASE OF THE FETUS AND NEWBORN OTHER THAN ANTI-D

Any IgG antibody is capable of causing HDFN, if the fetal red cells possess the antigen and the antigen is well developed at birth. Anti-c and anti-K are the next most common antibodies to cause HDFN after anti-D.[5] Less commonly reported antibodies include

TABLE 11-1	Comparison of ABO and Rh Hemolytic Disease of the Fetus and Newborn	
	ABO HDFN	**Rh HDFN**
Clinical findings		
Jaundice	Mild to moderate	Moderate to severe
Edema	No	Mild to severe
Serologic results		
ABO and D type	Mother: O	Mother: D-negative
	Baby: A or B	Baby: D-positive
Direct antiglobulin test	Negative or weakly positive	Positive
Antibody	Anti-A, anti-B, anti-A,B	Anti-D
Hematology results		
Anemia	Mild	Moderate to severe
Reticulocyte count	Mild increase	Greatly increased
Morphology	Spherocytes	Macrocytes, hypochromia
Nucleated RBC	Mild increase	Greatly increased
Chemistry results		
Bilirubin	Mild increase, peaks at 24-48 hours after birth	Moderate to severe

Data from McKenzie SB: *Textbook of hematology,* ed 2, Baltimore, 1996, Williams &Wilkins.
HDFN, Hemolytic disease of the fetus and newborn; *RBC,* red blood cell.

anti-k, anti-Kp^a, anti-Kp^b, anti-Js^a, anti-Js^b, anti-Jk^a, anti-Fy^a, anti-Fy^b, anti-S, anti-s and anti-U. Antibodies to low-frequency antigens, such as Js^a and Kp^a, may not be detected when using screening or panel cells. If evidence of HDFN is present, testing paternal cells with the mother's serum may demonstrate a positive reaction not detected with reagent red cells. Agglutination reaction with paternal cells would provide a clue to the presence of an antibody to a low-frequency antigen, and further testing with selected cells could be used to identify the specificity. See Chapter 7 for more information on low-frequency antigens.

SECTION 3
PREDICTION OF HEMOLYTIC DISEASE OF THE FETUS AND NEWBORN

Prenatal or antepartum testing serves the following two purposes:
- To identify D-negative women who are candidates for RhIG (see Section 5 on Prevention of Hemolytic Disease of the Fetus and Newborn)
- To identify women with antibodies capable of causing HDFN, which helps assess potential risk to the fetus

Prenatal testing should be performed in the first trimester and should include ABO and D phenotyping. Testing the mother for weak D antigen is not required according to AABB standards.[6] An antibody screen using separate screening cells to detect clinically significant IgG alloantibodies is performed. If the antibody screen is positive, antibody identification should be performed. Women with clinically significant IgG antibodies require careful management to monitor risk to the fetus. Table 11-2 outlines recommended laboratory testing to identify women at risk of HDFN.

MATERNAL HISTORY

An accurate obstetric and transfusion history is essential in predicting the course of a sensitized pregnancy. For a woman with a history of HDFN secondary to anti-D, a subsequent D-positive fetus has a much greater chance of being affected. A history of a previously affected infant can be useful in predicting the prognosis for future pregnancies.

ANTIBODY TITRATION

Antibody titration can be helpful in decisions regarding the performance and timing of procedures such as amniocentesis, ultrasound, color Doppler ultrasonography, and cordocentesis. The baseline antibody titer should be determined during the first trimester, and the specimen should be frozen for future testing. Testing should be repeated at 4- to

TABLE 11-2	Prenatal Testing: Tests to Identify Women at Risk of Hemolytic Disease of the Fetus and Newborn
Initial visit	ABO/D (weak D test is optional) Screen for IgG antibodies If antibody screen is positive, perform antibody identification Antibody titration for IgG antibodies to establish baseline
Follow-up visits (if IgG antibody was identified)	Selected reagent red cell panel should be run to exclude other clinically significant antibodies Perform antibody titration in parallel with initial sample at 2- to 4-week intervals
26-28 weeks	Confirm D typing

From Judd WJ: Practice guidelines for prenatal and perinatal immunohematology, revisited, *Transfusion* 41:1445, 2001.

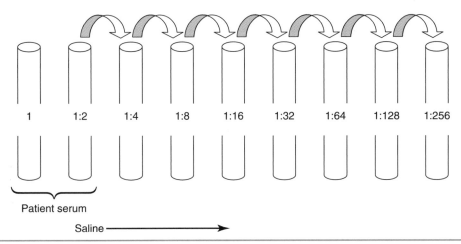

Fig. 11-2 Twofold serial dilutions of the serum containing the antibody are prepared with saline as the diluent. Saline is first added to tubes 1:2→1:256. Serum is then added to tube 1 and 1:2. The serum is transferred from 1 to 1:2 and then to 1:4 continuing to the last tube, changing pipette tips to prevent carryover. The red cell selected for testing is usually homozygous and tested by the antiglobulin technique using anti-IgG. The titer is reported as the reciprocal of the highest dilution that gives a 1+ reaction.

Sample	Dilution Strength								
	1:1	1:2	1:4	1:8	1:16	1:32	1:64	1:128	1:256
#1	2+	2+	1+	(1+)	0	0	0	0	0
#2 (4 weeks later)	3+	3+	2+	1+	1+	(1+)	0	0	0

Fig. 11-3 Example of parallel testing for monitoring antibody increases during pregnancy. Sample #1 titer is reported as "8." Sample #2 titer is reported as "32." In this example, the increase of two tubes is noted (fourfold increase) and is considered to be significant.

6-week intervals thereafter. A titer rising by two dilutions or greater is generally considered a significant change.[5] To ensure the validity of a rising titer, successive titrations should be performed using the same methods and test cells. Some facilities use a scoring method that combines titer and agglutination strength for the endpoint value. Titration methods are discussed in the AABB *Technical Manual* and should be carefully validated and used consistently at each facility.[5]

Testing previously frozen samples in parallel with the current specimen ensures that any change in the titer is not the result of technical variables. Critical titers for anti-D and other Rh system antibodies should be determined by each facility's medical director and is usually 16 or 32 at the antihuman globulin (AHG) phase.[5] The critical titer for anti-K is generally lower because of the K-antigen presence on early red cell precursors.[7] See Fig. 11-2 for an explanation of the titration technique and Fig. 11-3 for an example.

ULTRASOUND TECHNIQUES

Fetal anemia caused by hemolysis of red cells during pregnancy can be detected by ultrasound techniques, specifically color Doppler ultrasonography, which can be used to measure blood flow velocity.[5] An increased cardiac output and a decreased blood viscosity are associated with fetal anemia. Evaluation of the peak systolic velocity in the middle cerebral artery of the fetus with color Doppler ultrasonography can determine the severity of fetal anemia without invasive procedures. Before the development of color Doppler ultrasonography, the severity of HDFN was measured by amniocentesis, which is described next.

Fig. 11-4   Plot taken at 35 weeks of the optical density (absorbance) reading of amniotic fluid from a woman immunized to the D antigen. The difference between the baseline optical density at the 450-nm wavelength and the reading of the amniotic fluid is measured. The result in this case is 0.206, the change in optical density or ΔOD is plotted on a Liley graph to determine the correct course of treatment according to the period of gestation. (From Mollison PL, Engelfriet CP, Contreras M: *Blood transfusion in clinical medicine,* ed 9, London, 1993, Blackwell Scientific.)

AMNIOCENTESIS

Amniocentesis: process of withdrawal of amniotic fluid by aspiration for the purpose of analysis.

One measure of red cell destruction and the severity of HDFN is the level of bilirubin pigment found in amniotic fluid. Amniotic fluid is obtained by **amniocentesis,** or the insertion of a needle through the mother's abdominal wall and uterus and extraction of fluid from the amniotic sac. The aspirated fluid is scanned spectrophotometrically from 350 to 700 nm. The change in optical density (ΔOD) above the baseline at 450 nm is a measure of the bilirubin pigments (Fig. 11-4).

Liley graph: graph used to predict severity of HDFN during pregnancy by evaluation of the amniotic fluid.

The ΔOD is plotted on the **Liley graph** according to gestational age, from 27 to 40 weeks (Fig. 11-5, *A*). This graph defines three zones to estimate the severity of HDFN. The upper zone correlates with severe HDFN and fetal death, the lower zone indicates a mildly affected or unaffected fetus, and the middle zone correlates with moderate disease and necessitates repeat testing to establish a trend. Queenan et al described a graph similar to the Liley graph, which includes four zones and begins at 14 weeks of gestation (Fig. 11-5, *B*).[5]

Based on amniotic fluid analysis, three alternatives exist:
1. Allow the pregnancy to continue to term.
2. Perform intrauterine transfusion (see Section 6 on Treatment of Hemolytic Disease of the Fetus and Newborn).
3. Induce early labor.

Respiratory distress syndrome: inability to maintain stable pulmonary alveolar structures, caused by low levels of surfactant, lecithin, and other pulmonary lipids in premature infants.

If labor is induced, fetal lung maturity must be determined to avoid **respiratory distress syndrome.** Lecithin and phosphatidylglycerol are biochemical components of surfactant, a mixture of phospholipids that allows the exchange of gases in the lungs. A **lecithin/sphingomyelin (L/S) ratio** of greater than 2:1 is generally considered evidence of lung maturity.

Lecithin/sphingomyelin (L/S) ratio: ratio of lecithin to sphingomyelin that indicates lung maturity.

CORDOCENTESIS

Cordocentesis is a useful diagnostic and therapeutic technique. Using an ultrasound-guided needle, the umbilical vein is punctured near the point of placental insertion. A fetal blood sample is aspirated, which can be used to measure hematologic (hemoglobin/hematocrit) or biochemical (bilirubin) variables directly. Before testing, the specimen must be determined to be fetal and not maternal in origin. This distinction is made by

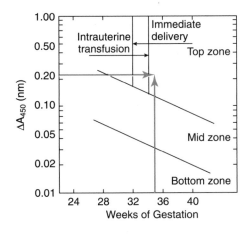

A. Liley Graph: arrows indicate where the reading of 0.206 (ΔOD 450) would fall in this graph

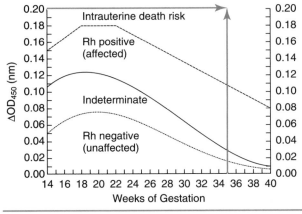

B. Queenan et al: arrows indicate where the reading of 0.206 (ΔOD 450) would fall in this graph

Fig. 11-5   Liley graph and Queenan et al modification. **A,** Liley graph for evaluating data from spectrophotometric analysis of amniotic fluid. The change in optical density at 450 (ΔOD 450) and weeks of gestation are plotted to estimate the severity of HDFN. A reading of 0.206 at 35 weeks correlates with severe HDFN, which may necessitate immediate delivery. **B,** Modification by Queenan et al. of the Liley graph to include four zones beginning at 14 weeks of gestation. (From McCullough J: *Transfusion medicine,* ed 2, Philadelphia, 2005, Saunders.)

measuring fetal hemoglobin. Red cell genotyping by molecular methods can be performed to determine the presence of an antigen on the fetal red cells if the mother has an IgG antibody. The fetal mortality rate associated with this technique is reported to be between 1% and 2%.[5] In cases of severe HDFN, cordocentesis also can be used for direct intravascular transfusion to the fetus (see Section 6 on Treatment of Hemolytic Disease of the Fetus and Newborn).

Fetal Genotyping

Molecular typing of fetal DNA can be performed on maternal plasma during the second trimester.[9,10] Fetal genotyping for blood groups, particularly the D antigen, can assist in predicting the risk that the antibody present during pregnancy could cause HDFN. The prediction of fetal genotype could potentially avoid amniocentesis or cordocentesis, if the fetus lacks the antigen for the maternal antibody.

SECTION 4

POSTPARTUM TESTING

After delivery, it is desirable to collect a sample of cord blood from newborns when there is a risk of HDFN. The specimen should be properly labeled and can be stored for 7 days. The sample can remain available for testing if the mother is D-negative or if the newborn develops signs or symptoms of HDFN. Cord blood should be washed several times before testing to avoid false-positive test results because of contamination with Wharton's jelly, a gelatinous substance found in the umbilical cord. Cord blood samples collected using a needle and a syringe avoids contamination with Wharton's jelly, eliminating the need for additional washing.[5]

POSTPARTUM TESTING OF INFANTS AND MOTHERS

D Testing

All infants born to D-negative mothers should be tested for the D antigen, including a test for weak D antigen.[6] D-negative mothers whose infants are found to be D-positive (including weak D–positive) are candidates for RhIG therapy (see Section 5 on Prevention of Hemolytic Disease of the Fetus and Newborn).

Testing for the D antigen on the cord cells or newborn's blood sample must be performed and interpreted carefully. In cases of HDFN, the baby's red cells may have a positive DAT, which can lead to false-positive or false-negative D-testing results. To ensure the validity of a D-positive test result, it is essential to include appropriate Rh controls. In cases where the mother is demonstrating anti-D in her serum and HDFN is suspected, the fetal red cells may type as D-negative. This false-negative D result may be due to a **blocking phenomenon**, where the D antigen sites are blocked by antibody. An elution performed on the fetal red cells demonstrates anti-D. Washing the cells several times with warm saline and retesting is suggested.[5] A false-positive D typing may occur if the weak D test is performed on red cells that are coated with antibodies. Antibodies coating the cells when testing for weak D should be suspected if the Rh control and anti-D are positive at the antiglobulin phase.

A diagnosis of HDFN is based on medical history, physical examination of the newborn, and results of laboratory testing on both the mother and the infant. Table 11-3 lists the tests that should be performed on the maternal and cord blood (or newborn's sample) to determine if RhIG is needed and in cases of suspected HDFN.[7]

Blocking phenomenon: The D antigen phenotype on cord blood may be falsely negative if the cells are heavily coated with maternal anti-D.

TABLE 11-3	Testing at Delivery (Postpartum Testing)	
SAMPLE	TEST	INDICATION
Maternal blood	ABO/D typing	To determine if RhIG is needed, pretransfusion testing, or suspected ABO HDFN Weak D test is not required if test for D is negative
	Antibody screen	If transfusion is necessary or HDFN is suspected
	Antibody ID	If screen is positive
	Fetal screen (rosette)	If mother is D-negative and baby is D-positive
	Kleihauer-Betke	If fetal screen (rosette) is positive, to determine dosage of RhIG
Cord or infant blood	ABO/D typing	To determine if RhIG is needed for the mother or if ABO HDFN is suspected Weak D test is required if test for D is negative
	DAT	Performed routinely or in suspected cases of HDFN
	Elution	If DAT is positive; test eluate against A cells, B cells, panel cells, or paternal cells, as indicated if HDFN is suspected

HDFN, Hemolytic disease of the fetus and newborn; *DAT*, direct antiglobulin test.

ABO TESTING

When ABO phenotyping is performed on newborns, only the ABO forward grouping is tested because ABO antibodies are not yet produced. ABO reverse grouping results can lead to misinterpretation or delays because of discrepancies. In addition, it is important to follow manufacturer's directions carefully because ABO antigens might not be fully developed and might demonstrate weaker results than expected in an adult.

ABO typing on cord blood and newborn samples should include forward grouping only.

Direct Antiglobulin Test

The DAT must be performed carefully because the result may be weak, especially in cases of ABO HDFN. In cases of a positive DAT, performing an elution is optional unless there are clinical indications or if the mother's antibody has not been identified.[7] If a maternal sample is unavailable, testing the eluate may be useful to confirm HDFN and determine the cause.

If the maternal antibody screen is negative and the DAT is positive, ABO incompatibility should be suspected. ABO HDFN can be confirmed by performing an elution. The eluate should be tested against group A_1, B, and O cells (screening cells) using an antiglobulin technique. Positive results with group A_1 or B cells (or both) and negative results with the screening cells are indicative of ABO HDFN. If the eluate is negative with all red cells, an antibody to a low-frequency antigen should be suspected. The maternal serum or eluate from the baby's red cells should be tested against the paternal red cells.

Intrauterine Transfusions

ABO and D phenotypes and DATs should be interpreted with extreme caution in newborns who have received intrauterine transfusions. Because group O, D-negative blood is used for intrauterine transfusions, cord blood test results may be misleading. Depending on the number of transfusions, the infant may phenotype as group O, D-negative or demonstrate weak mixed-field reactions with ABO and anti-D antisera. The DAT likewise may be falsely negative or only weakly positive.

SECTION 5
PREVENTION OF HEMOLYTIC DISEASE OF THE FETUS AND NEWBORN

As discussed previously, the production of IgG antibodies (particularly anti-D) can have life-threatening consequences for the fetus. Once a woman is alloimmunized and produces antibodies, the condition cannot be reversed. Therefore, accurate testing must ensure that alloimmunization in women of childbearing age is prevented whenever possible. RhIG is available and prevents alloimmunization in D-negative mothers exposed to D-positive red cells. RhIG was developed during the early 1960s and licensed for administration in 1968. Since its introduction, there has been a dramatic decrease in the incidence of HDFN caused by anti-D. Before the use of RhIG, 13% of D-negative women became sensitized after pregnancy. The routine postpartum administration of RhIG has reduced the probability of immunization to 11 cases per 10,000 births, with severe disease in less than 1 per 20,000 births.[8]

RhIG is a concentrate of IgG anti-D prepared from pools of human plasma. The product is given to D-negative women at 28 weeks of gestation (antepartum) and again within 72 hours of delivery (postpartum) of a D-positive infant. A D-negative woman must not have produced anti-D. Different preparations of RhIG are available for either intravenous or intramuscular administration. RhIG suppresses the immune response after exposure to D-positive fetal red cells and prevents the mother from producing anti-D. The mechanism of antibody suppression is not clearly understood, but it may involve the removal of D-positive cells by macrophages causing the release of cytokines that suppress the immune system response.[5] Antepartum and postpartum criteria for RhIG administration are outlined in Table 11-4.

TABLE 11-4	Decisions for Rh Immune Globulin Administration		
TEST RESULTS		**RhIG?**	**CONSIDERATIONS**
Antepartum RhIG Administration			
Mother: D-positive		No	RhIG not indicated
Mother: D-negative		Yes	Weak D test is optional
Mother: D-negative; anti-D in serum		No	Review patient history to ensure anti-D is not from RhIG administration and is immune anti-D
Postpartum RhIG Administration			
Mother: D-positive Cord: D-negative		No	RhIG not indicated
Mother: D-negative Cord: D-negative		No	Perform weak D test on cord cells
Mother: D-negative Cord: D-positive		Yes	Calculate dose
Mother: D-positive Cord: D-positive		No	RhIG not indicated
Mother: D-negative Cord: D-negative Anti-D in mother's serum		No*	Check records to verify that anti-D is not from antepartum RhIG administration

*Consider "blocking phenomenon," where the baby's D-positive red cells are blocked by maternal anti-D, giving a false-negative result.

ANTEPARTUM ADMINISTRATION OF Rh IMMUNE GLOBULIN

Antepartum administration of RhIG reduces the formation of anti-D during gestation from about 1.5% to 0.1%.[5] The American College of Obstetricians and Gynecologists recommends initial dosage of RhIG to unsensitized D-negative mothers at 28 weeks. Indications for additional doses of RhIG during pregnancy include invasive procedures such as amniocentesis, cordocentesis, intrauterine transfusions, inversion of a breach fetus, or abdominal trauma.[5]

Criteria for antepartum administration include D-negative mothers when the fetus is either D-positive or unknown. A D-negative mother whose infant is known to be D-negative or has been previously immunized to D is not a candidate for RhIG. D-positive mothers are also not candidates for RhIG. Weak D testing is not required. Mothers with red cells that are clearly weak D–positive should be considered D-positive and not receive RhIG.[5] The decision to perform the weak D test and its interpretation with regard to administration of RhIG is made by the medical director.[6]

As mentioned previously, all women should be phenotyped for ABO and D antigens and tested for alloantibodies during the first trimester of pregnancy. The antibody screen should be repeated at 26 to 28 weeks of gestation for all D-negative women. If the antibody screen remains negative for anti-D, RhIG should be administered. Other alloantibodies (e.g., anti-K, anti-E) should *not* prevent a woman from receiving RhIG. RhIG does not prevent immunization of antibodies other than D.

POSTPARTUM ADMINISTRATION OF Rh IMMUNE GLOBULIN

Cord blood from infants born to D-negative mothers should be tested for the D antigen, including the test for weak D.[5] A nonimmunized D-negative woman who delivers a D-positive infant should receive a full dose of RhIG within 72 hours of delivery. If the delivering hospital has a verified record of a negative antibody screen during the current pregnancy, the screen does not need to be repeated before administration of postpartum

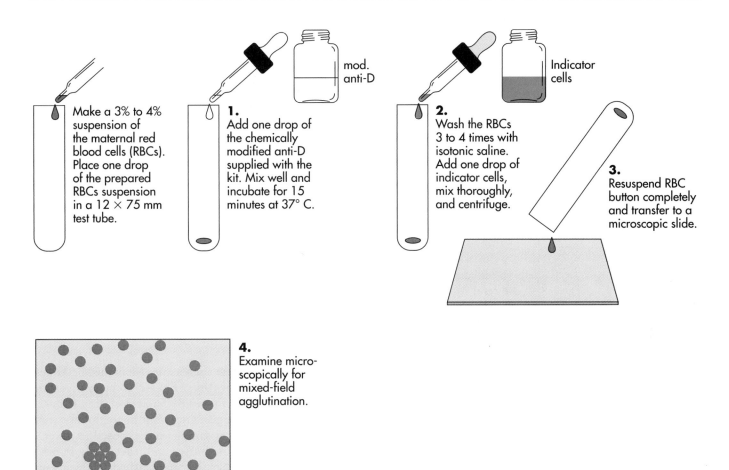

Make a 3% to 4% suspension of the maternal red blood cells (RBCs). Place one drop of the prepared RBCs suspension in a 12 × 75 mm test tube.

mod. anti-D

1. Add one drop of the chemically modified anti-D supplied with the kit. Mix well and incubate for 15 minutes at 37° C.

Indicator cells

2. Wash the RBCs 3 to 4 times with isotonic saline. Add one drop of indicator cells, mix thoroughly, and centrifuge.

3. Resuspend RBC button completely and transfer to a microscopic slide.

4. Examine microscopically for mixed-field agglutination.

Feto-Maternal Hemorrhage:
< 1 rosette per 3 lpf: one dose of RhIG
> 1 rosette per 3 lpf: quantitate bleed

Fig. 11-6 Rosette test for detection of fetomaternal hemorrhage. *RhIG,* Rh immune globulin; *lpf,* low power field. (Modified from Immucor, Norcross, Ga.)

RhIG. When the antibody screen is repeated at delivery, results must be interpreted with caution. A weak antibody to D may be detected because of prenatal administration of RhIG. If a check of the patient's history reveals administration of RhIG at 28 weeks, a full postpartum dose of RhIG still should be administered. Differentiating between active and passive anti-D by titration is not necessary.[7]

Screening for Fetomaternal Hemorrhage

A full 300-μg dose of RhIG provides protection for up to 15 mL of D-positive red cells (approximately 30 mL of fetal whole blood). If a woman experiences FMH exceeding 30 mL of D-positive fetal red cells, it is essential that she receive more than one dose of RhIG. All postpartum RhIG candidates should have a postpartum specimen tested for significant FMH.[3]

The most frequently used method to screen for FMH at the present time is the rosette test (Fig. 11-6). In this method, a suspension of the maternal red cells (containing D-negative maternal red cells and a small number of D-positive fetal red cells) is incubated with anti-D. During incubation, anti-D binds to the D-positive fetal red cells. The suspension is washed thoroughly, and D-positive indicator red cells are added, which bind to the anti-D and form a rosette around the D-positive fetal red cells. The blood suspension is placed on a slide and examined microscopically for the appearance and number of rosettes. Appropriate positive and negative controls should be run concurrently to ensure valid test results. A positive test indicates significant FMH and the potential need for more than one dose of RhIG. The rosette test detects a bleed of only 10 mL.[5] Because

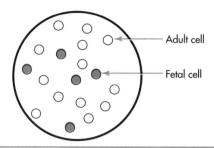

Fig. 11-7   Acid elution test for determination of hemoglobin F. After staining, fetal red cells appear dark pink, and adult cells appear as pale ghost cells. Fetal hemoglobin resists acid elution and remains intact, whereas the adult cells lose the hemoglobin and do not take up the stain.

the rosette assay is a screening test only, a method to quantify the number of fetal red cells should be performed.

The fetal cells must be D-positive and the mother must be D-negative for the rosette test to be valid. A false-positive result can occur if the mother is weak D–positive. A false-negative result can occur if the fetus is positive for weak D.

Quantifying Fetomaternal Hemorrhage

In patients with a positive rosette test, a quantitative test such as the Kleihauer-Betke test or flow cytometry is performed to calculate the dose of RhIG. Flow cytometry measures fetal hemoglobin or D-positive red cells or both.[11] Kleihauer-Betke acid elution is based on the fact that fetal hemoglobin is resistant to acid elution and adult hemoglobin is not. A blood smear is prepared from a postpartum maternal sample and exposed to an acid buffer. Hemoglobin from adult red cells leaches into the buffer and leaves only stroma, whereas the fetal red cells retain their hemoglobin. Smears are washed, stained, and examined under oil immersion. Adult red cells appear as "ghosts," and fetal cells appear pink (Fig. 11-7). Results are reported as the percentage of fetal red cells (number of fetal red cells divided by total red cells counted).

The volume (in milliliters of whole blood) of the FMH uses the percentage of fetal red cells counted or determined by flow cytometry. This percentage is multiplied by the mother's blood volume. The mother's blood volume can be calculated based on her height and weight or the average of 5000 mL used. Because a full dose of RhIG protects against 30 mL of whole blood, the volume of FMH is divided by 30 to determine the number of doses of RhIG. Fig. 11-8 provides an example.

To obtain a whole number, if the number to the right of the decimal point is less than 0.5, one rounds down. If the number to the right of the decimal is greater than or equal to 0.5, one rounds up. Because the accuracy and precision of this method are poor, a safety margin should be provided to ensure adequate protection by adding one dose of RhIG to the final number calculated.

> The fetal screen (rosette test) is a screening or qualitative test, whereas the Kleihauer-Betke and flow cytometric methods are quantitative tests for determining dosage of RhIG.

SECTION 6

TREATMENT OF HEMOLYTIC DISEASE OF THE FETUS AND NEWBORN

IN UTERO TREATMENT

Intrauterine transfusions are given to correct anemia in utero and prevent potential heart failure. Intrauterine transfusions historically have been administered by the intraperitoneal route. In an intraperitoneal transfusion, a needle is inserted into the mother's abdomen and into the peritoneal cavity of the fetus. The red cells are infused into the peritoneal cavity and absorbed into the fetal circulation through the lymphatics. Drawbacks of this procedure include the inability to perform the procedure before 25 weeks and variable absorption of red cells (particularly in hydropic fetuses). More recently cordocentesis has been used to provide direct intravascular transfusion into the umbilical

	Steps	Explanation	Example
1.	Estimate the volume of fetal blood in maternal circulation	Determine the percentage of fetal cells counted in 2000 total cells Percentage of fetal cells × maternal blood volume = fetal whole blood (mL)	16 fetal cells/2000 = .008% .008 × 5000 = 40 mL of fetal whole blood
2.	Calculate how many vials are needed: each 300-μg dose of RhIG protects against a **30** mL whole blood bleed	Divide the mL of fetal whole blood by **30**	40/30 = 1.3
3.	Round up or down to obtain a whole number	Round the calculated dose **up** if ≥ 0.5 following decimal point or **down** if < 0.5	1.3 → 1 (rounded down)
4.	Add 1 vial of RhIG to calculated dose to provide a safety margin	Calculated dose + 1	1 → 2 (add one)

Fig. 11-8 Calculating the dosage of RhIG. (From Roback JD, editor: *Technical manual,* ed 17, Bethesda, Md, 2011, AABB.)

vein. Benefits of this procedure include the ability to obtain blood for blood typing, DAT, antigen typing, hemoglobin, hematocrit, and bilirubin.

Blood for intrauterine transfusion should be:
- Group O, D-negative
- Red blood cells (RBCs) collected within 7 days
- Irradiated to prevent graft-versus-host disease
- Cytomegalovirus (CMV)-reduced-risk: CMV seronegative or leukocyte reduced
- Hemoglobin S–negative

Red cells with a hematocrit of 75% to 80% are used to avoid volume overload. Group O, D-negative is used because the ABO and D typing of the fetus are usually not known. If the mother has an alloantibody, the blood selected should be negative for the corresponding antigen. Fresh blood is necessary to ensure longer viability, higher 2,3-diphosphoglycerate (for release of oxygen to the tissues), and lower potassium (to avoid cardiac arrhythmias). Irradiation is necessary to prevent graft-versus-host disease in the fetus. Donor red cells are crossmatched using the maternal serum.

POSTPARTUM TREATMENT

Phototherapy

Phototherapy is performed as an initial treatment for hyperbilirubinemia. Exposure of newborns to fluorescent blue light in the 420-nm to 475-nm range can successfully treat physiologic jaundice and mild cases of HDFN, particularly ABO HDFN. Bilirubin, when exposed to light, undergoes photoisomerization to form photobilirubin. These isomers of bilirubin are carried by the plasma to the liver and excreted in the bile without the need for conjugation. Cases of hyperbilirubinemia that fail to respond to phototherapy require exchange transfusion.

Exchange Transfusion

As mentioned previously, newborns with HDFN are at risk of anemia and hyperbilirubinemia. If left untreated, elevated levels of indirect bilirubin can result in damage to the CNS. Exchange transfusion that involves the replacement of one to two whole blood volumes is primarily used to treat excessively high levels of unconjugated bilirubin.

TABLE 11-5 Selection of Blood for Exchange Transfusion
• Group O (or ABO-compatible) D-negative blood
• RBCs <7 days old, resuspended in group AB FFP
• CMV-reduced-risk components: CMV-seronegative donors or leukocyte reduced
• Irradiated blood
• Hemoglobin S–negative blood
• Blood lacks antigen corresponding to maternal antibody
• Compatible crossmatch with maternal serum or eluate prepared from newborn's red cells

RBCs, Red blood cells; *FFP,* fresh frozen plasma; *CMV,* cytomegalovirus.

Exchange transfusion accomplishes the following:
• Corrects anemia without expanding blood volume
• Removes a sensitized newborn's red cells and replaces them with antigen-negative cells
• Reduces the level of bilirubin to prevent kernicterus
• Reduces the level of maternal antibody

Many variables enter into the decision to perform exchange transfusion. A bilirubin level of 18 to 20 mg/dL historically has been used as the level at which kernicterus is a serious risk and exchange transfusion is necessary. However, complications such as low birth weight, sepsis, acidosis, or signs of CNS deterioration can affect the threshold level and indicate the need for exchange at levels much less than 20 mg/dL. For these reasons, premature infants may require exchange transfusions at lower bilirubin levels and more often than do full-term infants. Many physicians consider the rate of increase in the bilirubin level to be a better predictor of the need for exchange transfusion.[5]

Selection of Blood and Compatibility Testing for Exchange Transfusion

Before the initial exchange transfusion, infant cells must be tested to determine the ABO and D phenotype. Repeat ABO and D typing is not necessary for the remainder of the infant's hospital admission.[6] Serum or plasma from the infant or the mother may be used for the antibody screen. Maternal serum is used most commonly because it is readily available and has a high concentration of antibodies. If the antibody screen is positive, the red blood cells (RBCs) to be transfused must lack the antigen corresponding to the maternal antibody and be crossmatch compatible by the antiglobulin technique. If maternal serum is not available, the newborn's serum or an eluate from the newborn's red cells can be used for antibody detection and compatibility testing.

Many institutions simplify the procedure of selecting blood for exchange transfusion by using group O, D-negative RBCs for all exchange transfusions, but this is not always necessary. If the mother and the infant are ABO identical, type-specific RBCs can be used.

Fresh frozen plasma (FFP) is used to reconstitute the RBCs to a hematocrit between 45% and 60%.[5] Plasma must be ABO compatible (or group AB) with the RBCs. FFP restores albumin and coagulation factors. Additional requirements for CMV-seronegative blood and irradiation are commonly due to the immunocompromised status of newborns. Hemoglobin S–negative blood should be provided to avoid any possibility of intravascular sickling.[5] Table 11-5 summarizes the criteria to consider when selecting blood for exchange.

CHAPTER SUMMARY

HDFN is prevented, monitored, and treated with the help of tests performed in the laboratory. Understanding the physiology of HDFN is important in choosing the correct tests to perform and detecting early indicators of hemolytic disease. Important points to remember when performing these tests are outlined.
1. HDFN occurs when:
   • Fetal red cells, carrying antigens inherited from the father, stimulate the mother to produce IgG antibodies.
   • Maternal IgG antibodies destroy fetal red cells.

2. Hemolytic processes can cause the following:
   - In utero, this destruction can cause severe anemia, which can result in heart failure and possibly death.
   - After delivery, red cell destruction continues with the increase of bilirubin, causing jaundice and possible damage to the CNS (kernicterus).

3. HDFN can be caused by ABO, Rh, or other IgG antibodies:
   - ABO HDFN is the most common type of HDFN and occurs most commonly in group O mothers who deliver group A or B babies.
   - HDFN caused by anti-D is the most severe type of HDFN; it occurs in D-negative women with anti-D who deliver D-positive infants.
   - Any IgG antibody can cause HDFN if the child inherits the antigen from the father and the red cell antigen is well developed on the fetal red cells. Anti-c and anti-K are most frequently reported after anti-D.

4. Laboratory tests to predict, prevent, or monitor HDFN before delivery include:
   - ABO/D phenotype and antibody screen are performed on the mother.
   - D-negative mothers should receive prenatal RhIG.
   - Titration of the maternal antibody can be helpful in deciding when to perform diagnostic and invasive procedures.
   - Spectrophotometric analysis of the amniotic fluid and use of the Liley graph can aid in predicting the severity of HDFN.

5. After delivery, HDFN is monitored, prevented, and treated by:
   - Cord blood testing determines whether a D-negative mother should receive postpartum RhIG.
   - RhIG dosage is determined by the fetal screen (rosette) and Kleihauer-Betke test performed on the mother.
   - If HDFN is suspected, ABO and D phenotype and DAT should be performed; hemoglobin and bilirubin levels should also be closely monitored.
   - Depending on the severity of HDFN, treatment can begin in utero or after delivery.
   - After delivery, exchange transfusion is used to correct anemia, remove sensitized red cells, and reduce levels of maternal antibody and bilirubin.
   - Blood for exchange and intrauterine transfusion should be less than 7 days old, irradiated, CMV-reduced-risk, hemoglobin S–negative, and negative for the antigen corresponding to the maternal antibody. Group O, D-negative RBCs resuspended in AB plasma are used most often.

CRITICAL THINKING EXERCISES

EXERCISE 11-1

R.T. was seen by her OB-GYN for her initial visit at 9 weeks of gestation. This is her first pregnancy.
1. What tests should be run for her initial prenatal work-up?

Additional Testing

Results of prenatal testing indicate R.T. is group A, D-negative with a negative antibody screen.
2. Does R.T. need any additional laboratory testing during her pregnancy? If so, when should the testing be performed, what tests are needed, and why?

Additional Testing

R.T. was seen again by her OB-GYN at 28 weeks. Her antibody screen is repeated and found to be negative. Based on these test results, she received a 300-μg dose of RhIG. R.T. delivered a healthy 6 lb, 4 oz boy 12 weeks later.
3. What testing, if any, needs to be performed at the time of delivery?

Additional Testing

Results of the cord blood from R.T.'s infant indicate phenotype of group A, D-positive with a negative DAT.

4. Is R.T. a candidate for postpartum RhIG?
5. What additional test needs to be performed on R.T. before RhIG is given?

EXERCISE 11-2

J.M. is seen at the outpatient clinic for her first prenatal visit at 15 weeks of gestation. Obstetric history indicates one ectopic pregnancy (no RhIG given) and one full-term pregnancy (RhIG given). The last child required phototherapy. Results of prenatal testing indicate group O, D-negative with a positive antibody screen.

1. What additional testing needs to be performed?

Additional Testing

An antibody panel identifies anti-D. Parallel titers were performed on the sample from 15 weeks and 20 weeks of gestation. The following results were obtained:

	Dilution Strength								
Sample	**1:1**	**1:2**	**1:4**	**1:8**	**1:16**	**1:32**	**1:64**	**1:128**	**1:256**
#1 (15 weeks)	2+	2+	2+	1+	1+	0	0	0	0
#2 (20 weeks)	3+	3+	2+	2+	1+	1+	1+	+w	0

2. What is the purpose of performing antibody titration?
3. Are the results shown in the table significant, and how is this reported?
4. Why is parallel testing recommended?

Additional Testing

Amniocentesis performed at 24 weeks shows a ΔOD of 0.10.

5. Using the Liley graph, what outcome might be expected for this pregnancy given this result and the patient history?

Additional Testing

J.M. continues to be closely monitored throughout her pregnancy. She delivered a 4 lb, 10 oz girl at 37 weeks. Results of cord blood testing were as follows:

Anti-A	Anti-B	Anti-D	Weak D	D control	DAT
3+	0	0	2+	2+	2+

The hemoglobin is 13 g/dL; bilirubin is 5.2 mg/dL.

6. What is the ABO and D type interpretation?
7. What additional tests are necessary to resolve the D typing?
8. Does this infant have HDFN? If so, what is the cause? Use laboratory data to support your conclusions.

Additional Testing

The following evening, J.M.'s infant has a bilirubin value of 17.4 mg/dL, and an exchange transfusion is requested.

9. What ABO/D type blood should be selected, and how should it be tested?
10. What are the special requirements for blood selected for exchange transfusion?

EXERCISE 11-3

B.W. was seen by her OB-GYN at 10 weeks of gestation with her first pregnancy. Results of her prenatal work-up indicate she is group O, D-negative with a negative antibody screen. Repeat testing at 28 weeks continues to indicate a negative antibody screen, and she is given 300 µg of RhIG. The pregnancy proceeds normally, and she delivers a 7 lb, 2 oz boy at 39 weeks of gestation. Results of cord blood tests are as follows:

Anti-A	Anti-B	Anti-D	Weak D	D control	DAT	Screen cells
3+	0	0	1+	1+	1+	Weak positive

Infant hemoglobin is 17.3 g/dL, and bilirubin is 0.6 mg/dL.
1. Does this infant have HDFN? If so, what is the most probable cause?
2. What could be causing the positive screen result? How would you confirm this?

Additional Testing
An elution is performed. The eluate is tested against A_1, B, and O reagent red cells, incubated at 37° C, and tested at the AHG phase:

	A_1	B	O
Eluate	1+	1+	Negative

3. What do these results indicate?
4. What type of treatment most likely would be recommended for this infant?
5. Is B.W. a candidate for postpartum RhIG? If so, are any additional tests necessary?

Additional Testing
A rosette screen performed on B.W. yields a positive result.
6. What test needs to be performed and why?

Additional Testing
A Kleihauer-Betke stain is performed on B.W.'s postpartum specimen to quantify the amount of FMH. There were 19 fetal cells counted in a total of 2000 cells.
7. How many doses of RhIG should B.W. receive?

EXERCISE 11-4
M.K., a 26-year-old mother of two, is admitted to labor and delivery. No prenatal records are available. The antibody screen is positive at the AHG phase:

Anti-A	Anti-B	Anti-D	Rh control	Weak D	Weak D control	A_1 cells	B cells	Interpretation
0	4+	0	0	0 ✓	0 ✓	4+	0	?

The antibody identification is performed, and a weak anti-D is identified. Cord blood test results follow:

Anti-A	Anti-B	Anti-D	D control	DAT	Interpretation
0	0	0	0	0 ✓	?

DAT, Direct antiglobulin test; ✓, check cells reacted.

1. Based on these results, is M.K. a candidate for postpartum RhIG?

STUDY QUESTIONS

1. Objectives for performing an exchange transfusion include all of the following *except* to:
   a. decrease the level of maternal antibody
   b. reduce the level of indirect bilirubin
   c. provide platelets to prevent disseminated intravascular coagulation
   d. provide compatible RBCs to correct anemia

2. The greatest danger to the fetus (before delivery) affected by HDFN is:
   a. kernicterus
   b. anemia
   c. hyperbilirubinemia
   d. hypertension

3. A 300-μg dose of RhIG covers a maximum FMH of how many milliliters of whole blood?
   a. 10 mL
   b. 15 mL
   c. 30 mL
   d. 50 mL

4. RhIG should be administered within how many hours of delivery?
   a. 6
   b. 48
   c. 72
   d. 96

5. An often fatal condition characterized by general edema that results from anemia is:
   a. kernicterus
   b. DIC
   c. erythroblastosis fetalis
   d. hydrops fetalis

6. HDFN occurs when:
   a. maternal antigens react with fetal antibodies
   b. fetal antibodies react with maternal antibodies
   c. maternal antibodies react with fetal antigens
   d. fetal antigens react with maternal antigens

7. The greatest danger to the newborn affected by HDFN is:
   a. kernicterus
   b. anemia
   c. conjugated bilirubin
   d. low L/S ratio

8. Which of the following women should receive postpartum RhIG?

Mother's ABO/D phenotype	Mother's antibody screen	Newborn's ABO/D phenotype
a. A, D-negative	Negative	O, D-positive
b. O, D-negative	Negative	A, D-negative
c. A, D-positive	Negative	B, D-negative
d. B, D-negative	Immune anti-D	B, D-positive

9. Which of the following antibodies carries no risk of HDFN?
   a. anti-Le^a
   b. anti-C
   c. anti-K
   d. anti-S

10. Which of the following is *not* a characteristic of ABO HDFN?
    a. may occur in first pregnancy
    b. usually treated with phototherapy
    c. strongly positive DAT
    d. most frequent in babies born to group O mothers

11. Which of the following requirements is important when selecting blood for exchange transfusion to avoid high levels of potassium?
    a. irradiated blood
    b. CMV-negative blood
    c. leukocyte-reduced blood
    d. blood less than 7 days old

12. A mother is group A, D-negative with anti-D in her serum. Which of the following units should be selected for an intrauterine transfusion?
    a. group O, D-negative
    b. group O, D-positive
    c. group A, D-negative
    d. group A, D-positive

13. The rosette test is:
    a. performed on a cord blood sample
    b. used to screen for FMH
    c. a quantitative test used to calculate the volume of FMH
    d. an acid elution used to estimate the volume of FMH

14. Which of the following tests is *not* necessary when testing a cord blood sample?
    a. ABO   c. DAT
    b. D   d. antibody screen

15. The Liley method of predicting the severity of HDFN is based on the:
    a. resistance of fetal hemoglobin to acid elution
    b. ratio of lecithin to sphingomyelin
    c. change of optical density of amniotic fluid measured at 450 nm
    d. direct bilirubin evaluation of a cord blood sample

16. A titer was performed on a prenatal sample from a D-negative woman with anti-D. The sample was tested 4 weeks later in parallel with a current sample. The following results were obtained:

	1:1	1:2	1:4	1:8	1:16	1:32	1:64	1:128	1:256
Week 24:	2+	1+	1+	0	0	0	0	0	0
Week 28:	3+	2+	2+	2+	1+	1+	0	0	0

How would the titer results be interpreted?
    a. an intrauterine transfusion is necessary
    b. early induction of labor should be considered
    c. color Doppler ultrasonography should be considered
    d. RhIG should be administered

17. A group A, D-negative mother demonstrating anti-D antibodies delivered a group O, D-negative baby with a positive DAT (2+), elevated bilirubin (18 mg/dL), and low hemoglobin (8 g/dL). Which is the most probable explanation for these test results?
    a. ABO hemolytic disease of the newborn
    b. hemolytic disease of the newborn with a false-negative D typing due to blocking antibodies
    c. large fetomaternal hemorrhage causing discrepancy in the blood type
    d. prenatal RhIG administration

18. The appearance of spherocytes in a baby's blood smear after delivery is usually associated with:
    a. ABO HDFN
    b. HDFN caused by anti-D
    c. HDFN caused by other IgG antibodies
    d. normal physiologic anemia detected in newborns

19. The purpose of irradiation of blood selected for an exchange transfusion is to prevent:
    a. formation of HLA antibodies   c. graft-versus-host disease
    b. sepsis from bacterial contamination   d. transmission of viruses

20. The rosette test used for screening for a fetomaternal hemorrhage can detect a bleed as small as:
    a. 5 mL   c. 20 mL
    b. 10 mL   d. 30 mL

21. A Kleihauer-Betke stain performed on a postpartum blood sample demonstrated 10 fetal cells in a field of 2000. What is the estimated blood volume of the fetomaternal hemorrhage expressed as whole blood?
    a. 25 mL
    c. 45 mL
    b. 30 mL
    d. 100 mL

22. A rosette test performed on a D-negative mother who delivered a D-positive baby demonstrated two rosettes per three fields observed. The correct course of action is to:
    a. submit the sample for a Kleihauer-Betke test
    b. recommend two vials of RhIG
    c. suggest that RhIG is not necessary because records indicate that the mother received prenatal RhIG
    d. recommend one vial of RhIG because it is below the cutoff for the fetal screen

23. The principle of the Kleihauer-Betke test is that:
    a. fetal hemoglobin resists acid elution
    b. adult hemoglobin resists acid elution
    c. fetal red cells lose hemoglobin under alkaline conditions
    d. adult red cells accept dye under alkaline conditions

24. Results of a Kleihauer-Betke test determine there was a fetomaternal hemorrhage of 35 mL of whole blood during delivery. What is the correct dosage of RhIG?
    a. one vial
    c. three vials
    b. two vials
    d. four vials

25. A weakly reactive anti-D test was identified in a postpartum sample from a D-negative woman who gave birth to a D-positive baby. What is the most likely cause?
    a. immune anti-D produced from exposure during the first pregnancy
    b. immune anti-D produced from exposure during the current pregnancy
    c. antenatal RhIG given
    d. error in antibody identification or D typing

REFERENCES

1. Reid ME, Lomas-Francis C: *The blood group antigen facts book*, ed 2, San Diego, 2004, Elsevier Academic Press.
2. Chavez GF, Mulinare J, Edmonds LD: Epidemiology of Rh hemolytic disease of the fetus and newborn in the United States, *JAMA* 265:3270, 1991.
3. Mollison PL, Engelfriet CP, Contreras M: *Blood transfusion in clinical medicine*, ed 9, London, 1993, Blackwell Scientific.
4. McKenzie SB: *Textbook of hematology*, ed 2, Baltimore, 1996, Williams &Wilkins.
5. Roback JD: *Technical manual*, ed 17, Bethesda, MD, 2011, AABB.
6. Carson TH: *Standards for blood banks and transfusion services*, ed 27, Bethesda, MD, 2011, AABB.
7. Judd WJ: Practice guidelines for prenatal and perinatal immunohematology, revisited, *Transfusion* 41:1445, 2001.
8. McCullough J: *Transfusion medicine*, ed 2, Philadelphia, 2005, Saunders.
9. Faas BHW, et al: The detection of fetal RhD-specific sequences in maternal plasma, *Lancet* 352:1196, 1998.
10. Finning K, Martin P, Summers J, et al: Fetal genotyping for the K (Kell) and Rh, Cc, and E blood groups on cell-free fetal DNA in maternal plasma, *Transfusion* 47:2126, 2007.
11. Radel DJ, Penz CS, Dietz AB, et al: A combined flow-cytometry-based method for fetomaternal hemorrhage and maternal D, *Transfusion* 48:1886, 2008.

Donor Selection and Phlebotomy

CHAPTER OUTLINE

LEARNING OBJECTIVES

On completion of this chapter, the reader should be able to:

1. Describe the required donor registration information and why it is necessary.
2. Explain the importance and discuss the content of the "Blood Donor Educational Materials."
3. Compare the donor medical history criteria intended for protecting the donor with questions that protect the recipient.
4. Analyze health history examples that could cause a permanent, indefinite, or temporary deferral.
5. List the physical examination criteria for allogeneic blood donation.
6. Apply the physical examination guidelines to potential blood donor situations.
7. Determine eligibility status of donors when common medications and recent vaccines are part of the donor history.

8. Select eligible donors and identify donors for deferral.
9. List possible adverse donor reactions and appropriate treatment.
10. Compare and contrast allogeneic and autologous donor criteria.
11. List various forms of autologous donations.
12. Describe the apheresis procedure, the products that can be collected, and the donor requirements for each.
13. Discuss the reason for directed donation and the donor criteria.
14. Define therapeutic phlebotomy, and state the conditions for which it is used.

Blood centers and transfusion services are responsible for providing an adequate and safe blood supply to the patients they serve. Criteria for acceptable blood donors are established by the U.S. Food and Drug Administration (FDA) through the Code of Federal Regulations (CFR), guidance documents, or memoranda to the industry. The AABB, a voluntary accrediting agency, has established guidelines for blood donation, which are written in the *Standards for Blood Banks and Transfusion Services.* In an effort to provide uniformity and clarity for determining the eligibility criteria for volunteer blood donors,

The current donor history questionnaire and related materials are available from the AABB website at http://www.aabb.org/resources/donation/questionnaires/Pages/dhqaabb.aspx

the AABB Donor History Questionnaire (DHQ) was developed. This document meets FDA requirements for donor screening, and an updated version can be found on the FDA and AABB websites.[1,2]

Maintaining an adequate blood supply begins with educating the public about the need for volunteer donations. After recruiting donors, the safety of the blood supply depends on thorough and accurate donor screening and processing or testing of each unit collected. This chapter discusses donor screening, and Chapter 13 discusses the testing performed on donated blood.

SECTION 1
DONOR SCREENING

The screening of each donor can be divided into three phases: registration, health history interview, and physical examination.

REGISTRATION

The donor registration process includes documenting information that fully identifies the donor on an individual donation registration record. Questions regarding name changes or nicknames are important for correct identification. Registration should also include prescreening for donor eligibility status. With the exception of first-time donors, access to past donation history, usually through computerized databases, allows the staff to confirm that:
- Donor information is correct
- Sufficient time has passed since the last donation
- The donor has not been deferred from a donation based on previous history questions or test results

Correct identification of the donor is essential to prevent collection from a donor who is not qualified and to ensure that the donor can be contacted with test results or other relevant information. Donation records include the following:
- Donor's full name
- Permanent address/contact information
- Date of birth (donor must be at least 16 years old; if the state considers 16-year-olds to be minors, parental consent is required)
- Gender
- Date of last donation
  - 8 weeks must elapse between whole blood donations
  - 16 weeks must elapse after 2-unit red cell collection
  - 4 weeks must elapse after infrequent plasmapheresis
  - 2 days or more must elapse after plasmapheresis, plateletpheresis, or leukapheresis
  Additional useful information includes the following:
- Unique identification number: such as Social Security number or driver's license number
- Positive identification: usually entails photo identification
- Race: can be useful in selecting donor units for patients requiring certain phenotypes
- Intended use of the donation: **allogeneic donation, directed donation, autologous donation,** or **apheresis donation.**

The above-mentioned special donation processes are described later in this chapter.

Allogeneic donation: donation for use by the general patient population.

Directed donation: donation reserved for use by a specific patient.

Autologous donation: donation by a donor reserved for the donor's later use.

Apheresis donation: donation of a specific component of the blood; parts of the whole blood that are not retained are returned to the donor.

EDUCATIONAL MATERIALS

Before donating, all prospective donors must be given educational materials describing the donation process and donor eligibility. Specific information is provided regarding risks of infectious diseases transmitted by blood transfusion, including the signs, symptoms, and high-risk behaviors associated with the human immunodeficiency virus (HIV) and acquired immunodeficiency syndrome (AIDS) (Fig. 12-1). Prospective donors should be

---

Blood Donor Educational Materials:
MAKING YOUR BLOOD DONATION SAFE

Thank you for coming in today! This information sheet explains how **YOU** can help us make the donation process safe for yourself and patients who might receive your blood. **PLEASE READ THIS INFORMATION <u>BEFORE</u> YOU DONATE! If you have any questions now or anytime during the screening process, please ask blood center staff.**

ACCURACY AND HONESTY ARE ESSENTIAL!
Your **complete honesty** in answering all questions is very important for the safety of patients who receive your blood. **All information you provide is confidential.**

DONATION PROCESS:
To determine if you are eligible to donate we will:
– Ask questions about health, travel, and medicines
– Ask questions to see if you might be at risk for hepatitis, HIV, or AIDS
– Take your blood pressure, temperature, and pulse
– Take a small blood sample to make sure you are not anemic
If you are able to donate we will:
– Cleanse your arm with an antiseptic. **(If you are allergic to iodine, please tell us!)**
– Use a new, sterile disposable needle to collect your blood

DONOR ELIGIBILITY – SPECIFIC INFORMATION
Why we ask questions about sexual contact:
Sexual contact may cause contagious diseases like HIV to get into the bloodstream and be spread through transfusions to someone else.
Definition of "sexual contact":
The words "have sexual contact with" and "sex" are used in some of the questions we will ask you, and apply to <u>any</u> of the activities below, whether or not a condom or other protection was used:
1. Vaginal sex (contact between penis and vagina)
2. Oral sex (mouth or tongue on someone's vagina, penis, or anus)
3. Anal sex (contact between penis and anus)

HIV/AIDS RISK BEHAVIORS AND SYMPTOMS
AIDS is caused by HIV. HIV is spread mainly through sexual contact with an infected person OR by sharing needles or syringes used for injecting drugs.

DO NOT DONATE IF YOU:
– **Have AIDS or have ever had a positive HIV test**
– Have ever used needles to take drugs, steroids, or anything not prescribed by your doctor
– Are a male who has had sexual contact with another male, even once, since 1977

– Have ever taken money, drugs, or other payment for sex since 1977
– Have had sexual contact in the past 12 months with anyone described above
– Have had syphilis or gonorrhea in the past 12 months
– In the last 12 months have been in juvenile detention, lockup, jail, or prison for more than 72 hours
– Have any of the following conditions that can be signs or symptoms of HIV/AIDS:
  • Unexplained weight loss or night sweats
  • Blue or purple spots in your mouth or skin
  • Swollen lymph nodes for more than one month
  • White spots or unusual sores in your mouth
  • Cough that won't go away or shortness of breath
  • Diarrhea that won't go away
  • Fever of more than 100.5° F for more than 10 days
Remember that you <u>CAN</u> give HIV to someone else through blood transfusions even if you feel well and have a negative HIV test. This is because tests cannot detect infections for a period of time after a person is exposed to HIV. **If you think you may be at risk for HIV/AIDS or want an HIV/AIDS test, please ask for information about other testing facilities. *PLEASE DO NOT DONATE TO GET AN HIV TEST!***

Travel to or birth in other countries
Blood donor tests may not be available for some contagious diseases that are found only in certain countries. If you were born in, have lived in, or visited certain countries, you may not be eligible to donate.

What happens after your donation:
To protect patients, your blood is tested for hepatitis B and C, HIV, certain other infectious diseases, and syphilis. If your blood tests positive, it will not be given to a patient. You will be notified about test results that may disqualify you from donating in the future. **Please do not donate to get tested for HIV, hepatitis, or any other infections!**

Thank you for donating blood today!
(Donor Center Name)
(Telephone Number)

Fig. 12-1 Blood Donor Educational Materials (version 1.3, May 2008). (Courtesy AABB, Bethesda, Md.)

given ample opportunity to read the material and ask questions and understand that they are excluded from donating blood if they have experienced any of the signs or symptoms explained in the material. Information regarding the tests that are to be performed on the donor blood and state requirements that often exist to report positive test results to government agencies must be made available. This preinterview material also describes the possible side effects and risks associated with the donation process. Communication of this information must be available for donors who are not fluent in English or who are hearing or vision impaired.

HEALTH HISTORY INTERVIEW

Medical directors: designated physicians responsible for the medical and technical policies of the blood bank.

The health history is used to protect both the donor during the donation process and the patient receiving the blood. Questions are asked in an environment that provides confidentiality and encourages the donor to answer truthfully. Self-administered interview formats have been shown to yield more information regarding HIV high-risk behavior.[3] The interviewer should document and evaluate all responses to determine suitability for donation.

Although the use of the DHQ (Fig. 12-2) developed by AABB and approved by the FDA is recommended, **medical directors** have the option to add questions as appropriate for their center, based on demographics or questions not addressed by the FDA. These questions must be placed at the end of the DHQ.

An abbreviated donor history questionnaire for qualified frequent donors has been approved by the FDA for use in a few blood centers.[3] This abbreviated questionnaire is intended to improve the donation process for donors who donate several times a year as well as to maintain safety of the blood supply.

Questions generally can be divided into two categories: questions intended to protect the donor and questions intended to protect the recipient. An explanation of some of the questions from the DHQ follows (see Fig. 12-2).

Donors may be deferred indefinitely, permanently, or temporarily based on medical history or prior tests. An *indefinite deferral* is sometimes due to current regulatory requirements that may change in the future. An example is a donor who states that he lived in England for 1 year between 1980 and 1996. A *permanent deferral* is required based on a high-risk behavior or a positive test result, such as for hepatitis C. Table 12-1 lists indefinite and permanent deferrals. A *temporary deferral* is recommended if the donor would be eligible at a specific time in the future. An example of a temporary deferral is potential contact with hepatitis from body piercing, tattoos, or living with a person with symptomatic viral hepatitis, which necessitates a 12-month deferral. The temporary deferral allows for viral screening tests to detect a developing antibody or the presence of the virus.

Questions for Protection of the Donor

Properly trained blood bank personnel are required to ask specific questions to determine donor eligibility, such as questions regarding general health, previous surgeries, heart and lung disease, bleeding problems, cancer, and pregnancy. Donors with cold or influenza symptoms, headache, or nausea should be temporarily deferred. Donors who are currently pregnant or have been pregnant in the last 6 weeks are also deferred. The medical director of the facility must evaluate donors with a history of cancer because there are no U.S. federal regulations or professional standards that address donor eligibility regarding cancer.[4]

TABLE 12-1   Conditions for Indefinite or Permanent Deferral
• History of viral hepatitis after eleventh birthday
• Confirmed positive test for hepatitis B surface antigen
• Reactive test to antibodies to hepatitis B core on more than one occasion
• Present or past clinical or laboratory evidence of infection with hepatitis C virus, human T-cell lymphotropic virus, or HIV
• History of babesiosis or Chagas disease
• Family history of CJD
• Recipient of dura mater or human pituitary growth hormone
• Risk of vCJD
• Use of a needle to administer nonprescription drugs

Data from Roback JD, editor: *Technological manual*, ed 17, Bethesda, MD, 2011, AABB.
HIV, Human immunodeficiency virus; *CJD,* Creutzfeldt-Jakob disease; *vCJD,* variant Creutzfeldt-Jakob disease.

Full-Length Donor History Questionnaire

	Yes	No	
Are you			
1. Feeling healthy and well today?	❏	❏	
2. Currently taking an antibiotic?	❏	❏	
3. Currently taking any other medication for an infection?	❏	❏	
Please read the Medication Deferral List.			
4. Are you now taking or have you ever taken any medications on the Medication Deferral List?	❏	❏	
5. Have you read the educational materials?	❏	❏	
In the past 48 hours			
6. Have you taken aspirin or anything that has aspirin in it?	❏	❏	
In the past 6 weeks			
7. Female donors: Have you been pregnant or are you pregnant now? (Males: check "I am male.")	❏	❏	❏ I am male
In the past 8 weeks have you			
8. Donated blood, platelets, or plasma?	❏	❏	
9. Had any vaccinations or other shots?	❏	❏	
10. Had contact with someone who had a smallpox vaccination?	❏	❏	
In the past 16 weeks			
11. Have you donated a double unit of red cells using an apheresis machine?	❏	❏	
In the past 12 months have you			
12. Had a blood transfusion?	❏	❏	
13. Had a transplant such as organ, tissue, or bone marrow?	❏	❏	
14. Had a graft such as bone or skin?	❏	❏	
15. Come into contact with someone else's blood?	❏	❏	
16. Had an accidental needle-stick?	❏	❏	
17. Had sexual contact with anyone who has HIV/AIDS or has had a positive test for the HIV/AIDS virus?	❏	❏	
18. Had sexual contact with a prostitute or anyone else who takes money or drugs or other payment for sex?	❏	❏	
19. Had sexual contact with anyone who has ever used needles to take drugs or steroids, or anything <u>not</u> prescribed by their doctor?	❏	❏	
20. Had sexual contact with anyone who has hemophilia or has used clotting factor concentrates?	❏	❏	
21. Female donors: Had sexual contact with a male who has ever had sexual contact with another male? (Males: check "I am male.")	❏	❏	❏ I am male
22. Had sexual contact with a person who has hepatitis?	❏	❏	
23. Lived with a person who has hepatitis?	❏	❏	
24. Had a tattoo?	❏	❏	
25. Had ear or body piercing?	❏	❏	
26. Had or been treated for syphilis or gonorrhea?	❏	❏	
27. Been in juvenile detention, lockup, jail, or prison for more than 72 hours?	❏	❏	
In the past 3 years have you			
28. Been outside the United States or Canada?	❏	❏	
From 1980 through 1996,			
29. Did you spend time that adds up to three (3) months or more in the United Kingdom? (Review list of countries in the U.K.)	❏	❏	
30. Were you a member of the U.S. military, a civilian military employee, or a dependent of a member of the U.S. military?	❏	❏	

Fig. 12-2 Donor History Questionnaire (version 1.3, May 2008). (Courtesy AABB, Bethesda, Md.)   *Continued*

		Yes	No
From 1980 to the present, did you			
31.	Spend time that adds up to five (5) years or more in Europe? (Review list of countries in Europe.)	❑	❑
32.	Receive a blood transfusion in the United Kingdom or France? (Review list of countries in the U.K.)	❑	❑
From 1977 to the present, have you			
33.	Received money, drugs, or other payment for sex?	❑	❑
34.	Male donors: had sexual contact with another male, even once? (Females: check "I am female.")	❑	❑
Have you **EVER**			
35.	Had a positive test for the HIV/AIDS virus?	❑	❑
36.	Used needles to take drugs, steroids, or anything <u>not</u> prescribed by your doctor?	❑	❑
37.	Used clotting factor concentrates?	❑	❑
38.	Had hepatitis?	❑	❑
39.	Had malaria?	❑	❑
40.	Had Chagas' disease?	❑	❑
41.	Had babesiosis?	❑	❑
42.	Received a dura mater (or brain covering) graft?	❑	❑
43.	Had any type of cancer, including leukemia?	❑	❑
44.	Had any problems with your heart or lungs?	❑	❑
45.	Had a bleeding condition or a blood disease?	❑	❑
46.	Had sexual contact with anyone who was born in or lived in Africa?	❑	❑
47.	Been in Africa?	❑	❑
48.	Have any of your relatives had Creutzfeldt-Jakob disease?	❑	❑

For question 34: ❑ I am female

Use this area for additional questions	Yes	No

Fig. 12-2, cont'd

Deferring donors for any reason should be handled tactfully. Donors should be provided with a full explanation of the reason for the deferral and information on whether they can donate in the future.

Questions for Protection of the Recipient

Donors are thoroughly questioned regarding possible exposure to diseases that could be transmitted through the blood supply. Medications, vaccinations, and high-risk activities are carefully evaluated to protect recipients of blood transfusions from risks. The list of donor questions in this category is updated frequently to reflect current knowledge of blood-borne pathogen and medication issues.

Although viral marker testing has increased the safety of the blood supply, questions to determine potential exposure to certain transmissible diseases are also necessary. Many viral markers may be below detectable limits on donation, and an available screening test may not currently exist for some blood-borne diseases, such as malaria or Creutzfeldt-Jakob disease (CJD). Questions regarding potential exposure through travel may be the only method to prevent transmission through the blood supply.

Transmissible spongiform encephalopathies are degenerative brain disorders caused by prions, which are believed to be infectious proteins. Two forms of transmissible spongiform encephalopathies include classic CJD and variant Creutzfeldt-Jakob disease (vCJD). Both forms are potentially transmitted by blood transfusion. Because there are no current tests to screen donors, donor history questions are critical to avoid transmission. Current deferral criteria for vCJD and CJD as directed by the FDA can be found on the Web.[5] The FDA document outlines the research and current restrictions regarding residing in the United Kingdom, France, and Europe. In addition, receipt of human pituitary growth hormone, history of familial CJD, or dura mater transplant has been associated with transmission of CJD.

TABLE 12-2	Deferral Periods for Potential Transfusion-Transmitted Infections
INFECTIOUS DISEASE	**HEALTH HISTORY DEFERRAL**
Malaria (*Plasmodium* spp.)	History of malaria: 3 years Lived in endemic country for 5 consecutive years: 3 years from departure Travel to endemic area: defer for 1 year from departure
Babesiosis *(Babesia microti)*	History of babesiosis: indefinite deferral
Chagas disease *(Trypanosoma cruzi)*	History of Chagas disease: indefinite deferral
Leishmaniasis	Travel to Iraq: defer for 1 year from departure
vCJD	Indefinite deferral by geographic regions: Lived ≥3 months in United Kingdom from 1980-1996 Lived ≥5 years in Europe from 1980 to present
CJD	Family history of CJD, dura mater transplant, human pituitary-derived growth hormone: indefinite deferral

Data from Roback JD, editor: *Technological manual,* ed 17, Bethesda, MD, 2011, AABB.
CJD, Creutzfeldt-Jakob disease; *vCJD,* variant Creutzfeldt-Jakob disease.

TABLE 12-3	Medications Commonly Accepted for Blood Donation

- Hypnotics used at bedtime
- Blood pressure medications (if patient is free of side effects and cardiovascular symptoms)
- Over-the-counter bronchodilators
- Decongestants
- Oral contraceptives
- Replacement hormones
- Weight-reduction drugs
- Mild analgesics
- Vitamins
- Tetracyclines and other antibiotics taken for acne

Malaria, Chagas disease, leishmaniasis, and babesiosis are parasitic infections that can be transmitted through transfusion. Malaria is caused by several species of the protozoan genus *Plasmodium.* Chagas disease is endemic in South and Central America and is caused by the parasite *Trypanosoma cruzi. Leishmania* species are transmitted by the sandfly (*Phlebotomus* species) and have been reportedly found in personnel stationed in Iraq. Infected deer ticks in the northeastern United States can spread the parasite *Babesia microti,* which causes babesiosis. An important method of screening for these diseases is by questioning donors regarding travel or immigration from endemic areas. A summary of deferrals related to travel is presented in Table 12-2.

Certain medications may cause deferrals based on the nature of the disease process for which they are being used, not because of the drug's properties. Antibiotics, anticonvulsants, anticoagulants, insulin, and antiarrhythmic drugs are prescribed for conditions that generally exclude donors. Medications such as finasteride (Proscar), dutasteride (Avodart), isotretinoin (Accutane), etretinate (Tegison), and acitretin (Soriatane) can cause birth defects if in a high enough level and transfused to a pregnant woman. Aspirin and aspirin-containing medications inhibit platelet function. For this reason, donors who are the only source of platelets for a patient (e.g., apheresis donors) are deferred for 2 days. Commonly used medications that are acceptable for donation are listed in Table 12-3. Medications requiring deferrals are listed in Table 12-4.

Donors receiving vaccinations that are prepared from toxoids or killed organisms do not require deferral if the donor is free of symptoms. With the exception of receiving an

TABLE 12-4   Medication Deferrals

MEDICATION	PRIMARY USE	DEFERRAL
Finasteride (Proscar)	Benign prostatic hyperplasia	1 month
Finasteride (Propecia)	Male baldness	1 month
Dutasteride (Avodart, Jalyn)	Benign prostatic hyperplasia	6 months
Isotretinoin (Accutane, Amnesteem, Claravis, Sotret)	Severe acne	1 month
Acitretin (Soriatane)	Severe psoriasis	3 years
Etretinate (Tegison)	Severe psoriasis	Permanent
Warfarin (Coumadin)	Prevention of blood clots	1 week
Bovine insulin	Diabetes	Indefinite deferral
Aspirin and piroxicam (Feldene)	Nonsteroidal antiinflammatory	2 days for platelet donors
Clopidogrel (Plavix), ticlopidine (Ticlid)	Prevention of blood clots	14 days for platelet donors
Hepatitis B immune globulin	Exposure to hepatitis B	1 year

Data from Roback JD, editor: *Technical manual,* ed 17, Bethesda, MD, 2011, AABB.

TABLE 12-5   Temporary Deferrals

DEFERRAL TIME	REASON FOR DEFERRAL
2 weeks	Measles (rubeola) vaccine Mumps vaccine Polio (oral) vaccine Typhoid (oral) vaccine Yellow fever vaccine
4 weeks	German measles (rubella) vaccine Varicella-zoster (chickenpox) vaccine
28 days	Hepatitis B vaccine
6 weeks	Conclusion of pregnancy
12 months	Tattoos or permanent makeup (unless applied by a state-regulated facility with sterile needles and ink that is not reused) Mucous membrane or skin penetration exposure to blood Sexual contact with an individual at high risk for HIV Incarceration in a correctional institution for >72 hours Completion of therapy for syphilis Transfusion of blood, components, human tissue, plasma-derived clotting factor concentrates Human diploid cell–rabies vaccine after animal bite

HIV, Human immunodeficiency virus.

intranasal live attenuated flu vaccine, the use of attenuated viral and bacterial vaccines generally necessitates a temporary deferral as indicated in Table 12-5. Recombinant vaccines such as for human papillomavirus vaccine do not require deferral. A 12-month deferral is necessary if the donor was exposed to an animal that resulted in the need for a rabies vaccination.

A 12-month deferral is necessary if a prospective donor has had a positive test for syphilis or has been treated for syphilis or gonorrhea.[6] The likelihood of transmitting syphilis through a transfusion is improbable. The potential high-risk behavior that makes transmission of other infectious diseases more likely is the main reason for deferral.

Questions regarding high-risk behavior associated with transmission of HIV are required. Donors must understand the activities that might be considered high risk, and they must be deferred if they are donating for the purpose of HIV testing. Alternate-site testing should be offered to individuals seeking HIV testing. Donors must also be informed of local requirements and policies that necessitate notification to governmental agencies of the donor's HIV status. A 12-month deferral is required for donors who have had sexual contact with anyone who:

* Has used a needle to take drugs not prescribed by a physician
* Has taken clotting factor concentrates for a bleeding problem
* Has HIV/AIDS or has had a positive test for HIV

In addition, men who have had sex with other men since 1977 are permanently deferred.[7] Women who have had sexual contact with a man who has had sex with another man are deferred for 12 months. The donor's responses to these questions could lead to additional questions or to a temporary, indefinite, or permanent deferral from donating.

PHYSICAL EXAMINATION

General Appearance

The prospective donor should appear to be in generally good health. Donors should be deferred if alcohol or drug use is suspected.

Hemoglobin or Hematocrit Determination

Blood for the hemoglobin or hematocrit test is obtained from venipuncture or finger stick. For whole blood donation, the minimum hemoglobin level is 12.5 g/dL (125 g/L) or minimum hematocrit is 38%.[8] This requirement ensures a sufficient hemoglobin level to allow the removal of a maximum of 525 mL, including samples drawn for testing without harming the donor.

The spun hematocrit is determined by centrifugation of a capillary tube filled with blood. The hemoglobin can be estimated by the use of copper sulfate ($CuSO_4$) or determined by spectrophotometric methods. The $CuSO_4$ method is based on the fact that blood dropped into a $CuSO_4$ solution becomes encased in a sac of copper proteinate and the specific gravity of the drop is not changed for about 15 seconds. If the specific gravity of the blood is higher than the specific gravity of the solution, the drop sinks within 15 seconds. If the specific gravity of the blood is less than the specific gravity of $CuSO_4$, it remains suspended or rises to the top. A specific gravity of 1.053 corresponds to a hemoglobin concentration of 12.5 g/dL. State regulations regarding the disposal of $CuSO_4$, which is an environmental and biological hazard, have restricted its use.[3]

Temperature

Body temperature should not exceed 37.5° C (99.5° F).[9] An elevated temperature could indicate a possible infection in the donor, which could pose a danger to the recipient.

Blood Pressure

There are no specific AABB requirements for **systolic blood pressure** and **diastolic blood pressure** for donors. FDA guidelines require that "systolic and diastolic blood pressures are within normal limits."[10] Previous guidelines were 180/100 mm Hg or less. The medical director establishes the normal range for each facility and the appropriate deferral when the donor does not meet the requirement.

Systolic blood pressure: contraction of the heart; the first sound heard while taking a blood pressure.

Diastolic blood pressure: filling of the heart chamber; the second sound heard while taking a blood pressure.

Pulse

For whole blood donors, there are no specific requirements in the AABB standards or by the FDA for pulse rates. The pulse should be between 50 and 100 beats per minute for source plasma donors according to FDA guidelines.[11]

Weight

AABB standards permit collection of 10.5 mL of blood per kilogram (kg) of the donor's weight for each donation.[4] Donors weighing a minimum of 110 lb (50 kg) can tolerate

TABLE 12-6	Physical Examination Requirements
CRITERIA CHECKED	**ACCEPTABLE LIMIT**
Appearance	In good health
Hemoglobin	≥12.5 g/dL (125 g/L)
Hematocrit	≥38%
Blood pressure	Normal limits (defined by medical director)
Temperature	≤37.5° C (99.5° F)
Pulse	No restrictions for whole blood donors
Weight	>100 lb (45 kg); collection adjusted to weight if <110 lb; maximum whole blood collection of 10.5 mL/kg donor weight, including samples
Age	Conform to applicable state law or >16 years

a maximum withdrawal of 525 mL, including samples drawn for processing. Donors who weigh less are not restricted from donating, but a proportionally smaller amount of blood should be removed. For example, a donor who weighs 100 lb (45 kg) can donate 473 mL. The physical examination criteria for blood donation are summarized in Table 12-6.

INFORMED CONSENT

Before donation, the donor must sign a written informed consent to allow blood to be collected and used. The donor is asked to read and sign a statement that shows an understanding of all the donor information presented, including what high-risk behaviors are included. The donor is also asked whether he or she has additional questions. The donor is informed about the infectious disease tests to be run on the blood and that he or she will be notified if testing indicates that the blood presents a risk for transmitting disease; his or her name is then placed on a list to defer future donations. If units are to be used for reasons other than transfusion, such as research, informed consent must address this as well.

SECTION 2
PHLEBOTOMY

IDENTIFICATION

The donor's identity should be confirmed at each step of the donation process. The phlebotomist is often different from the person taking the donor's health history; therefore, he or she needs to confirm the identity of the donor before beginning the venipuncture. Next, the antecubital area of both donor arms needs to be inspected. This inspection gives the phlebotomist the opportunity to select the arm with the best vein and to check for skin lesions and intravenous drug use.

BAG LABELING

The primary bag used for blood collection, all attached satellite bags, sample tubes, and the donor registration form must be labeled with a unique identification number. The label consists of both numbers and letters readable by the phlebotomist and bar codes used for computer scanning. The use of identical numbers allows the collected blood, prepared components, and blood samples used for testing to be traced back to the original donor registration record.

ARM PREPARATION AND VENIPUNCTURE

Blood is usually drawn from the antecubital area. After an appropriate vein has been selected, the skin needs to be prepared for the venipuncture. Skin cannot be sterilized, but several methods are acceptable for disinfecting the drawing site.

The venipuncture site is scrubbed with a 0.7% aqueous scrub solution of iodophor compound to remove surface dirt and bacteria and begin germicidal action. Next, a preparation solution of 10% povidone-iodine is applied beginning at the intended venipuncture site and continuing outward in a concentric spiral. The area is allowed to air dry for 30 seconds before being covered with sterile gauze. For donors sensitive to these solutions, another method should be designated by the blood bank physician, such as chlorhexidine (ChloraPrep 2%) and 70% isopropyl alcohol.[3]

> Two solutions for the preparation of the venipuncture site are iodophor compound to remove surface dirt followed by a solution of 10% povidone-iodine.

A tourniquet or blood pressure cuff inflated to 40 to 60 mm Hg makes the vein more prominent for venipuncture. A 16-gauge needle attached to a primary blood bag is inserted into a large, firm vein free of skin lesions. The usual donation time for a unit of whole blood is 8 to 12 minutes. Units requiring more than 15 minutes draw time may not be suitable for the preparation of platelets, fresh frozen plasma (FFP), or cryoprecipitated antihemophilic factor (CRYO). Frequent mixing of the blood during donation with the anticoagulant/preservative in the bag is critical to avoid blood clots and can be performed manually or with a mechanical mixing devise. A balance system or electronic scale is used to monitor the volume of blood drawn. Either before or after donation, two to four specimen tubes used for testing along with the segments are filled before the needle is removed. After the needle is removed, pressure is applied to the venipuncture site over the gauze and the arm is elevated (elbow straight). The needle is disposed of in an appropriate biohazard container.

To prevent potential contamination with epidermal cells and potential bacteria entering the donor unit, AABB standards require the use of collection containers that divert the first 10 to 20 mL of blood into a "diversion pouch" when platelet products are to be prepared from whole blood donations (Fig. 12-3).[4]

ADVERSE DONOR REACTIONS

Donors usually tolerate the donation process, but adverse reactions do occur. Most reactions are vasovagal, which may include sweating, rapid breathing, dizziness, nausea, and syncope (fainting). Whether caused by the actual loss of blood or the sight or thought of donating blood, the tourniquet and needle are removed, and immediate treatment is initiated at the first sign of a reaction. Instructions for handling donor reactions, including procedures for emergency medical treatment, must be available to the staff and part of their training. Table 12-7 summarizes possible donor reactions and appropriate treatment.[12]

POSTDONATION INSTRUCTIONS AND CARE

The donor is given postphlebotomy instructions as follows:
*   Contact the donor center if there are any concerns regarding the safety of the blood or if you believe the blood should not be transfused.
*   Avoid smoking for 30 minutes; avoid alcohol until something has been eaten.
*   Drink more fluids than usual in the next 4 hours.
*   If dizziness or fainting occurs, lie down or sit with the head between the knees.
*   Caution donors who work at certain occupations who will be returning to work immediately (involving heights, construction, or machine operators).
*   Remove the bandage after a few hours.
*   Inform the blood center if any symptoms persist.

Postdonation fluid replacement begins in the donor room. Donors should not be released until checked by a staff member. Total fluid-volume replacement is usually restored within 72 hours of donation. Iron replacement takes substantially longer; a whole blood donor must wait 56 days to be eligible to donate again.

Used for test tube sample collection following donation

Diversion pouch

Empty attached bags used for component preparation

Scale designed to indicate when bag is full

Blood bag for whole blood collection

Fig. 12-3 Diversion pouch. The sample diversion pouch automatically diverts the initial volume of whole blood into a pouch to reduce the incidence of bacterial contamination. The diverted blood is subsequently used for collection of test samples.

TABLE 12-7	Adverse Donor Reactions and Appropriate Treatment
SYMPTOMS	**TREATMENT**
Weakness, sweating, dizziness, pallor, nausea and vomiting	Remove needle and tourniquet; elevate legs above head; apply cold compresses to forehead and back of neck
Syncope (fainting)	Cold compresses on back of neck
Twitching, muscle spasms	Have donor cough
Hematoma	Apply pressure for 7-10 minutes; apply ice to area for 5 minutes
Convulsions	Call for help; prevent donor from falling from the donor chair or injuring himself or herself; ensure donor's airway is adequate
Cardiac difficulties	Begin cardiopulmonary resuscitation; call for emergency help

TABLE 12-8	Advantages and Disadvantages of Autologous Donations
ADVANTAGES	**DISADVANTAGES**
Prevention of transfusion-transmitted diseases	Inventory control
Prevention of alloimmunization	Preoperative anemia
Supplementing blood supply	Increased cost
Prevention of febrile and allergic reactions	High wastage
Reassurance of patient	Increased incidence of adverse reactions to donation

SECTION 3
SPECIAL BLOOD COLLECTION

AUTOLOGOUS DONATIONS

A voluntary donation of blood for use by the general patient population is called allogeneic. Any donation of blood reserved for the donor's own use at a later time is considered an autologous donation. Risk of disease transmission, transfusion reactions, or alloimmunization to red blood cells, platelets, white blood cells, or plasma proteins is significantly reduced. Requirements for autologous donors are significantly different from the requirements for allogeneic donors and are described in the following section. Advantages and disadvantages of autologous donations are summarized in Table 12-8.

Three general types of autologous procedures exist: preoperative collection, normovolemic hemodilution, and blood recovery. Preoperative autologous donation is the most common and necessitates careful tracking and handling to ensure units are available for surgery. Each category is summarized in the following sections.

Preoperative Collection

In preoperative collection, the blood is drawn and stored before the anticipated transfusion. This procedure is used for stable patients scheduled for surgical procedures likely to necessitate blood transfusion. It is especially useful for patients with rare antibodies that make crossmatching allogeneic units difficult or for patients whose religious beliefs do not allow allogeneic transfusions. Patients being treated for bacteremia are ineligible to be autologous donors.

The preoperative blood collection process begins with a written order from the patient's physician. Informed consent must be obtained from the patient (donor) with written notification that all test results are released to the patient's physician. Criteria for donor selection do not include high-risk questions. The collecting facility's medical director establishes guidelines concerning the autologous donor's health for donation eligibility. Donors are not restricted by age; the ability of younger patients to donate is determined more by the size of the patient. For patients weighing less than 110 lb, the volume of blood collected and the amount of anticoagulant used should be proportionately less. The patient (donor) hemoglobin concentration should be no less than 11 g/dL. The hematocrit should be no less than 33%.[4] Blood collection should be completed more than 72 hours before surgery. In addition to the routine labeling of the blood bag, the name of the donor, the identification number, the blood group, and the name of the hospital must be included.[3]

The ABO and D phenotype must be determined at the collecting facility. If the blood is transfused outside the collecting facility, infectious disease testing must be performed before shipping.[3] At a minimum, the first unit shipped within each 30-day period must be tested.[13] A repeatedly reactive viral test does not necessarily mean that the unit is destroyed as allogeneic units are. With permission of the patient's physician and the receiving facility's transfusion service, units can ship after a biohazard label has been

Fig. 12-4   A and **B,** Intraoperative cell recovery instrument. (**A** courtesy COBE Cardiovascular, Arvada, Colo. **B** with permission from Haemonetics Corp., Braintree, MA.)

affixed. Autologous units that are not used cannot be crossed over to the general inventory because they do not meet the same donation and testing requirements as allogeneic donations.

Normovolemic Hemodilution

Normovolemic hemodilution involves removing 1 or more units of blood at the beginning of surgery. The blood removed is replaced with crystalloid or colloid solutions to restore fluid volume. The blood is stored for reinfusion during or at the end of surgery. This process is sometimes referred to as acute normovolemic hemodilution.

Blood Recovery

Blood recovery is the collection and reinfusion of shed blood. A medical device is used to collect shed blood from the operative field. The process can include collecting and directly reinfusing the blood using a device that washes, filters, and concentrates it. Washing does not remove bacteria; intraoperative blood collection should not be used if the operative field has bacterial contamination. Fig. 12-4 shows an intraoperative cell recovery instrument.

DIRECTED DONATIONS

The public's concern for the safety of the blood supply led to demands from potential recipients to choose their own donors. Although no substantial evidence exists that directed donations provide safer blood than allogeneic donations, most blood centers and hospitals participate in a directed-donor program. Donor requirements and testing must meet the same criteria as allogeneic donations. The donor collection, health history, and testing requirements are the same for directed donors as for routine blood donors. Policies regarding crossover to the general patient population, determination of the ABO phenotype before collection, additional fees, and time for unit availability vary among institutions. The 56-day interval between donations may be waived with the medical director's approval.

APHERESIS

Apheresis is a category of procedures in which whole blood is removed from a donor or patient, a component is separated by mechanical means, and the remainder of the blood is returned. The following terms describe the portion that is removed and the donor requirements:

- *Leukapheresis:* white blood cells are removed

  Collection of sufficient granulocytes for a therapeutic dose requires drugs or sedimenting materials be given to the donor before collection. Donor consent to the use of these treatments is required.

- *Plateletpheresis:* platelets are removed

  At least 48 hours must elapse between donations, and donors should not undergo plateletpheresis more than twice a week or more than 24 times per year.[4] Plateletpheresis donors must have a platelet count of at least 150,000 μL before collection if the interval between donations is less than 4 weeks.

- *Plasmapheresis:* plasma is removed

  Collection of plasma by apheresis is designated as either frequent or infrequent. For an infrequent plasmapheresis program, donors do not donate more often than once every 4 weeks. The donor must weigh at least 110 lb. Plasmapheresis more often than once every 4 weeks necessitates that total plasma protein, IgG, and IgM levels be monitored at 4-month intervals.[14]

- *Red cell apheresis:* 2 units of red blood cells (RBCs) are removed

  Donors who meet certain criteria levels may have 2 units of RBCs removed by apheresis. Current FDA guidelines require donors to be larger and have higher hematocrit values than for single RBC donations.[15] For male donors, the minimum weight is 130 lb, and minimum height is 5 feet 1 inch; female donors must weigh at least 150 lb and be 5 feet 5 inches tall. Both male and female donors must also have a hematocrit of 40% or higher. Donors are also deferred for 16 weeks following a double RBC donation. Saline infusion is used to minimize volume depletion.[3]

These procedures are used with donors to collect a greater quantity of a specific component than can be obtained from single whole blood donations. The procedure in patients is used to treat various diseases (**therapeutic apheresis**); this is described in more detail in Chapter 15.

Apheresis was originally performed manually. The process involved removing a unit of whole blood, centrifuging it, removing the desired component, and returning the remaining blood before removing the next unit. At the present time, apheresis is routinely performed with a cell-separator machine (Fig. 12-5). Centrifugal force is used to separate the blood into components based on their specific gravity. The blood flows directly from the donor's arm into the centrifuge bowl, a specific component is removed, and the remainder of the blood is returned to the donor; all of this occurs within a closed system. Depending on the procedure and the equipment used, the process can take 30 minutes to 2 hours. The procedure can be performed by intermittent or continuous flow. An intermittent flow process involves one venipuncture; blood is removed, centrifuged, and returned in alternating steps. A continuous flow procedure necessitates a venipuncture in both arms; blood is removed from one arm, centrifuged, and returned in the other arm.

Therapeutic apheresis: blood is removed from a patient and the portion that might be contributing to a pathologic condition is retained; the remainder is returned along with a replacement fluid such as colloid or fresh frozen plasma.

THERAPEUTIC PHLEBOTOMY

Therapeutic phlebotomy is performed to withdraw blood from a patient for medical reasons. Although the removal of blood does not cure the disease, it can help treat the patient's symptoms. Common indications for therapeutic phlebotomy include polycythemia, hemochromatosis, and porphyrias. Blood collected from donors with hereditary hemochromatosis, which is a disorder of iron metabolism, can be put into the blood supply if the blood center meets certain FDA criteria.[3] The FDA has permitted variances regarding labeling and frequency of collection. The service to the donor for phlebotomy must be free of charge, regardless of the donor's eligibility. Donor centers that provide this service are available on the FDA website.[16]

Fig. 12-5 Example of apheresis machine.

CHAPTER SUMMARY

- Careful donor selection by trained phlebotomy personnel is the most important element in ensuring a safe blood supply.
- Criteria for acceptable blood donors are established by the FDA through the Code of Federal Regulations (CFR), guidance documents or memoranda to the industry, and AABB *Standards*.
- Registration and donor identification determine whether sufficient time has elapsed for donating and whether the donor was previously deferred.
- Donors must be informed of high-risk behavior and discouraged from donating if they have the potential of transmitting infection through the blood supply.
- Blood is not tested for certain diseases, such as malaria and Creutzfeldt-Jakob disease; therefore, questions regarding exposure and travel are important for screening purposes.
- The safety of the donor and the recipient are important elements of the screening process, which includes medical history questions and a brief physical examination to determine eligibility.
- Arm preparation to avoid contamination with bacteria involves a two-step disinfecting procedure and a "diversion pouch" for platelet collection.
- Signs of adverse donor reactions during phlebotomy, although uncommon, must be recognized and responded to quickly.
- Postdonation instructions to the donor regarding concerns about the safety of their donation, activities to avoid, and the importance of increasing fluid intake complete the donation process.
- Special donations, such as autologous, directed, apheresis, and therapeutic phlebotomy, are important donor and patient services that necessitate unique policies and procedures.

CRITICAL THINKING EXERCISES

EXERCISE 12-1

A potential donor is questioned regarding her previous medical history, and she states that she has been in Ethiopia (a malarial area) for 1 year doing Peace Corps activities. She just returned last week. Can she donate? If not, how long must she wait?

EXERCISE 12-2

A potential donor has the following results on a physical examination:

Hemoglobin: 14 g/dL
Temperature: 98.9° F
Weight: 150 lb

She states she has had aspirin for a headache that day and received hepatitis B immune globulin for a needle stick 3 months ago. Can she donate? Is there a deferral time?

EXERCISE 12-3

A 15-year-old girl would like to donate blood for her relative. She weighs 108 lb, and her temperature and hemoglobin are within acceptable limits.
1. Is she an eligible donor?
2. Are exceptions made for directed donations?
3. If she were donating for herself for a planned surgery, could she donate?
4. What are some of the issues surrounding directed donations?

EXERCISE 12-4

An 18-year-old student donated for the first time at a blood drive at his high school. Concerned that he may have contracted HIV before the donation, what instructions should he follow to prevent his unit from being transfused? Why are questions regarding HIV important even when there are tests performed to detect the virus?

EXERCISE 12-5

While scrubbing a donor's arm, the phlebotomist was distracted by another donor's reaction and did not use the second cleansing solution. What potential problems could this cause? Would it affect the donor or the recipient of those blood products?

STUDY QUESTIONS

For questions 1 through 12, determine the best course of action based on the information for potential whole blood allogeneic donors. Indicate whether you would:

    A = Accept
    TD = Temporarily defer (indicate when donor is eligible)
    PD = Permanently or indefinitely defer

1. A 28-year-old woman; 112 lb; hemoglobin, 12.5 g/dL; miscarried 2 weeks ago

2. A 56-year-old man; 168 lb; hematocrit, 44%; took aspirin 4 hours ago for arthritis pain

3. A 35-year-old woman; copper sulfate screen, blood drop sinks in 5 seconds; 115 lb; temperature, 37° C

4. A 17-year-old female high-school student; taking isotretinoin (Accutane) for acne

5. A 75-year-old male donor center volunteer; first-time blood donor; contracted hepatitis 20 years ago following surgery

6. A 22-year-old male; received tattoo while in the service 4 months ago, just before he returned from Iraq

7. A 65-year-old female; has instructions from physician to donate for upcoming surgery; had syphilis and was treated 40 years ago; hematocrit, 37%; temperature, 99° F

8. A 38-year-old male; received recombinant hepatitis B vaccine as a new employee 3 months ago

9. A 19-year-old male first-time donor; received human growth hormone 12 years ago

10. A 24-year-old female with a history of a positive test for hepatitis C from another blood center

11. A 52-year-old businessman who lived in England for 1 year in 1993

12. A 130-lb, 5 feet 1 inch female; hematocrit, 40%; would like to donate 2 units by apheresis

13. Which of the following is a cause for temporary deferral of a whole blood donor?
    a. intranasal influenza vaccine
    b. antibiotics taken for acne
    c. oral polio vaccine 4 weeks ago
    d. rubella vaccine 2 weeks ago

14. A donor with a physician's request to donate for planned surgery in 3 weeks has a hemoglobin value of 10 g/dL. She is:
    a. permitted to donate as an autologous donor
    b. deferred because of low hemoglobin
    c. permitted to donate with the approval of the blood bank's medical director
    d. permitted to donate a smaller unit of blood

15. Plateletpheresis donors cannot donate more than:
    a. twice a week
    b. 24 times a year
    c. every 48 hours
    d. all of the above

True or False

____ 16. Viral marker tests are not required on autologous blood to be used within the collection facility.

____ 17. Autologous units may be given to other patients if they are not used for the patient who donated the units.

____ 18. A unit donated therapeutically from a person with hereditary hemochromatosis cannot be used for transfusion purposes.

____ 19. Donor centers are authorized to release positive test results to their state health department if the donor signs a consent form.

____ 20. According to the FDA, prospective donors with a history of cancer are not permitted to donate blood.

REFERENCES

1. AABB Blood Donor History Questionnaire. http://www.aabb.org/resources/donation/questionnaires/Pages/dhqaabb.aspx. Accessed Dec. 2011.
2. Full-Length Donor History Questionnaire Documents, Version 1.3, May 2008. http://www.fda.gov/BiologicsBloodVaccines/BloodBloodProducts/ApprovedProducts/LicenseProductsBLAs/BloodDonorScreening/ucm164185.htm. Accessed Dec. 2011.

3. Roback JD, editor: *Technical manual*, ed 17, Bethesda, MD, 2011, AABB.

4. Carson TH: *Standards for blood banks and transfusion services*, ed 27, Bethesda, MD, 2011, AABB.

5. U.S. Food and Drug Administration: *Guidance for industry: revised preventative measures to reduce the possible risk of transmission of Creutzfeldt-Jakob disease (CJD) and variant Creutzfeldt-Jakob disease (vCJD) by blood and blood products (May 2010)*, Rockville, MD, 2010, CBER Office of Communication, Outreach and Development.

6. U.S. Food and Drug Administration: *Memorandum: clarification of FDA recommendations for donor deferral and product distribution based on the results of syphilis testing (Dec. 12, 1991)*, Rockville, MD, 1991, CBER Office of Communication, Outreach and Development.

7. U.S. Food and Drug Administration: *Memorandum: revised recommendations for the prevention of human immunodeficiency virus (HIV) transmission by blood and blood products (April 23, 1992)*, Rockville, MD, 1992, CEBR Office of Communication, Training Outreach and Development.

8. U.S. Food and Drug Administration: *Code of federal regulations*, 21 CFR 640.3(b)(3), Washington, DC, 2011, U.S. Government Printing Office (revised annually).

9. U.S. Food and Drug Administration: *Code of federal regulations*, 21 CFR 640.3(1), Washington, DC, 2011, U.S. Government Printing Office (revised annually).

10. U.S. Food and Drug Administration: *Code of federal regulations*, 21 CFR 640.3(2), Washington, DC, 2011, U.S. Government Printing Office (revised annually).

11. U.S. Food and Drug Administration: *Code of federal regulations*, 21 CFR 640.63(c), Washington, DC, 2011, U.S. Government Printing Office (revised annually).

12. Brecher ME, editor: *Technical manual*, ed 15, Bethesda, MD, 2005, AABB.

13. U.S. Food and Drug Administration: *Code of federal regulations*, 21 CFR 640.40(d).

14. U.S. Food and Drug Administration: *Code of federal regulations*, 21 CFR Part 640, Subpart G—Source Plasma, Washington, DC, 2010, U.S. Government Printing Office (revised annually).

15. U.S. Food and Drug Administration: *Guidance for industry: recommendations for collection red blood cells by automated apheresis methods (January 30, 2001: Technical Correction February 2001)*, Rockville, MD, 2001, CEBR Office of Communication, Training Outreach and Development.

16. U.S. Food and Drug Administration: *Guidance for industry: variances for blood collection from individuals with hereditary hemochromatosis (August 22, 2001)*, Rockville, MD, 2001, CEBR Office of Communication, Training Outreach and Development.

13

Testing of Donor Blood

CHAPTER OUTLINE

LEARNING OBJECTIVES

On completion of this chapter, the reader should be able to:

1. List the required tests performed on allogeneic and autologous donor blood.
2. Describe the enzyme-linked immunosorbent assay (ELISA).
3. Differentiate among sandwich, indirect, and competitive ELISA techniques.
4. Describe the principle of nucleic acid testing for testing donor blood samples.
5. Compare and contrast internal and external controls in ELISA testing.
6. Compare and contrast test sensitivity with test specificity.
7. Discuss the theory and evaluate the Western blot test as a confirmatory test.
8. Describe when cytomegalovirus screening is performed.
9. State the frequency of positive tests on blood donated for allogeneic transfusion.
10. Define look-back and the Food and Drug Administration (FDA) requirements with regard to hepatitis C virus and human immunodeficiency virus testing on blood donors.
11. State the reason for performing bacterial detection tests on plateletpheresis products.

SECTION 1

OVERVIEW OF DONOR BLOOD TESTING

The laboratory testing of donor blood follows careful donor screening as described in Chapter 12. The interview process with the prospective donor asks questions to identify a donor who may potentially be at a higher risk for exposure to infectious agents. Some of these agents, such as malaria and prions, do not have screening tests to identify exposure. Other infectious agents, such as hepatitis and human immunodeficiency virus (HIV), have blood tests that can identify donors with potential exposure. With each donation, the donor's blood undergoes testing for a battery of infectious agents to ensure the safety of the blood products. This screening process is critical to the blood transfusion process because many blood components are administered to the recipient without undergoing treatment to inactivate any infectious agent. An infectious agent in the donor's blood not detected by the screening process would directly affect the recipient.

Before the distribution of blood components, a sample of donor blood is tested using tests licensed by the Food and Drug Administration (FDA). All testing must be performed in accordance with the manufacturer's instructions following specimen and quality control requirements. Test results must be recorded and maintained to ensure traceability to a specific donor unit or blood component. Test results are confidential and cannot be released to anyone without the donor's written consent. At donation, donors sign a consent form that informs of the release of positive infectious disease test results to public health agencies if required by state or other laws.

REQUIRED TESTING ON ALLOGENEIC AND AUTOLOGOUS DONOR BLOOD

The goal of donor testing is to improve the safety of the blood supply. Tests can be divided into two categories:
1. Immunohematologic testing to determine ABO and D phenotype and antibody screen
2. Infectious disease screening

The scope and characteristics of the testing will be modified as new tests are licensed and new regulatory requirements are imposed on the blood bank industry. The testing required to be performed on allogeneic donor blood at the present time is outlined in Table 13-1.[1,2]

With an autologous donation, the intended recipient is the blood donor. Autologous donations are phenotyped for ABO and D antigens and are tested for unexpected antibodies. Blood collection facilities are not required to perform infectious disease testing on autologous blood products that are not shipped. However, many facilities perform the infectious disease testing on these donor units and attach a biohazard label if any test is positive.

SECTION 2
IMMUNOHEMATOLOGIC TESTING OF DONOR UNITS

ABO AND D PHENOTYPE

In determination of the ABO group, red cells are tested with reagent anti-A and anti-B to detect the presence of A or B antigens. Serum or plasma is tested with reagent A_1 and

TABLE 13-1   Required Donor Blood Tests

TESTING FOR	TESTING PERFORMED
RBC antigens	ABO and D phenotype
Clinically significant RBC antibodies	Antibody screen
Hepatitis	HBsAg Anti-HCV Anti-HBc HCV NAT
HIV-1/2	Anti-HIV-1/2 HIV NAT
HTLV-I/II	Anti-HTLV-I/II
Syphilis	Rapid plasma reagin or hemagglutination
WNV	WNV NAT
Trypanosoma cruzi (Chagas disease)	IgG antibody to *T. cruzi* (one-time testing for donor screening)

RBC, Red blood cell; *HBsAg,* hepatitis B surface antigen; *anti-HBc,* antibody to hepatitis B core; *anti-HCV,* antibody to hepatitis C virus; *HCV,* hepatitis C virus; *HIV,* human immunodeficiency virus; *HTLV,* human T-cell lymphotropic viruses; *WNV,* West Nile virus; *NAT,* nucleic acid test.

See Chapter 4 for a review of the ABO blood group system and testing.

B cells to detect anti-A or anti-B. Test methods used for the ABO phenotype include tube, microplate, solid phase adherence, and gel test. The results of ABO testing are compared with previous ABO results, if available. Discrepancies between red cell and serum testing or with previous ABO determinations must be resolved before labeling the donor unit.

Routine D typing for donors involves testing with reagent anti-D. If the initial D antigen typing is negative, an additional test for weak D is performed. If the initial test or the test for weak D is positive, the unit is labeled as D-positive. When tests for both D and weak D are negative, the unit is labeled as D-negative. Test methods used for the D phenotype include tube, microplate, solid phase adherence, and gel test. AABB standards mandate weak D testing on donor blood.[3]

See Chapter 5 for a review of the Rh blood group system and testing.

In donor collection facilities, ABO and D typing are often performed on automated equipment using methods such as solid phase adherence, microplate, or gel technology because of the large volume of samples tested on a daily basis.

ANTIBODY SCREEN

The antibody screen detects unexpected blood group antibodies in the donor's plasma. Anti-A and anti-B are expected antibodies and are not detected by this test. The antibodies considered most important are antibodies produced after exposure to red cells from transfusion or pregnancy. Although this test is required only on donors with a history of transfusion or pregnancy, most donor collection facilities test all donor samples rather than sort samples.

See Chapter 2 for a discussion of reagent red cells used in antibody screening methods.

The method used to perform the antibody screen should demonstrate antibodies considered clinically significant. Donor samples can be tested separately or in pools. The screening cells can be separate or pooled. Standard tube, gel technology, solid phase adherence, and microplate techniques are used in addition to automated techniques.

If a clinically significant antibody is present, the plasma and platelet components are not used for transfusion because the antibody is present in the plasma. Red blood cell (RBC) products that have not been washed, frozen, or deglycerolized contain minimal amounts of the donor's plasma. If these blood products are used for transfusion, the antibody interpretation is required on the label of the RBC component.

SECTION 3
INFECTIOUS DISEASE TESTING OF DONOR UNITS

SEROLOGIC TESTS FOR SYPHILIS

Serologic testing for syphilis has been performed on donor samples for more than 60 years. This test was the first infectious disease screening performed on blood donations. The FDA mandated donor testing for syphilis in the 1950s. Syphilis is a venereal disease caused by the spirochete *Treponema pallidum*. Although the most common method of transmission is direct sexual contact, at least one case of transmission has occurred through transfusion.[4] The routine storage of RBCs at refrigerated temperatures limits the survival of *T. pallidum*, but platelets stored at room temperature could transmit the organisms. Donated blood can be tested by various methods, including rapid plasma reagin (RPR) or hemagglutination tests.

Rapid Plasma Reagin Test

The RPR test is a common screening test, even though it is not specific for antibodies to *T. pallidum*. This test detects reagin, an antibody-like substance in the blood directed against cardiolipin, a widely distributed lipoidal antigen. Cardiolipin antibodies routinely develop in individuals who have had untreated syphilis infection; however, they may also develop after the appearance of other infections. In an RPR test, the donor's serum is placed onto a card and mixed with cardiolipin-coated charcoal particles. The particles serve as an indicator by making the antigen-antibody reaction visible.

Hemagglutination Test for *Treponema pallidum* Antibodies

Hemagglutination is performed in microtiter plates for detection of the antibodies to *T. pallidum*. The test uses fixed chicken erythrocytes sensitized with components of *T. pallidum*. Hemagglutination occurs in the presence of antibodies to *T. pallidum* and is read photometrically.[5] Hemagglutination tests for *T. pallidum* have gained wide acceptance since their emergence in the mid-1960s.[6] Automation has enhanced the value of the test by significantly reducing the time and labor needed to perform the assay.[7]

Confirmatory Testing for Syphilis

Most positive screening tests for syphilis do not indicate an active syphilis infection. Biological false-positive results are commonly observed. Hemagglutination tests are positive in previously treated individuals because of the presence of the antibodies to *T. pallidum*. If either of the syphilis screening tests is reactive, a test for the specific antibody to *T. pallidum* is performed for confirmation. Fluorescent treponemal antibody absorption is the procedure of choice. This test is used to guide the management of donors and components. The FDA has permitted the release of donor units with reactive screening test results and negative confirmatory test results, provided that test results are labeled on the donor unit.[8] A positive confirmatory test result defers the donor for at least 12 months.

PRINCIPLES OF VIRAL MARKER TESTING

Infectious disease testing involves a variety of methods. This section provides a general overview of the theory for enzyme-linked immunosorbent assay (ELISA) technology, nucleic acid testing (NAT), and chemiluminescence. These methods are viewed as the state of the art in viral marker testing and are widely used to detect viral antigens and antibodies.

Enzyme-Linked Immunosorbent Assay

ELISA technology, sometimes referred to as enzyme immunoassay (EIA), is used to detect the presence of small amounts of antigen or antibody. ELISA tests use a solid object such as a plastic bead in a tray or the well of a plastic microplate, coated with either antigen or antibody (Fig. 13-1). Although each test varies, the general principles of the test are the same. The **indirect ELISA** technique detects antibodies, whereas the **sandwich ELISA** technique detects antigen. **Competitive ELISA** can be used to detect antigen or antibody. Fig. 13-2 illustrates the principle of these ELISA techniques. Table 13-2 defines terminology commonly used in ELISA testing.

As an example of ELISA, hepatitis B surface antigen (HBsAg), a hepatitis viral marker, is detected using a bead or microplate (solid phase) coated with unlabeled antiserum against the antigen. An antibody, labeled with an enzyme, is used as an indicator of the antigen-antibody reaction. If the unknown serum contains the HBsAg, it binds to the solid phase antibody. The indicator antibody binds to the HBsAg. A substrate is added to the test, and an enzymatic color change is measured with absorbance values.

Indirect ELISA: enzyme-linked immunosorbent assay technique used to determine the presence or quantity of an antibody.

Sandwich ELISA: enzyme-linked immunosorbent assay technique used to determine the presence or quantity of an antigen.

Competitive ELISA: enzyme-linked immunosorbent assay technique used to determine the presence or quantity of an antigen or an antibody; in this test, a lower absorbance indicates detection of the marker.

✵ = Antigen or antibody on the bead or well

Fig. 13-1 Enzyme-linked immunosorbent assay methodologies. Enzyme-linked immunosorbent assay tests are performed either in a microplate well *(right)* or in a tray containing wells with beads *(left)*. The well or the bead contains the antigen or antibody that combines with the antibody or antigen being detected (if present).

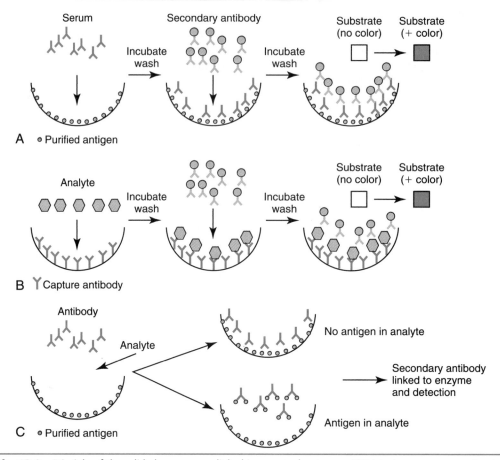

Fig. 13-2 Principle of the solid phase enzyme-linked immunosorbent assay. ELISA tests use enzyme conjugates to detect the viral marker through a colored end product that is read spectrophotometrically. **A,** Indirect ELISA. **B,** Sandwich ELISA. **C,** Competitive ELISA. (From Roback JD, editor: *Technical manual,* ed 17, Bethesda, Md, 2011, AABB.)

TABLE 13-2	Enzyme-Linked Immunosorbent Assay Test Terms and Definitions
TERM	**DEFINITION**
Internal controls	Validation materials provided with assay kit
External controls	Reagents or materials that are not part of test kit used for surveillance of test performance
Cutoff value	Absorbance value unique to each test run that determines a positive or negative result; calculated from internal controls
Conjugate	Enzyme, usually horseradish peroxidase, labeled antibody or antigen
Substrate	Color developer, usually o-phenylenediamine

Interpretation of the results obtained on completion of the sandwich or indirect ELISA test is summarized as follows:

- Specimens with absorbance values less than the cutoff value are considered nonreactive; further testing is not required.
- Specimens with absorbance values greater than or equal to the cutoff value are defined as initially reactive.
- All initially reactive tests are repeated in duplicate; if both repeat tests are negative, the sample is considered nonreactive, and the donor unit is acceptable for transfusion;

if one or both of the repeat tests are positive, the sample is considered reactive, and the unit is discarded.

- If a confirmatory test is available, it is routinely performed on tests that are positive after repeat testing.
- If a sample is repeatedly reactive, whether or not the confirmatory test is positive, the blood is not used for allogeneic transfusion.

Nucleic Acid Testing

NAT technology is based on the amplification of nucleic acids of infectious agents and identifies the presence of viral ribonucleic acid (RNA) in donor blood samples.[9] The technique requires the extraction of nucleic acid from donor plasma followed by amplification to detect the viral genetic sequences. The advantage of NAT is the detection of very low numbers of viral copies in the bloodstream before the appearance of antibodies. The possibility of detecting the virus during the serologic window period—the period from time of infection to detection of antibody in serologic laboratory assays—is enhanced with NAT technology.

These test systems were first introduced in 1999 for screening of HIV and hepatitis C virus (HCV) RNA. Plasma samples were tested in minipools of 16 to 24 donors. The sensitivity of NAT allowed for the pooling of these donors. If a minipool NAT result was negative, all donations in that pool were considered negative for HIV and HCV RNA. A positive minipool NAT result required further separation of donor plasma samples to identify the source of the positive test. Donations nonreactive on additional testing were released for transfusion. Donations that reacted positive at the individual sample level were regarded as positive for the viral nucleic acid and could not be released for transfusion.

Fully automated systems are now available for donor viral nucleic acid testing.[9] These systems use multiplex assay platforms that can detect HIV RNA, HCV RNA, and hepatitis B virus (HBV) deoxyribonucleic acid (DNA) in a single reaction chamber. The FDA has approved the systems for testing individual samples or pools of 6 to 16 donor plasma samples. The FDA requires permanent deferral for any donor who has a reactive result on NAT screen for HIV or HCV using an individual sample.

The RNA viruses routinely tested using this technology are HIV, HCV, and West Nile virus (WNV).[9,10] Testing for HBV DNA is not required by the FDA. Polymerase chain reaction (PCR) testing and transcription-mediated amplification are two examples of testing procedures using NAT. Chapter 3 describes the principle of the PCR test, and a source of information on current NAT viral marker screening for blood donors is provided in the Suggested Readings in this chapter.

> Because of its increased sensitivity, NAT has reduced the window period for detection of HIV to 9 days and detection of HCV to 7.4 days.[9]

Chemiluminescence

Chemiluminescence is the emission of light from a chemical reaction. In chemiluminescence, an excited electron state is created by a chemical treatment of the luminescent compound. When the electrons move from this "excited" or more energetic state back to their more natural "relaxed" state, they release energy in the form of light.

Chemiluminescent labels can be attached to an antigen or an antibody, depending on the assay format. The light from the label is emitted in the form of a flash lasting 1 to 5 seconds. The highest intensity is used for the measurement. The detection device for analysis is a photomultiplier tube used to detect emitted light. Chemiluminescence has the advantage of being stable, relatively nontoxic, and very sensitive. Reagent use is less than ELISA, and because the reactions are quick, turnaround time is faster.

Controls

Internal Controls

Viral marker testing is performed in donor testing facilities with "kits," which contain specific reagents for each assay, licensed by the FDA. Internal controls are the validation materials that accompany the licensed assay kit. These controls are used to demonstrate that the test was performed as expected.

External Controls

The **Clinical Laboratory Improvement Act** regulations state that a positive and a negative control must be tested with each run of patient specimens. The same rule applies to donor testing. Controls provided by a test kit manufacturer are considered calibration material if they are used to calculate the cutoff value. If the negative control from the reagent kit is used to calculate the assay cutoff, a separate negative control, external to the test kit, needs to be included. External controls are not a component of the test kit. They can be purchased separately or are developed by the institution.

External control results not within the acceptable stated range may "invalidate" ELISA testing and necessitate that all samples be retested. The FDA has issued strict guidelines regarding the interpretation of reactive test results when the testing performed is invalid because of external controls.[11]

Sensitivity and Specificity

Sensitivity is the ability of an assay to identify samples from infected individuals as positive.

$$\text{Sensitivity percentage} = \frac{100 \times \text{Number of positive individuals detected in an infected population}}{\text{Total number of infected individuals tested}}$$

Specificity is the ability of an assay to identify samples from noninfected individuals as negative.

$$\text{Specificity percentage} = \frac{100 \times \text{Number of negative individuals in a noninfected population}}{\text{Total number of infected individuals tested}}$$

To provide a safe blood supply, viral marker screening tests are designed to have the highest possible sensitivity and to detect all infected donors. Testing is not yet 100% sensitive, but it is close. Sensitivity and specificity are inversely proportional; samples from noninfected donors may occasionally give a false-positive reaction. Because of this limitation, reactive samples must be retested, and confirmatory or supplemental testing must follow.

VIRAL HEPATITIS

Hepatitis Viruses

Hepatitis is inflammation of the liver that can be caused by bacteria, drugs, alcohol, toxins, and several different viruses, including hepatitis A, B, C, D, and E. Data from the U.S. Centers for Disease Control and Prevention confirm that viral hepatitis is the leading cause of liver cancer and the most common reason for liver transplantation. An estimated 4.4 million Americans have chronic hepatitis; most do not know they are infected. About 80,000 new infections are acquired each year.[12]

The hepatitis viruses are compared in Table 13-3. Hepatitis B and hepatitis C are transfusion-transmitted diseases and are linked to development of most posttransfusion hepatitis cases. Both viruses can establish prolonged carrier states in donors with accompanying viremia and absence of symptoms.

Hepatitis A

Hepatitis A, also known as infectious hepatitis, is usually transmitted by fecal contamination and oral ingestion. The hepatitis A virus (HAV) circulates in the bloodstream only during the initial phase of infection, when an individual is usually too ill to donate; however, if blood is collected while the virus is circulating, it can be transmitted by

TABLE 13-3	Hepatitis Viruses				
	A	**B**	**C**	**D**	**E**
Transmission	Enteric; oral and fecal	Parenteral; sexual; perinatal	Parenteral; sexual; perinatal	Parenteral; sexual; perinatal	Enteric; oral and fecal
Incubation (days)	15-50	60-150	14-300	30-50	21-42
Classification	Picornavirus	Hepadnavirus	Flavivirus	Satellite	Calicivirus
Nucleic acid	RNA	DNA	RNA	RNA	RNA
Tested for	No	Yes	Yes	No	No

RNA, Ribonucleic acid; *DNA,* deoxyribonucleic acid.

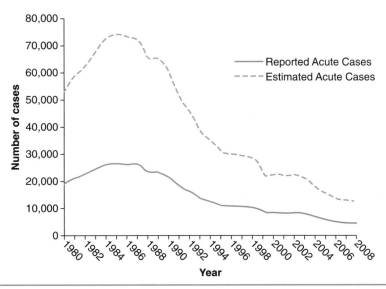

Fig. 13-3 Incidence of HBV by year in the United States, 1980-2008. (Courtesy Division of Viral Hepatitis, Centers for Disease Control and Prevention, Atlanta, Ga.)

transfusion. Because transfusion transmission is extremely rare, donated blood is not tested for hepatitis A antigen or antibody.

Hepatitis B

Originally called serum hepatitis, HBV was the first known hepatitis virus transmitted by blood transfusion. It can also be transmitted **parenterally,** by sexual contact, and **perinatally.** The rate of new HBV infections has declined by approximately 82% since 1991. The decline has been greatest among children born since 1991, when routine vaccination of children was first recommended.[12] See Fig. 13-3 for incidence of acute HBV from 1980-2008.

The serology and clinical patterns observed in hepatitis B infections are illustrated in Fig. 13-4. During HBV infection, the viral envelope material, the surface antigen or HBsAg, is detected in the blood before the antibody to the core antigen (anti-HBc) is produced. The FDA requires donor screening for both HBsAg and anti-HBc.

Hepatitis C

Posttransfusion hepatitis persisted after hepatitis B testing was implemented owing to hepatitis C virus (HCV).[13] HCV is transmitted by the same modes as HBV.

Hepatitis D

Although hepatitis D virus (HDV) is also transmitted by blood, the concurrent presence of HBV is necessary to cause disease. HDV is a defective virus found only in HBV

Parenterally: by routes other than the digestive tract, including needle stick and transfusion.

Perinatally: exposure before, during, or after the time of birth.

The window period for detection of HBV is estimated at 38 days with current testing excluding HBV DNA.[9]

Fig. 13-4   Serologic and clinical patterns observed in hepatitis B. *HBsAg,* Hepatitis B surface antigen; *anti-HBc,* antibody to hepatitis B core; *HBV,* hepatitis B virus; *HBeAg,* hepatitis B e antigen; *anti-HBe,* antibody to hepatitis B e antigen; *ALT,* alanine aminotransferase; *SGPT,* serum glutamate pyruvate transaminase. (From Hollinger FB, Dreesman GR: In Rose RN, Friedman H, editors: *Manual of clinical immunology,* ed 2, Washington, DC, 1980, American Society for Microbiology.)

carriers. Blood is not screened for HDV because testing for HBV is sufficient to avoid hepatitis D transmission.

Hepatitis E

Hepatitis E is spread in much the same way as hepatitis A, through an oral-fecal route. Therefore, donated blood is not tested.

Hepatitis G

Hepatitis G virus (HGV) is a virus that might not even cause hepatitis. HGV is an RNA virus similar to, but distinct from, HCV. The transmission routes of hepatitis G are not well known other than through infected blood products. HGV was discovered in the mid-1990s. A flavivirus similar to HCV, HGV was originally found in a person with liver disease, which associated the virus with hepatitis.

Hepatitis Tests

To prevent the transmission of hepatitis by transfusion, four tests are currently performed on donor blood: HBsAg, anti-HBc, antibody to HCV (anti-HCV), and NAT to detect the RNA of HCV. HBV DNA testing is optional.[9]

Hepatitis B Surface Antigen

Studies published in 1965 by Blumberg et al[14] described an antigen in the blood of Australian Aborigines later named HBsAg. HBV comprises intact viral particles and excess noninfectious forms of the antigen consisting of the outer surface of the virus. HBsAg is a protein on the surface of HBV. The presence of HBsAg indicates that an individual is infectious. The body normally produces antibodies to HBsAg as part of the normal immune response to infection. The period between exposure and the emergence of HBsAg is estimated at 30 to 38 days.[9] See Fig. 13-4 for the serology and clinical symptoms. Symptoms typically last several weeks but can persist for 6 months. HBsAg is the antigen used to make hepatitis B vaccine. Because of the large amount of HBsAg present, it is possible to test for the antigen directly. By the mid-1970s, donor screening for HBsAg was implemented. ELISA and chemiluminescent assays, described earlier in this chapter, are used to screen donors.

The HBsAg confirmatory assay uses the principle of specific antibody neutralization to confirm the presence of HBsAg. In the neutralization procedure, antibody to HBsAg is incubated with the donor's serum. If HBsAg is present in the serum, the antibody binds the antigen. The neutralized HBsAg is blocked from binding to the antibody-coated solid medium. If the neutralization causes the reaction to disappear or diminish by at least 50%, the original result is considered positive for HBsAg.[9]

Antibody to Hepatitis B Core

In 1986, anti-HBc and alanine aminotransferase (ALT) were added as **surrogate markers.** Anti-HBc is an antibody to the inner portion or core of the hepatitis B antigen. These antibodies generally appear after HBsAg is detected but before the manifestation of hepatitis symptoms (see Fig. 13-4). Anti-HBc can persist at detectable levels for many years after infection and has been demonstrated in individuals who have transmitted other types of hepatitis. No specific confirmatory test for anti-HBc exists. The FDA and AABB no longer require ALT testing. Anti-HBc was licensed and required by the FDA in 1991.

Surrogate markers: disease markers such as antibodies or elevations in enzymes that can be used as indicators for other potential infectious diseases; often used when direct testing is not available.

Antibody to Hepatitis C Virus

In 1989, the existence of hepatitis C was demonstrated, and a test was developed and implemented for donor screening by 1990. Antibody to hepatitis C virus (anti-HCV) is detectable by third-generation ELISAs and chemiluminescent assays approximately 10 weeks after infection.[9] After the ELISA test for anti-HCV was added to routine donor blood testing, the incidence of posttransfusion hepatitis dramatically decreased.[15]

A recombinant immunoblot assay (RIBA) is used as a supplemental test to determine the specificity of the antibody to HCV. If the ELISA test is positive, this assay uses a nitrocellulose strip to which recombinant HCV antigens have been immobilized. During incubation, the anti-HCV, if present, reacts with the bound antigen.[16] A positive test strongly correlates with infectivity and is used with the donor's clinical condition to diagnose HCV.

Nucleic Acid Testing to Detect Ribonucleic Acid of Hepatitis C Virus

In 1999, NAT for HCV RNA was implemented to screen donor blood in minipools of samples from 16 to 24 whole blood donations. Sensitive NAT techniques for HCV RNA even in pooled donor samples has reduced the window period for HCV detection to 7.4 days.[9]

HUMAN RETROVIRUSES

Retroviruses contain reverse transcriptase, which allows the virus to copy its RNA onto DNA and to integrate this DNA into the DNA of the host cell. Three subfamilies of retroviruses exist: lentivirus (HIV types 1 and 2), oncornavirus or oncovirus (human T-cell lymphotropic virus [HTLV] types I, II, and V), and spumavirus (no association with human disease).[17]

Fig. 13-5 illustrates the incidence of HIV infection in the United States. In 2009, the 50 states and 5 U.S. dependent areas estimated the rate of diagnosis of HIV infection was 17.4 per 100,000 population. The estimated rates of diagnosis of HIV infection ranged from 0.0 per 100,000 in American Samoa and the Northern Mariana Islands to 33.0 per 100,000 in Florida.[18]

Three tests are currently used as a screen for retroviruses in donated blood: antibody to HIV type 1 or type 2 (anti-HIV-1/2), NAT to detect RNA of HIV-1 and antibody to HTLV types I and II (anti-HTLV-I/II). The first donor screening test for HIV antibodies

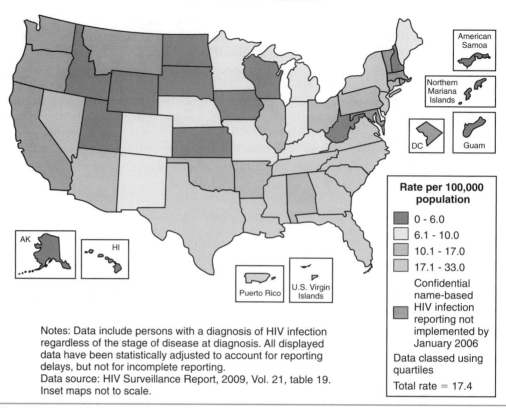

Fig. 13-5   Rates of diagnoses of HIV infection, 2009—50 states and 5 U.S. dependent areas. (From Centers for Disease Control and Prevention: *CDC HIV/AIDS.* www.cdc.gov/HIV. Accessed September 10, 2011.)

was implemented in 1985 followed by the anti-HTLV-I test in 1988. In 1992, the anti-HIV-1/2 test was licensed with improved detection of early infection and an expanded range of detection to include HIV-2. This test was closely followed in 1996 by the HIV-1 p24 antigen test. This test detected HIV-1 infection 6 days earlier than the antibody screen and reduced the window period. New anti-HTLV-I/II antibody tests expanded the detection to include HTLV-II in addition to HTLV-I in 1997-1998. As stated previously, HIV-1 NAT was initially implemented in 1999 as investigational assays and received FDA licensure in 2002.[9] Screening tests for HIV are designed to possess high sensitivity to low-titer antibody and variant forms of the virus. This assay design concept is driven by the adverse outcome of missing even one truly infected individual in the donor population.

Human Immunodeficiency Virus Types 1 and 2

HIV-1 was the first virus designated as the causative agent of acquired immunodeficiency syndrome (AIDS) in 1984. The virus infects CD4-positive T lymphocytes (helper T cells). Viremia is first detectable in plasma 10 days to 3 weeks after infection.[9] Approximately 60% of acutely infected individuals develop a flulike illness during this phase. The disease enters a clinically latent stage on appearance of HIV-1 antibodies. The long incubation period before immunosuppression symptoms appear promotes the spread of the disease by sexual contact and exposure to blood products.

A second type of HIV, HIV-2, was discovered in 1985 and also causes AIDS. This form of the virus is more common in Africa than in the United States, and it appears to produce a less severe disease. Both forms of HIV are spread by sexual contact, perinatal breast-feeding, and parenteral exposure to blood.

Testing for the antibody to HIV-1 has been included in donor blood testing since 1985. In 1992, anti-HIV-2 was added to the requirements for donor testing. Most donor collection facilities use a combination test that detects anti-HIV-1 and anti-HIV-2. Because

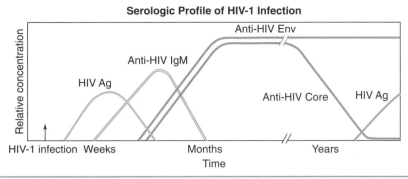

Fig. 13-6 Serologic profile of HIV-1 infection. (From Babu R: *HIV technologies ELISA and Western blot, Centers for Disease Control and Prevention.* www.cdc.gov/dls/ila/cd/india/Jan21/2.00-3.00%20Rames. Accessed September 10, 2011.)

this test detects antibody, a 22- to 25-day window exists between the time a person is infected and the time the antibody is measurable.[19]

Nucleic Acid Testing for Ribonucleic Acid of Human Immunodeficiency Virus Type 1

In 1999, NAT for the RNA of HIV antigen type 1 was added to the test for anti-HIV required on all donor blood. The FDA and AABB no longer require HIV-1-antigen testing as long as licensed HIV-1 NAT is in place. With its increased sensitivity, the implementation of HIV NAT for donor testing has reduced the window period for HIV to 9 days.[9] The HIV NAT has also reduced the number of false-positive tests with increased test specificity. A serologic profile of HIV-1 infection is presented in Fig. 13-6.[20]

Human T-Lymphotropic Virus Types I and II

HTLV-I has been associated with adult T-cell leukemia, a rare neoplasm, and tropical spastic paraparesis and HTLV-I–associated myelopathy, a semiprogressive neurologic disease.[21,22] The first reported patients with HTLV-II infections showed an atypical T-cell variant of hairy cell leukemia. At the present time, HTLV-II is assumed to be associated with large granular lymphocyte leukemia[23] and leukopenic chronic T-cell leukemia.[24] HTLV-I and HTLV-II are transmitted through cellular blood products, breast milk, sexual contact, and contaminated needles.

In 1997, the requirement to test for antibody to HTLV-II was added to the requirement to test for antibody to HTLV-I. The two are combined into one assay.

Western Blotting

The Western blot is the most common confirmatory test for both anti-HIV-1/2 and anti-HTLV-I/II. Viral antigen is separated into bands according to molecular weight by polyacrylamide gel electrophoresis in the presence of sodium dodecyl sulfate.[25] The separated bands are transferred to nitrocellulose membrane strips by blotting. Antibodies in the test serum are tested for reaction with the individual protein bands (antigen) on the strips. Enzyme-labeled conjugate detects the antibodies bound to the specific proteins on the strip. The pattern of distinct bands is visually compared with a strip that has been tested for reaction with a specimen containing antibodies to *all* HIV proteins. Each licensed Western blot has specific interpretation criteria. For example, a sample is defined as anti-HIV-positive if at least two of the following bands are present: p24, gp41, and gp120/160 in current FDA and Centers for Disease Control and Prevention criteria. No bands are present in negative Western blot results. Samples producing band patterns that do not fit the criteria for positivity are classified as indeterminate. See Fig. 13-7 for the details of the HIV-1 proteins and glycoproteins.[20] Fig. 13-8 demonstrates the Western blot banding results for HIV-1 proteins and glycoproteins.[20]

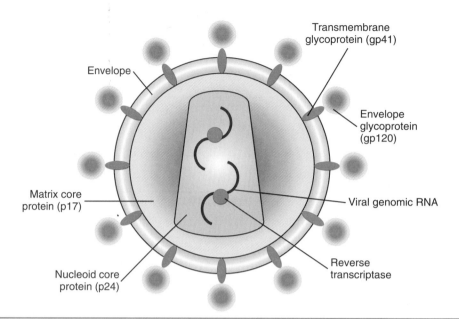

Fig. 13-7 Structure of HIV-1 virus particle. (From Babu R: *HIV technologies ELISA and Western blot, Centers for Disease Control and Prevention.* www.cdc.gov/dls/ila/cd/india/Jan21/2.00-3.00%20Rames. Accessed September 10, 2011.)

Fig. 13-8 Western blot banding of HIV-1 proteins and glycoproteins. Certain band patterns that represent specific antibodies must be present for confirmation of HIV-1. If a definite band pattern does not exist, the sample is indeterminate. (From Babu R: *HIV technologies ELISA and Western blot, Centers for Disease Control and Prevention.* www.cdc.gov/dls/ila/cd/india/Jan21/2.00-3.00%20Rames. Accessed September 10, 2011.)

WEST NILE VIRUS

WNV is a mosquito-borne flavivirus that manifests symptoms ranging from a mild febrile illness to encephalitis, coma, and death. Before 2002, the human infection was generally believed to occur via infected mosquitoes. In 2002, transfusion transmission was identified as the cause of WNV infection in at least 21 people. The persistent low-level transmission of WNV by transfusion continued in 2003 and led to the implementation of nationwide donor screening for WNV using NAT in 2003.[9] In 2009, the FDA recommended NAT testing of individual donations rather than minipools at times of increased geographic WNV activity. Donor blood screening for WNV has improved blood safety.

RECIPIENT TRACING (LOOK-BACK)

Look-back constitutes a series of actions taken by a blood establishment when donor test results indicate infection with hepatitis, HIV, HTLV, or WNV. These steps are performed on prior donations from that donor. These prior blood products were possibly donated during the window period of infection when screening tests were negative, but infectious agent was present in the donor's blood.

Look-back activities within the blood collection facility may include the following actions[26]:

* Quarantine of prior collections from that donor that remain in inventory
* Notification of facilities (e.g., hospitals, clinics) that received these products to quarantine prior collections
* Further testing of the donor
* Destruction or relabeling of potentially infectious prior collections
* Notification of transfusion recipients who received human blood or blood components from the donor, when appropriate

Responsibilities of the transfusion service in the look-back process are as follows:

* Process to identify recipients, if appropriate, of blood or components from donors subsequently found to have, or be at risk for, relevant transfusion-transmitted infections
* Notification, if appropriate, of the recipient's physician or recipient as specified in FDA regulations and recommendations[3]

> **Look-back:** identification of persons who have received seronegative or untested blood from a donor subsequently found to be positive for disease markers.

ADDITIONAL TESTS PERFORMED ON DONOR BLOOD

Cytomegalovirus

Cytomegalovirus (CMV) is a widespread infection that can be transmitted through transfusion. Transmission occurs through the transfusion of intact white cells contained in cellular blood components. In most individuals, CMV infection is asymptomatic, but mononucleosis-like symptoms are occasionally reported. For immunosuppressed patients, including premature infants, exposure to CMV may cause motor disabilities, mental retardation, and even death. In addition, CMV-seronegative recipients of organ or hematopoietic cell transplants are also at increased risk of transfusion-transmitted CMV infection.[9]

Tests to detect antibody to CMV are not required for blood donors and are usually performed only on a portion of the blood collected. Units that test negative for CMV are set aside for intrauterine transfusion or blood replacement for premature infants and immunocompromised adults. CMV testing for antibodies can be performed by ELISA, latex agglutination, or hemagglutination.

CMV-reduced-risk blood products can also be achieved by leukocyte reduction because the virus resides within intact white cells. The estimated transmission of CMV by antibody negative is 1% to 2% compared with a 2% to 3% risk with leukocyte reduction.[9]

Chagas Disease

Chagas disease, or American trypanosomiasis, is a disease endemic in Central and South America caused by the protozoan parasite *Trypanosoma cruzi*. Infection usually results after contact with feces of infected reduviid bugs. Transmission is also possible by transfusion. Infected individuals can experience severe heart or intestinal problems, which usually occur many years after the initial infection.

Because cases of transfusion-transmitted Chagas disease have been reported in the United States, some blood collection facilities with many immigrants from endemic areas perform an ELISA or chemiluminescent assay test to detect the antibodies to *T. cruzi*. The test is approved for screening donors of whole blood, plasma, and serum samples for cell, organ, and tissue donors (heart-beating).[27] In response to the availability of a licensed test, multiple large blood-collecting facilities implemented testing in 2007. The rarity of donor seroconversion in the United States prompted one-time testing of blood donors. In 2010, the FDA issued guidance that recommends one-time donor screening for *T. cruzi*.

Testing for Bacterial Contamination of Blood Components

In March 2004, the AABB added a new testing requirement for bacterial contamination in apheresis platelets and platelet concentrates. This requirement was implemented because bacterial contamination is an important cause of transfusion morbidity and mortality. This testing is performed on the blood products rather than on the donor blood samples. Despite careful attention to phlebotomy techniques, blood processing, and storage requirements, it is impossible to eliminate the possible contamination with microbial organisms. Bacteria originating from the donor during phlebotomy or an unsuspected bacteremia can multiply more readily in blood components stored at room temperature.

Platelet components are stored at 20° C to 24° C to maintain their viability and function. These products provide an excellent environment for the growth of any bacteria. Normal skin flora account for the most common source of contamination isolated from platelet components. Severe transfusion reactions from bacterial contamination include fever, shock, and disseminated intravascular coagulation. Bacteria proliferate to a lesser extent in refrigerated RBCs.

Blood collection facilities have implemented two measures for the reduction of bacteria in blood components at the time of collection. Careful attention in the preparation of the donor's arm before blood collection serves as an important check in the prevention of contamination. Another prevention measure diverts the first few milliliters of donor blood after phlebotomy into a pouch attached to the donor collection bag.

AABB standards require a check for bacteria detection in platelet components by an FDA-approved method.[3] These methods require time for bacterial detection after platelet collection. The most commonly used culture system in the United States is the BacT/ALERT (bioMerieux, Marcy L'Etolie, France).[9] This system screens apheresis platelets and requires that platelet components be stored for 24 hours before sampling. If negative culture results are obtained at 12 hours and 24 hours, the component is released for transfusion. If cultures become positive after 24 hours, the blood center should recall the unit. Positive cultures should be processed for identification of the organism. Donors should be notified if positive results are unrelated to skin contaminants.

CHAPTER SUMMARY

Testing performed on blood samples from volunteer donors has increased from one viral test to nine tests within the last 20 years. These tests are also more specific and sensitive in detecting hepatitis, HIV, and HTLV diseases that could potentially be spread by transfusion. However, the safety of the blood supply continues to be a serious concern, and new testing methods and disease markers may be added in the future. The incorporation of NAT technology for HIV and HCV detection has increased the ability to detect recently infected donors and decreased the window period. The following table summarizes the donor disease marker testing requirements currently mandated by regulatory agencies including the confirmatory testing.

Donor Disease Marker Testing

Disease	Marker Detected	Test Method	Confirmatory Test
Hepatitis B	HBsAg IgG and IgM Anti-HBc	ELISA or ChLIA ELISA or ChLIA	Neutralization
Hepatitis C	IgG Anti-HCV HCV RNA	ELISA or ChLIA NAT	RIBA
HIV	IgG and IgM Anti–HIV-1/2 HIV RNA	ELISA or ChLIA NAT	Western blot or IFA
HTLV	IgG Anti–HTLV-I/II	ELISA or ChLIA	Immunoblot or IFA
Syphilis	Nontreponemal test or IgG/IgM Anti-*T. pallidum*	RPR or hemagglutination	*T. pallidum* antigen– specific IFA
West Nile	WNV RNA	NAT	
Chagas	IgG antibody to *T. cruzi*	ELISA or ChLIA	RIPA

HBsAg, Hepatitis B surface antigen; *Anti-HCV*, antibody to hepatitis C virus; *Anti-HBc*, antibody to hepatitis B core; *RIBA*, recombinant immunoblot assay; *HIV*, human immunodeficiency virus; *HTLV*, human T-cell lymphotropic virus; *RPR*, rapid plasma reagin; *NAT*, nucleic acid test; *WNV*, West Nile virus; *RIPA*, radioimmunoprecipitation assay; *IFA*, immunofluorescence assay; *ChLIA*, chemiluminescent assay; *ELISA*, enzyme-linked immunosorbent assay.

CRITICAL THINKING EXERCISES

EXERCISE 13-1

A test for the HIV-1/2 antibody contains an external control that did not fall into the range required. What is the correct procedure for this problem? Why are external controls tested?

EXERCISE 13-2

A donor's sample tests positive with the hemagglutination test for syphilis. The confirmatory test is negative, and the donor's history indicates no high-risk behavior. The donor is 68 years old and donating an autologous unit for surgery. Can this autologous unit be used?

EXERCISE 13-3

On completion of hepatitis testing using the ELISA procedure, an acid is added to stop the color development of the conjugate-substrate. On this particular day, a power failure results in equipment downtime, causing a delay. The acid is not added until 10 minutes past the allowable time. How might a delay in the addition of the acid affect the test results?

EXERCISE 13-4

A donor is identified with an anti-Le[a] in her serum. Can this donor's plasma be used for transfusion, or should it be discarded?

EXERCISE 13-5

Previous testing on a donor's computer record indicates CMV–antibody negative. The most recent donation demonstrates that antibodies are currently present. Can the donor still donate? Why has the CMV antibody test result changed? What patients require the transfusion of CMV-reduced-risk blood products? What alternatives exist in the provision of CMV antibody–negative blood?

STUDY QUESTIONS

1. Which disease has the highest potential for transmission through a transfusion?
   a. AIDS
   b. syphilis
   c. CMV
   d. hepatitis

2. Syphilis tests on donors are usually performed by which method or methods?
   a. RPR
   b. Venereal Disease Research Laboratory
   c. hemagglutination
   d. both a and c

3. HTLV-I/II is:
   a. transmissible by contaminated needles
   b. an oncornavirus
   c. found in patients with tropical spastic paraparesis
   d. associated with adult T-cell leukemia
   e. all of the above

4. The marker that demonstrates a previous exposure to hepatitis B that remains in convalescence is:
   a. anti-HCV
   b. anti-HBc
   c. anti-HAV
   d. HBsAg

5. Which of the following is the confirmatory test for a positive anti-HIV screen?
   a. Western blot
   b. RIBA
   c. PCR
   d. Southern blot

6. Which of the following conditions requires a thorough donor history because it is not a routinely tested disease?
   a. syphilis
   b. Creutzfeldt-Jakob disease
   c. hepatitis C
   d. HTLV-I

7. HAV transmission through a blood transfusion is unusual because it is:
   a. transmitted enterically
   b. an acute hepatitis
   c. not infective after 2 weeks
   d. all of the above

8. A donor who is positive for HBsAg is:
   a. temporarily deferred
   b. permanently deferred
   c. deferred if the antibody to HBc is also present
   d. deferred if ALT is elevated

9. Which of the following was a surrogate test for hepatitis that is no longer required?
   a. ALT
   b. CMV
   c. anti-HBc
   d. HBsAg

10. In a _____, a lower absorbance value indicates the detection of the viral marker.
    a. RIBA
    b. sandwich ELISA
    c. competitive ELISA
    d. Western blot

REFERENCES

1. AABB/America's Blood Centers/American Red Cross: *Circular of information for the use of human blood and blood components*, May 2011.
2. Food and Drug Administration: *Memorandum: West Nile Virus final guidance*, Rockville, MD, June 23, 2005, FDA.
3. Carson TH: *Standards for blood banks and transfusion services*, ed 27, Bethesda, MD, 2011, AABB.
4. Chambers RW, Foley HT, Schmidt PJ: Transmission of syphilis by fresh blood components, *Transfusion* 9:32, 1969.
5. Olympus PK-TP System: *Product insert*, Irving, Texas, 1990, Olympus.
6. Rathlev T: Hemagglutination tests utilizing antigens from pathogenic and apathogenic *Treponema pallidum*, World Health Organization Document Venereal Disease Testing/RES 77.65, 1965.

7. Cox PM, Logan LC, Norins LC: Automated quantitative microhemagglutination assay for *Treponema pallidum* antibodies, *Appl Microbiol* 18:485, 1969.
8. Code of Federal Regulations. *Title 21, CFR Parts 211 and 610.* Washington, DC, 2011, U.S. Government Printing Office (revised annually).
9. Roback JD, editor: *Technical manual*, ed 17, Bethesda, MD, 2011, AABB.
10. AABB: *Association bulletin No. 99-3: NAT implementation*, Bethesda, MD, February 8, 1999, AABB.
11. Food and Drug Administration: *Memorandum: Recommendations for the invalidation of test results when using licensed viral marker assays to screen donors*, Rockville, MD, January 3, 1994, Congressional and Consumer Affairs.
12. Centers for Disease Control and Prevention: *CDC viral hepatitis.* http://www.cdc.gov/hepatitis. Accessed September 10, 2011.
13. Smith DM, Dodd RY, editors: *Transfusion transmitted infections*, Chicago, 1991, American Association of Clinical Pathologists.
14. Blumberg BS, Alter HJ, Visnich S: A "new" antigen in leukemia sera, *JAMA* 191:541, 1965.
15. Busch MP: Let's look at human immunodeficiency virus look-back before leaping into hepatitis C virus look-back, *Transfusion* 31:655, 1991.
16. CHIRON/RIBA/HCV 3.0 Strip Immunoblot Assay (SIA): Product insert, Emeryville, CA, 1995, Chiron Corporation.
17. Murray PR, Kobayashi GS, Pfaller MA, et al: *Medical microbiology*, ed 3, St Louis, 1997, Mosby.
18. Centers for Disease Control and Prevention: *CDC HIV/AIDS.* www.cdc.gov/HIV. Accessed September 10, 2011.
19. Busch MP, Lee LL, Satten GA, et al: Time course of detection of viral and serologic markers preceding human immunodeficiency virus type 1 seroconversion: implications for screening of blood and tissue donors, *Transfusion* 35:91, 1995.
20. Babu R: *HIV technologies ELISA and Western blot, Centers for Disease Control and Prevention.* www.cdc.gov/dls/ila/cd/india/Jan21/2.00-3.00%20Rames. Accessed September 10, 2011.
21. McFarlin DE, Blattner WA: Non-AIDS retroviral infections in humans, *Annu Rev Med* 42:97, 1991.
22. Janssen RS, Kaplan JE, Khabbaz RF, et al: HTLV-I-associated myelopathy/tropical spastic paraparesis in the United States, *Neurology* 41:1355, 1991.
23. Loughran TP Jr, Coyle T, Sherman MP, et al: Detection of human T-cell leukemia/lymphoma virus, type II, in a patient with large granular lymphocyte leukemia, *Blood* 80:1116, 1992.
24. Sohn CC, Blayney DW, Misset JL, et al: Leukopenic chronic T cell leukemia mimicking hairy cell leukemia: association with human retroviruses, *Blood* 67:949, 1986.
25. Centers for Disease Control and Prevention: *Interpretation and use of Western blot assay for serodiagnosis of human immunodeficiency virus type 1 infection.* www.cdc.gov/mmwr/preview/mmwrhtml/00001431.htm. Accessed September 11, 2011.
26. Food and Drug Administration: *Guidance for industry: nucleic acid testing (NAT) for human immunodeficiency virus type 1 (HIV-1) and hepatitis C virus (HCV): testing, product disposition, and donor deferral and reentry*, July 2005, CBER.
27. AABB: *Association bulletin No. 06-08: Information concerning the implementation of a licensed test for antibodies to Trypanosoma cruzi*, Bethesda, MD, December 14, 2006, AABB.

SUGGESTED READINGS

AABB, Government/Regulatory Affairs: *Donor screening and testing.* http://www.aabb.org/resources/governmentregulatory/. Accessed September 10, 2011.

14

Blood Component Preparation and Therapy

CHAPTER OUTLINE

LEARNING OBJECTIVES

On completion of this chapter, the reader should be able to:

1. Explain the benefits of component separation.
2. Define storage lesion, and list the elements that change during blood storage.
3. Compare anticoagulant and preservative solutions with regard to expiration and content.
4. Illustrate the steps in blood component preparation.
5. Given certain clinical conditions, state the blood component most appropriate for the patient's transfusion needs.
6. State the storage temperature and storage limits for each blood component.

7. Given laboratory quality control test measurements, determine which component products meet acceptable AABB standards and Food and Drug Administration (FDA) guidelines.
8. Explain the intent and activities of the FDA in regulating blood component preparation, storage, and distribution.
9. List the International Society of Blood Transfusion (ISBT 128) labeling requirements common to all blood components.
10. Discuss the importance of monitored storage equipment for blood components and the alarm requirements.
11. Describe essential aspects of safe blood administration.

Whole blood: blood collected from a donor before separation into its components.

Components: parts of whole blood that can be separated by centrifugation; consists of Red Blood Cells (RBCs), Plasma, Cryoprecipitated Antihemophilic Factor (AHF), and Platelets.

Hemotherapy: treatment of a disease or condition by the use of blood or blood derivatives.

The separation of **whole blood** into its parts, or **components,** allows for optimal storage of each part and the ability to provide appropriate therapy for patients. Each unit of whole blood can be separated into several components that can be transfused into patients, depending on their medical requirements. The separation of blood into components maximizes a limited resource and allows for a method of transfusing patients who require a large amount of a specific blood component. The availability of blood components permits patients to receive specific **hemotherapy** that is more effective and usually safer than the use of whole blood.

The primary goal of facilities that prepare components is to provide a product of optimal benefit to the recipient. All staff involved in the collection, testing, separation,

Fig. 14-1 Blood collection bags. **A,** Quad-bag system. **B,** Triple-bag system.

labeling, storage, and distribution of blood and blood components must have an understanding of and adherence to Food and Drug Administration (FDA) **current good manufacturing practices** (cGMPs). Regulations regarding cGMPs and blood product manufacture can be found in the FDA *Code of Federal Regulations*[1,2] and are written to optimize the "safety, purity, and potency" of blood products. cGMPs are outlined in Chapter 16.

This chapter describes the preparation, labeling, and storage of blood components. A summary of the clinical indications for each component and general administration policies are also reviewed. Transfusion therapy specific for certain diseases and treatments are described in more detail in Chapter 15. The component names presented in this chapter reflect the International Society of Blood Transfusion (ISBT 128) terminology[3] and are used in the 27th edition of the AABB *Standards for Blood Banks and Transfusion Services*. A detailed and updated description of product codes and terminology can be found on the International Council on Commonality in Blood Banking Automation website at http://www.iccbba.org. Labeling requirements for blood products is described in more detail later in this chapter.

Current good manufacturing practices: methods used in, and the facilities or controls used for, the manufacture, processing, packing, or holding of a drug (including a blood product) to ensure that it meets safety, purity, and potency standards.

SECTION 1
BLOOD COLLECTION AND STORAGE

Blood is collected in a primary bag that contains an anticoagulant-preservative mixture. The entire blood collection set, including integrally attached satellite bags and tubing, is sterile and considered a **closed system.** Collection of blood in a closed system and using the integral satellite bags permits the maximal allowable storage time for all components. The sterile system becomes an **open system** when administration ports or other areas are exposed to air, and the allowable storage time is reduced because of potential bacterial contamination. Fig. 14-1 shows blood collection sets with integral satellite bags.

Anticoagulant-preservative solutions work together to prevent clotting and extend the storage of Red Blood Cells (RBCs). The volume of this solution in the primary collection bag is either 63 mL or 70 mL. The standard whole blood collection volume is 450 ± 45 mL for blood collected in a bag containing 63 mL of anticoagulant or 500 ± 50 mL for the larger volume bag containing 70 mL of anticoagulant-preservative. If collection is planned for less than 300 mL, the volume of anticoagulant-preservative solution should be reduced proportionately. Reducing the anticoagulant may be necessary if a unit of blood is collected from an individual weighing less than 110 lb. Fig. 14-2 shows this calculation for the proportion of anticoagulant reduction as well as the collection blood volume.

If the whole blood collection does not meet the volume requirements of the collection bag and the anticoagulant has not been adjusted, the RBCs prepared from the unit are labeled as "Red Blood Cells Low Volume." Other components such as Platelets, Fresh Frozen Plasma (FFP), and Cryoprecipitated AHF should not be prepared.[4]

Closed system: collection of blood in a sterile blood container.

Open system: collection or exposure to air through an open port that would shorten the expiration because of potential bacterial contamination.

"Red Blood Cells Low Volume" unit is defined as RBCs prepared from:
- 300 to 404 mL of whole blood collected into an anticoagulant volume calculated for 450 ± 45 mL
- 333 to 449 mL of whole blood collected into an anticoagulant volume calculated for 500 ± 50 mL

$$\frac{\text{Weight of patient}}{110\ \text{lb}} = \text{factor to use to reduce volumes (A)}$$

$$A \times 70\ \text{mL} = \text{amount of anticoagulant (B)}$$

$$70 - B = \text{amount of anticoagulant to remove}$$

$$A \times 500\ \text{mL} = \text{amount of blood that should be withdrawn}$$

Example: An 85-lb donor would yield a "factor" of .77 (A)
.77 × 70 = 54 mL anticoagulant should be used
70 − 54 = 16 mL should be removed
.77 × 500 = 385 mL blood should be drawn

Fig. 14-2   Calculation for adjusting anticoagulant and blood volume drawn. Donors who are below the acceptable weight limit can donate if the amount of blood and anticoagulant is adjusted.

Fig. 14-3   Storage lesion.

STORAGE LESION

Biochemical changes occur when blood is stored at 1° C to 6° C, which affects red cell viability and function. These changes are called the storage lesion. The biochemical changes that occur during storage of red cells are summarized in Fig. 14-3.

The purposes of the preservative solutions are to minimize the effects of the biochemical changes and to maximize the shelf life of the components. The storage limits and temperature criteria for each preservative solution are established by the FDA and are based on the blood container manufacturers' data to support that at least 75% of the original red cells be in the recipient's circulation 24 hours after transfusion, with less than 1% hemolysis.[5] Table 14-1 summarizes the function of the chemical elements in the preservative solutions.

Red cell glucose, adenosine triphosphate (ATP), and plasma pH decrease as red cells are stored. Storage also affects the level of red cell 2,3-diphosphoglycerate (2,3-DPG), which is important in the release of oxygen from hemoglobin. High levels of 2,3-DPG cause greater oxygen release, whereas lower levels increase the affinity of hemoglobin for oxygen. In red cells stored in citrate-phosphate-dextrose-adenine (CPDA-1) or additive solution, 2,3-DPG levels decrease significantly. After these cells are transfused, stored cells

TABLE 14-1	Anticoagulant-Preservative Composition: Purpose and Storage Limits

CHEMICAL	PURPOSE
Dextrose	Supports ATP generation by glycolytic pathway
Adenine	Acts as substrate for red cell ATP synthesis
Citrate	Prevents coagulation by chelating calcium, also protects red cell membrane
Sodium biphosphate	Prevents excessive decrease in pH
Mannitol	Osmotic diuretic acts as membrane stabilizer

ANTICOAGULANT/PRESERVATIVE	STORAGE LIMIT (DAYS)
CPD/citrate-phosphate-dextrose	21
CP2D/citrate-phosphate-2-dextrose	21
CPDA-1/citrate-phosphate-dextrose-adenine	35
AS-1 (Adsol); AS-5 (Nutricel)/dextrose, adenine, mannitol, saline	42
AS-3 (Optisol)/dextrose, adenine, saline, citrate	42

ATP, Adenosine triphosphate; *RBC,* Red Blood Cell.

regenerate ATP and 2,3-DPG to normal levels after about 12 to 24 hours.[5] Although the storage lesions seem significant, neonates may be the only group of patients requiring "fresh" RBC products.[6] RBC units for intrauterine transfusion and exchange transfusions are often fewer than 7 days old to maximize 2,3-DPG levels and to avoid high potassium levels and low pH.

TYPES OF ANTICOAGULANT-PRESERVATIVE SOLUTIONS

Anticoagulant-preservative solutions in the primary collection bag may be citrate-phosphate-dextrose (CPD), citrate-phosphate-2-dextrose (CP2D), or CPDA-1. Blood collected in CPD and CP2D is approved for storage for 21 days at 1° C to 6° C, whereas blood collected in CPDA-1 can be stored for 35 days at 1° C to 6° C. RBCs prepared from blood collected in CPDA-1 must have a hematocrit less than 80% to ensure sufficient plasma remains for red cell metabolism.[4] See Table 14-1 for chemical content and expiration limits of preservative solutions.

ADDITIVE SOLUTIONS

Additive solutions (AS-1, AS-3, or AS-5) are provided as an integral part of the collection bag system. After the whole blood is collected in CPD or CP2D and the plasma is separated from the RBCs, the additive "pouch" of normal saline, dextrose, and adenine is allowed to flow into the RBCs to enhance red cell survival and function. More plasma can be removed from the RBC units because the additive solution is added to maintain red cell metabolism during storage. The amount of additive solution is either 100 mL for a 450-mL whole blood collection or 110 mL for a 500-mL collection. AS-1 and AS-5 solutions contain mannitol along with saline, adenine, and dextrose. AS-3 contains additional sodium citrate and does not contain mannitol. These preservatives are designed to minimize hemolysis during storage to less than 1%.[5] The 100-mL additive solution must be added within 72 hours of the whole blood collection. In addition to extending the storage to 42 days from collection, the additive solution reduces the unit's red cell viscosity and improves the flow rate during administration because the hematocrit values of

| TABLE 14-2 | Storage Temperature, Expiration Limits, and Quality Control Requirements of Selected Blood Components |

COMPONENT	STORAGE TEMPERATURE	EXPIRATION LIMITS	QUALITY CONTROL: MINIMUM REQUIREMENTS
Whole blood	1-6° C; shipping: 1-10° C	CPD, CP2D: 21 days CPDA-1: 35 days	
RBCs	1-6° C; shipping: 1-10° C	CPD, CP2D: 21 days CPDA-1: 35 days AS-1, AS-3, AS-5: 42 days	Hematocrit: ≤80% in CPDA-1 units
Frozen RBCs	≤–65° C	10 yr	None
RBCs, deglycerolized or washed (open system)	1-6° C	24 hr	Visual hemoglobin check; method known to provide a ≥80% RBC recovery
Irradiated RBCs	1-6° C	28 days from irradiation or original outdate, whichever is first	Irradiator QC applied 2500 cGy in center of unit
RBCs leukocytes reduced	1-6° C	See above, depends on anticoagulant/ preservative	$<5 \times 10^6$ residual leukocytes and 85% of original red cells retained
Plasma, frozen within 24 hr (PF24)	≤–18° C	1 yr	None
FFP	≤–18° C ≤–65° C	1 yr 7 yr	None
FFP, PF24, thawed	1-6° C	24 hr	None
Thawed plasma	1-6° C	5 days from thawing	Not FDA licensed product
Cryoprecipitated AHF	≤–18° C	1 yr	Factor VIII: ≥80 IU and ≥150 mg fibrinogen
Pooled CRYO	20-24° C	4 hr	Factor VIII: ≥80 IU and ≥150 mg fibrinogen times number in pool
Platelets	20-24° C	5 days	$≥5.5 \times 10^{10}$ platelets in 75% of units tested; pH ≥6.2
Pooled platelets	20-24° C	4 hr	None
Apheresis platelets leukocytes reduced	20-24° C	5 days	$<5 \times 10^6$ residual leukocytes in 95% of units; $≥3 \times 10^{11}$ platelets in 75% of units tested; pH ≥6.2
Apheresis granulocytes	20-24° C	24 hr	$≥ 1 \times 10^{10}$ granulocytes in 75% of units tested

Data from *ISBT-128.* http://www.iccbba.org. Accessed February 2011; and Roback JD, editor: *Technical manual,* ed 17, Bethesda, MD, 2011, AABB. *CPD,* Citrate-phosphate-dextrose; *CP2D,* citrate-phosphate-2-dextrose; *CPDA-1,* citrate-phosphate-dextrose-adenine; *RBCs,* Red Blood Cells; *AS,* additive solution; *FFP,* Fresh Frozen Plasma; *CRYO,* Cryoprecipitated Antihemophilic Factor; *PF24,* plasma frozen within 24 hours of phlebotomy; *QC,* quality control.

these units range from 55% to 65%.[5] Table 14-2 summarizes the storage limits, expiration limits, and quality control requirements for components.

REJUVENATION SOLUTION

Although the procedure is not routine, it may be necessary to restore 2,3-DPG and ATP levels in RBC units collected in CPD or CPDA-1 during storage or up to 3 days after expiration with a solution containing pyruvate, inosine, phosphate, and adenine. The rejuvenation solution extends the expiration date for freezing or transfusing the RBC unit, which may be necessary when a rare or autologous unit is involved. Rejuvenated RBCs require washing to remove the inosine before transfusion because it may be toxic to the recipient.[7]

SECTION 2
BLOOD COMPONENT PREPARATION

The facility's inventory requirements and the drawing location usually determine the number of satellite bags or the "bag configuration" used for collecting blood from donors. The primary bag can have as many as four additional bags attached. Storage temperature and time constraints after collection also affect which components are to be prepared. For example, if platelets are to be prepared from the whole blood, the unit must not be allowed to cool below room temperature (20° C), and the platelets must be separated from the whole blood within 8 hours. If platelets are not to be separated from the whole blood, units are stored at 1° C to 6° C before component preparation.

Separation of components from the original whole blood unit is performed by centrifugation. Red cells move to the bottom because they are the heaviest component, whereas the platelets and plasma components remain on top. Variables that affect the yield of the product being prepared include speed of the centrifuge (revolutions per minute [RPM]) and length of time of centrifugation.

Each centrifuge used for preparing components is calibrated for optimal time and speed for each product made. Quality control measures are performed to evaluate the products and determine whether the centrifugation parameters are set for maximum product yield. A short centrifugation time at a low RPM is usually called a light spin, whereas a longer spin time at a higher RPM is called a heavy spin. Steps in the preparation of RBCs, FFP, Plasma, Platelets, and Cryoprecipitated AHF are outlined subsequently. This process varies according to the bag type and filter system the collection facility uses. Details regarding prestorage filtration are discussed in the sections addressing leukocyte reduction. The AABB *Technical Manual* provides detailed procedures for the preparation of blood components. Fig. 14-4 illustrates component separation.

- After the whole blood unit is centrifuged at a light spin, the platelet-rich plasma (PRP) is expressed or pushed through the attached tubing into an empty satellite bag. The RBCs remain in the original bag, and the tube between the plasma and red cells is heat sealed and cut.
- If collected in an additive system, the additive solution (AS-1, AS-3, or AS-5) is added to the RBCs. Prestorage leukocyte reduction may be performed at this step. The RBCs are sealed and split from the remaining bags and refrigerated at 1° C to 6° C.
- The PRP unit is centrifuged again at a heavy spin, which causes the platelets to sediment to the bottom of the bag. All but about 50 to 70 mL of plasma is removed from the platelets. The additional plasma that remains with the platelets is required to maintain a pH of 6.2 or higher during the storage period. The platelets are sealed and allowed to "rest" for a period of at least 1 hour before they are stored on a rotator that maintains continuous gentle agitation. Platelet concentrates are maintained at 20° C to 24° C for a maximum of 5 days.
- The plasma that had been expressed into another empty attached bag can be processed further as:
  - FFP: Plasma frozen within 8 hours of collection and stored at or below −18° C for up to 1 year or stored at or below −65° C for 7 years. FFP contains the labile coagulation factors (factors V and VII) and stable factors.[8]
  - Plasma frozen within 24 hours of phlebotomy (PF24): Contains similar coagulation factors as FFP, although factor VIII levels are reduced and factor V may be variable compared with FFP.[8] PF24 is stored at or below −18° C for up to 1 year. PF24 is referred to as FP24 in some literature.[6]
  - Recovered plasma for further manufacture, which is usually shipped to a fractionator for processing into derivatives such as albumin, immune globulin, and coagulation factor concentrates.

Light spin—short time, low RPM, yields PRP
Heavy spin—longer spin, high RPM, concentrates component

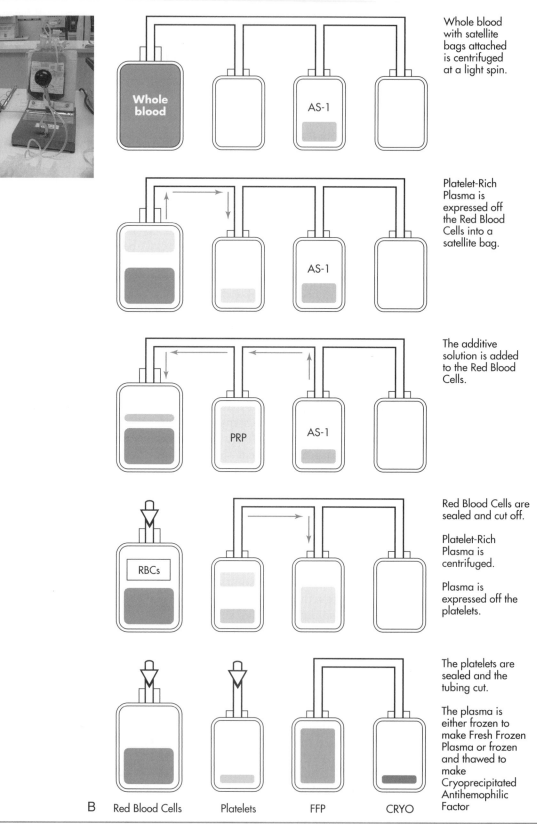

Fig. 14-4 Component production. **A,** Component equipment used to express the plasma supernatant into a satellite bag during component production. **B,** Preparation of RBCs, FFP, Cryoprecipitated AHF, and Platelets from a Whole Blood Unit. *AS,* Additive solution; *PRP,* Platelet-Rich Plasma; *RBCs,* Red Blood Cells; *FFP,* Fresh Frozen Plasma; *CRYO,* Cryoprecipitated Antihemophilic Factor. (**A,** Courtesy LifeSouth Community Blood Centers, Gainesville, Fla.)

- If FFP will be processed further into Cryoprecipitated AHF, an empty satellite bag is left attached to the FFP and frozen with it. The FFP is thawed at 1° C to 6° C. A white precipitate forms, and the plasma and satellite bag is centrifuged (heavy spin). All but about 10 to 15 mL of the supernatant plasma is expressed into the empty satellite bag. The CRYO remains in the bag that originally contained the FFP. It is relabeled as Cryoprecipitated AHF, refrozen within 1 hour of thawing, and stored at or below −18° C for up to 1 year from donation. The plasma that is expressed into the satellite bag is used as recovered plasma or prepared into "Plasma Cryoprecipitate Reduced." This plasma is refrozen at −18° C or colder and has a 12-month expiration date. It is used primarily as a replacement solution for therapeutic plasmapheresis for the treatment of thrombotic thrombocytopenic purpura.[6]

WHOLE BLOOD

Whole blood is the unmodified component, drawn from a donor, which consists of erythrocytes, leukocytes, platelets, and plasma proteins with the anticoagulant-preservative solution. Whole blood is stored in a monitored refrigerator at 1° C to 6° C for 21 days if collected in CPD or for 35 days if collected in CPDA-1. Additive solutions cannot be added to whole blood to increase the storage period.

Before development of the technology involved in blood component preparation, whole blood was the only blood product available. In the 1960s, when plastic replaced glass as the collection medium, separation of whole blood into its components became possible. Availability of whole blood declined, and whole blood was replaced with RBCs. Problems associated with whole blood transfusions include circulatory overload in patients who require only oxygen-carrying capacity from RBCs. Viable platelets are lost, and labile coagulation factors decrease within the first 24 hours of storage. Whole blood must also be ABO identical to the patient, limiting its flexibility in inventory management and in emergency situations. Therefore whole blood has a limited use in most clinical situations.[6]

Indications for Use

Whole blood is indicated for patients who are actively bleeding and who have lost more than 25% of their blood volume.[6] The use of whole blood in massively bleeding patients may limit donor exposures if given in place of RBCs and plasma. Whole blood increases the hemoglobin by about 1 g/dL or the hematocrit by about 3%. Whole blood must be ABO identical and crossmatched before administration. When whole blood is not available, RBCs administered with crystalloid solutions are usually effective in restoring both oxygen-carrying capacity and blood volume.[5] Reconstituted whole blood (RBCs reconstituted with type AB FFP from a different donor) is usually prepared for exchange transfusions in infants.

RED BLOOD CELL COMPONENTS

Indications for Use

RBCs contain hemoglobin, which transports oxygen through the bloodstream and to the tissues. RBC transfusions increase the mass of circulating red cells in situations where tissue oxygenation may be impaired by acute or chronic blood loss, such as in hemorrhage or anemia. Patients commonly requiring RBC transfusion therapy include (but are not limited to):
- Oncology patients undergoing chemotherapy or radiation therapy
- Trauma victims
- Patients undergoing cardiac, orthopedic, and other surgeries
- Patients with end-stage renal disease
- Premature infants
- Patients with sickle cell disease

The diseases and conditions that commonly necessitate component therapy are reviewed in Chapter 15. Transfusing 1 unit of RBCs usually increases the hemoglobin by about

1 g/dL and increases the hematocrit by about 3% in the average 70-kg adult. RBCs necessitate crossmatching before issue (see Chapter 8).

RBCs are often modified into additional products needed for specific patient requirements. The following section summarizes the preparation, storage, and use of leukocyte-reduced, frozen and deglycerolized, washed, and irradiated RBCs.

Red Blood Cells Leukocytes Reduced

Leukocytes remaining in RBC units have been implicated in adverse transfusion reactions and immunization to leukocyte antigens. A reaction caused by leukocytes can be extremely uncomfortable for a patient, causing shaking chills or an increase in temperature, or both, soon after initiating the RBC transfusion. In addition to the intact or fragmented membranes of the leukocytes, cytokines produced by leukocytes during RBC storage are also responsible for febrile reactions.[5] Reduction in leukocytes *before* RBC storage is optimal because it reduces the leukocyte fragments and cytokines that increase during storage. The use of leukocyte-reduced RBCs has become standard practice in many hospitals. The use of leukocyte-reduced RBCs for trauma patients, who may not benefit from these more expensive products, remains controversial.

The standard 170-μm blood filter does not remove leukocytes. White blood cell removal is best accomplished by the use of commercially available leukocyte removal or leukocyte reduction filters. Filtration can be performed by the following procedures:

- Using inline filters integral to the collection set allows blood to be filtered before storage (Fig. 14-5). The inline filter is designed to remove leukocytes from whole blood without removing platelets. This filter provides a mechanism for manufacturing both red cell and platelet products that are leukocyte reduced before storage.

Fig. 14-5 Leukocyte reduction filter. RBC units are filtered before storage at the blood center for optimal effectiveness. (Courtesy LifeSouth Community Blood Centers, Gainesville, Fla.)

Fig. 14-6   **Sterile connection device.** Applications of sterile connection devices[5]:
✓ Addition of a bag while preparing components
✓ Pooling of components
✓ Preparation of pediatric units
✓ Addition of leukocyte reduction filter
✓ Removing samples for testing

- Red cells that have been separated from the plasma can also be leukocyte reduced using inline filters. The manufacturer's instructions are followed regarding timing, priming with additive solutions, and the temperature of filtration.
- Sterile-connecting a leukocyte reduction filter to the RBCs and filtering before storage-FDA-approved sterile-connecting devices allow for the attachment of tubing from filters, from transfer pacts, and between units without creating an "open system" (Fig. 14-6).[9]
- A bedside leukocyte reduction filter can be used when the unit is transfused. This system is least optimal because standardization of leukocyte removal is difficult to attain, and leukocyte fragments and cytokines that accumulate from storage are not removed.

In addition to preventing reactions, the removal of leukocytes reduces the danger of transfusion-transmitted cytomegalovirus (CMV) because this virus resides in the cytoplasm of white blood cells.[5] The removal of leukocytes does not prevent graft-versus-host disease (GVHD), which is a serious potential transfusion reaction for immunocompromised patients and patients receiving units from blood relatives. Chapter 10 outlines these transfusion complications in more detail.

According to the AABB standards, leukocyte-reduced RBCs are prepared with a method known to retain at least 85% of the original RBCs and reduce the leukocyte number in the final component to less than 5×10^6 in each unit.[4]

Apheresis Red Blood Cells

Automated apheresis technology allows for the collection of 1 unit of RBCs and a second component such as Platelets and Plasma or 2 units of RBCs from one donor. The benefits to this method of red cell collection include the reduction of potential viral exposure to the recipient and reduction of pretransfusion viral marker testing and recruiting expenses.[5] Donor selection requirements differ from RBC collection with regard to donor weight and hematocrit and are outlined in Chapter 12. Donations can be collected every 16 weeks. Saline is used to replace the fluid lost to minimize volume depletion to the donor. The expiration date of the unit depends on the anticoagulant-preservative used. Apheresis red cells are drawn into acid-citrate-dextrose, which provides a 21-day storage limit. Depending on the instrument used, leukocyte reduction and the addition of an additive solution may be performed automatically by the instrument or manually using a sterile

Fig. 14-7   Frozen RBCs. RBCs can be frozen for 10 years at −65° C or below to preserve rare or autologous units. (Courtesy LifeSouth Community Blood Centers, Gainesville, Fla.)

connection device.[5] This step increases the outdate to 42 days. To be labeled as Apheresis Red Blood Cells Leukocytes Reduced, the method must be known to ensure a final component containing at an average hemoglobin of greater than 51 g/dL (or 153 mL red cell volume).[4] Less than 5×10^6 residual leukocytes per unit is also required.[4] The double unit is placed in the inventory as two separate units, and the indications and dosage are comparable to single units of RBCs obtained from whole blood donations.

Frozen Red Blood Cells

RBCs can be frozen for long-term preservation to maintain an inventory of rare units or extend the availability of autologous units. Freezing extends storage up to 10 years from collection when stored at or below −65° C. To prepare RBC units for freezing, glycerol is added as a **cryoprotective** agent to prevent cell dehydration and the formation of ice crystals, which causes cell hemolysis. Glycerol is slowly added to the unit for a final glycerol concentration of 40% weight per volume. The unit is transferred to a polyolefin or polyvinyl chloride bag and placed in a metal or cardboard canister to prevent breakage at low temperatures. Units can subsequently be stored at −65° C for up to 10 years from the date of collection (Fig. 14-7).[4]

Freezing can also be accomplished with a lower glycerol concentration if a liquid nitrogen freezer is used. This method is not as common for RBC storage. Glycerol concentration is approximately 20%, and the initial freezing temperature is −196° C. Maximum storage temperature is −120° C for 10 years.[4]

Deglycerolized Red Blood Cells

Frozen RBCs are thawed, and the glycerol is removed by the process of deglycerolization. After thawing in a 37° C dry warmer or water bath, the unit is washed in a series of saline solutions of decreasing osmolar solutions of saline. Saline solutions of 12% and 1.6% followed by 0.9% normal saline that contains 0.2% dextrose are used to draw the glycerol out of the cells. This process is usually performed on an instrument called a blood cell processor, which gradually adds preset saline volumes, mixes and centrifuges the cells, and removes supernatant automatically (Fig. 14-8). Because the process of glycerolization and deglycerolization involves entering the blood unit, the system is considered "open," and the product must be transfused within 24 hours. A visual check of the supernatant from the final wash is performed to ensure sufficient glycerol removal and minimal hemolysis.[5] Additional methods for quality control of Deglycerolized RBCs are explained in more detail in the AABB *Technical Manual* Method Section.

Cryoprotective: solution added to protect against cell damage that occurs at or below freezing temperatures.

Fig. 14-8 Deglycerolization process. Blood cell processor **(A)** and washed RBCs **(B)**. The blood processor is used to wash RBC and platelet components. It is also used to deglycerolize thawed RBCs. (Courtesy COBE Cardiovascular, Arvada, Colo.)

Washed Red Blood Cells

Washing RBCs with normal saline may be indicated for patients who react to the small amount of plasma proteins that remain in a unit of RBCs. Reactions can be allergic, febrile, or anaphylactic. A patient with IgA deficiency and clinically significant anti-IgA requires washed RBCs if a transfusion is necessary. Washed RBCs may also be used in infant or intrauterine transfusions.[8] Washing is accomplished with approximately 1000 mL of 0.9% saline using the automatic blood cell processor described for deglycerolizing frozen RBCs. Washing is associated with a loss of about 10% to 20% of the original RBCs and is no longer considered an effective method of removing leukocytes.

Red Blood Cells Irradiated

Viable T cells in cellular blood components may cause transfusion-associated GVHD, which is fatal in more than 90% of affected patients.[5] Factors that determine a patient's risk for transfusion-associated GVHD include whether, and to what degree, the patient is immunodeficient and the degree of similarity between donor and recipient regarding human leukocyte antigens (HLAs). Gamma irradiation of cellular blood components prevents proliferation of T cells that cause transfusion-associated GVHD. RBCs that have been leukocyte reduced by filtration do not prevent GVHD because some leukocytes remain in the final product. AABB standards require irradiation of cellular components (RBCs and platelets) if the donor unit is from a blood relative of the intended recipient or the donor unit is HLA-matched for the recipient.

Irradiation can be performed with a gamma irradiator (cesium-137 or cobalt-60 radioisotopes), linear accelerators, ultraviolet-A irradiation, and nonradioisotope equipment (x-rays). The required dose of irradiation is 2500 cGy, or 25 Gy, in the middle of the canister, and the lowest dose should be 1500 cGy. Periodic verification and documentation of dose delivery is required.[4]

Irradiation induces erythrocyte membrane damage that causes RBC units to have a higher plasma potassium level and a decrease in ATP and 2,3-DPG levels.[5] Cell activities that are not dependent on reproduction (notably platelet activation and oxygen delivery) are not significantly affected by irradiation. The expiration date of irradiated RBCs is changed to 28 days after irradiation if the available shelf life exceeds 28 days. If the irradiated cells are not given to the originally intended recipient, they can be returned to the inventory and transfused to another patient.

PLATELET COMPONENTS

Indications for Use

Normal platelet function and adequate numbers of circulating platelets are essential for hemostasis. Functions of platelets include:
- Maintenance of vascular integrity
- Initial arrest of bleeding by formation of platelet plug
- Stabilization of the hemostatic plug by contributing to the process of fibrin formation

Platelets are transfused to control or prevent bleeding associated with critically decreased circulating platelet numbers or functionally abnormal platelets.[8] Platelet transfusions are not usually effective or indicated for patients with destruction of circulating platelets caused by autoimmune disorders, such as idiopathic thrombocytopenic purpura. Patients requiring platelet transfusions typically include:
- Cancer patients undergoing chemotherapy or radiation therapy
- Recipients of hematopoietic progenitor cell transplants for a period following transplant
- Patients with postoperative bleeding

Refractory: unresponsive to platelet transfusions.

Corrected count increment: relative increase in platelet count adjusted for the number of platelets transfused and the size of the patient.

Because transfused platelets normally circulate with a life span of only 3 to 4 days, frequent transfusion support is often necessary for patients using platelets. Evaluation of the effectiveness of platelet transfusions is important in determining whether the patient is **refractory,** or unresponsive to the platelet transfusions. The **corrected count increment** (CCI), outlined in Fig. 14-9, determines the increase in platelet count adjusted for the number of platelets infused and the size of the patient.[8] Platelet counts should be

$$CCI = \frac{\textbf{posttransfusion} \text{ platelet count} - \textbf{pretransfusion} \text{ platelet count}}{\text{Number of platelets transfused (multiples of } 10^{11})} \times \textbf{BSA}$$

Example: Patient: BSA = 1.5 M^2
Precount: 2000/μL
Postcount: 29,000/μL
Platelets transfused: 4.5 × 10^{11}

$$CCI = \frac{29,000 - 2000}{4.5} \times 1.5 = 9000$$

A CCI of greater than 7500 indicates adequate platelet count increment at 10 min to 1 hr following transfusion.

To calculate the BSA, a nomogram is used. The height and weight of the patient are needed to determine the BSA.

Fig. 14-9 Platelet refractoriness and CCI. Platelet refractoriness may be due to immune or nonimmune causes. The CCI is used to calculate the effectiveness of platelet transfusions based on the number of platelets infused and the body surface area (BSA). *CCI,* Corrected count increment.

TABLE 14-3	Conditions Causing Platelet Refractoriness or Poor Response to Platelet Transfusions
Immune	
HLA alloantibodies	
Platelet alloantibodies	
Autoantibodies	
Nonimmune	
Splenomegaly	
Medications	
Sepsis	
Active bleeding	
Disseminated intravascular hemolysis (DIC)	
Fever	

performed before transfusion and within 1 hour after transfusion. In a clinically stable patient, a CCI less than 5000/μL at 10 minutes to 1 hour posttransfusion may indicate a refractory state to platelet therapy. Table 14-3 lists conditions associated with refractoriness. Platelets do not require crossmatching before issue and should be ABO compatible with the recipient's red cells whenever possible.

Platelets

Platelet concentrates prepared from a unit of whole blood, as described in the section on blood component preparation, contain at least 5.5×10^{10} platelets per unit and, under optimal conditions, should elevate the platelet count by about 5000 μL in a recipient weighing 75 kg.[5] Platelets prepared from whole blood are also referred to as random donor platelets or platelet concentrates.

Pooled Platelets

To achieve a therapeutic dose, platelet concentrates are pooled for transfusion in adults. This is accomplished by transferring the platelet concentrates into a transfer set, while being careful not to contaminate the ports. An approximate dose is 1 unit per 10 kg of patient body weight, yielding pools of 6 to 10 platelets. Because it is necessary to create an "open system" when pooling platelets, the expiration of the pooled product changes to 4 hours. The pooled platelets should be stored at 20° C to 24° C with gentle agitation until transfusion. Platelets can also be pooled using a commercial prestorage pooling bag, which maintains an expiration date of the oldest component in the pool, up to 5 days.[5]

Units selected for pooling should be type-specific or type-compatible owing to the presence of some RBCs in each unit. A unique pool number is placed on the final container, and the units' numbers in the pool must be recorded.

Apheresis Platelets

Apheresis is an effective method of harvesting a therapeutic dose of platelets from one individual donor (Fig. 14-10). During **plateletpheresis**, whole blood is collected from a donor using automated apheresis equipment, which separates whole blood into components. The platelets are retained, and the remaining elements are returned. The product is also referred to as single-donor platelets. Plateletpheresis donors may donate as often as twice a week or 24 times a year with an interval of 48 hours between procedures. A unit of platelets prepared by apheresis should contain a minimum of 3×10^{11} platelets in 90% of the sampled units, which is about the same as a pool of 5 to 6 platelets prepared from whole blood. Quality control must also include the pH, which must be greater than or equal to 6.2 at the end of the allowable storage period.[4]

Platelets display class I HLA. Class I antigens refer to the A, B, and C antigens. Platelets also demonstrate platelet antigens that can elicit an immune response from a patient receiving frequent platelet components. Patients who have developed antibodies to HLA

Apheresis: a method of blood collection where whole blood is removed from a donor or patient and separated into components; one or more of the components are retained, and the remainder is returned.

Plateletpheresis: collection of platelets by apheresis.

Fig. 14-10 Apheresis. **A,** Instrument used for apheresis procedures. **B,** Apheresis platelets. (Courtesy Baxter Healthcare Corp., Deerfield, Ill.)

or platelet antigens usually require platelets matched for HLA antigens or crossmatched to achieve satisfactory increment. Locating HLA-matched donors from previously typed HLA plateletpheresis donors requires a large donor base. Identical HLA-A and HLA-B antigen matching from unrelated donors is rare (1 in 5000 to 20,000).[5] However, less than perfect matching may be sufficient to overcome the refractory state. Chapter 1 discusses the HLA system.

Platelets Leukocytes Reduced

Leukocyte reduction can be achieved using certain apheresis devices and leukocyte reduction filters designed for bedside and prestorage filtration. Leukocyte reduction is indicated to prevent recurrent febrile nonhemolytic reactions and HLA alloimmunization for patients requiring long-term platelet support or eventual transplantation. As with leukocyte reduction in RBC products, leukocyte removal before storage also reduces cytokines and the potential febrile reactions they cause. Leukocyte-reduced platelets are also effective in preventing CMV infection.[5] Platelets collected by apheresis must have less than 5 × 10⁶ leukocytes in 95% of the units tested.[4]

PLASMA COMPONENTS

Fresh Frozen Plasma, Plasma Frozen within 24 Hours of Phlebotomy
Indications for Use

The process of coagulation involves a series of biochemical reactions that transform circulating plasma into an insoluble gel through conversion of fibrinogen to fibrin. This process requires certain plasma proteins or coagulation factors, phospholipids, and calcium. Impairment of the coagulation system can occur because of decreased synthesis of the coagulation factors or consumption of the factors. Defects in the plasma clotting factors may be due to congenital or acquired conditions.

FFP contains all the coagulation factors, including the **labile factors** V and VIII, which do not store well at temperatures greater than −18° C (Table 14-4).[5] PF24 may have reduced levels of factors V and VIII compared with FFP.[8] FFP and PF24 are indicated for the following situations[6]:

Labile factors: factors V and VIII, which are coagulation factors that deteriorate on storage.

- Management of bleeding in patients who require coagulation factors II, V, X, or XI, when the concentrates are not available or are not appropriate
- Abnormal coagulation assays resulting from massive transfusion
- Management of patients anticoagulated with warfarin who are bleeding or require emergency surgery
- Replacement solution for therapeutic plasmapheresis for the treatment of thrombotic thrombocytopenic purpura and hemolytic uremic syndrome (plasma cryoprecipitate reduced can also be used for these patients)
- Correction or prevention of bleeding complications in patients who have severe liver disease with multiple factor deficiencies
- Management of patients with disseminated intravascular coagulation when fibrinogen level is less than 100 mg/dL
- Management of patients with rare specific plasma protein deficiencies

TABLE 14-4 Coagulation Factors and Their Sources

FACTOR NAME	INDICATION	SOURCE
Factor I, fibrinogen	Fibrinogen deficiency	Fibrinogen concentrate, Cryoprecipitated AHF
Factor II, IX, X, prothrombin complex	Hemophilia B	Prothrombin Complex Concentrate
Protein C	Venous thrombosis, severe protein C deficiency	Protein C concentrate
Factor VIIa (recombinant)	Factor VII deficiency, hemophilia A or B with inhibitors	Recombinant factor VIIa concentrate
Activated prothrombin complex, factor II, IX, X (nonactivated), VII (activated)	Bleeding or prophylaxis before surgery for hemophilia A or B with inhibitors	Activated Prothrombin Complex Concentrate
Factor VIII, antihemophilic factor	Hemophilia A, von Willebrand's disease	Factor VIII concentrate, human and recombinant
Factor IX, Christmas factor	Hemophilia B	Factor IX concentrate, human and recombinant
Factor XI, plasma thromboplastin antecedent	Factor XI deficiency	Thawed plasma, FFP, PF24
Factor XIII, fibrin stabilizing factor	Factor XIII deficiency	Cryoprecipitated AHF or plasma
VWF, von Willebrand's factor	von Willebrand's disease	Factor VIII concentrate, Cryoprecipitated AHF, FFP

FFP, Fresh Frozen Plasma; *PF24,* plasma frozen within 24 hours of phlebotomy.

Units of FFP and PF24 are thawed before administration in a 30° C to 37° C water bath for approximately 30 to 45 minutes. Units should be placed in protective overwraps to prevent contamination of the administration ports or in a device that maintains the ports above water. Water baths with an agitator accelerate the thawing process. FDA-approved microwave ovens specially designed for plasma thawing also can be used by carefully following the manufacturer's instructions. Standard microwave ovens should never be used because they denature plasma proteins. After thawing, FFP is stored at 1° C to 6° C and should be transfused within 24 hours from thawing.

The dose of FFP or PF24 depends on the clinical situation and the underlying disease process. If coagulation factor replacement is necessary, the dose is 10 to 20 mL/kg (3 to 6 units in an adult).[6] Crossmatching is not necessary, but the plasma should be ABO compatible with the patient's red cells.

If not transfused within 24 hours, the product should be relabeled as "thawed plasma" and stored at 1° C to 6° C for up to 5 days after thawing. Thawed plasma should not be used for replacement of labile coagulation factor VIII. Thawed plasma is not licensed by the FDA, and the label should be modified to reflect this. Concentrations of all the coagulation factors have been shown to be comparable to FFP and clinically adequate for transfusion.[10,11]

Cryoprecipitated Antihemophilic Factor

Indications for Use

Cryoprecipitated AHF, also referred to as cryoprecipitate or CRYO, is the cold insoluble precipitate that forms when a unit of FFP is thawed between 1° C and 6° C. It contains, in a concentrated form, most of the coagulation factors that are found in FFP. These factors include:

- von Willebrand's factor (vWF), which is needed for platelet adhesion to damaged endothelium
- Fibrinogen, which is cleaved into fibrin in the presence of thrombin to form a clot
- Factor VIII, the procoagulant activity factor that is deficient in hemophilia A
- Fibronectin
- Factor XII

Once separated from FFP, CRYO is refrozen within 1 hour of preparation and stored at −18° C or colder for up to 1 year from the date of phlebotomy.

The primary clinical uses of CRYO are as a supplement for patients with deficiencies of factor XIII and fibrinogen. Because viral inactivated factor VIII concentrates are currently available for patients with hemophilia A, von Willebrand's disease, and factor VIII:C deficiency, CRYO is less commonly used for correcting or preventing bleeding in these patients. CRYO is the only concentrated fibrinogen product available and is used to treat patients with congenital or acquired fibrinogen defects. Dysfibrinogenemia, a condition in which fibrinogen is not functionally effective, is associated with severe liver disease.

> Cryoprecipitated AHF (CRYO) contains at least 150 mg of fibrinogen and 80 IU of factor VIII in each unit.

Quality control of CRYO must demonstrate greater than 150 mg of fibrinogen and 80 international units (IU) of factor VIII per unit tested. In facilities that pool CRYO before freezing, the final unit must have greater than 150 mg of fibrinogen and 80 IU of factor VIII times the number in the pool.

Plasma Cryoprecipitate Reduced

Following the removal of CRYO from FFP, the remaining plasma unit can be refrozen. The refreezing must occur within 24 hours of the thawing. The product is relabeled as "Plasma, Cryoprecipitate Reduced" and is stored at −18°C or lower for 1 year from the date of collection. The CRYO-poor plasma (CPP) is used primarily in the treatment of thrombotic thrombocytopenic purpura (TTP) because it contains ADAMTS13, the protein that is reduced in TTP. Albumin and coagulation factors II, V, VII, IX, X, and XI remain in the same concentrations as in FFP. Once thawed for use, this product has a 5-day expiration date and should be stored at 1° C to 6° C.

Cryoprecipitated Antihemophilic Factor, Pooled

Cryoprecipitated AHF is pooled into a transfer bag to achieve a therapeutic dose. The frozen units first must be thawed in a 30° C to 37° C water bath for up to 15 minutes using overwraps to prevent contamination of the ports. The contents of bags can be rinsed with 10 to 15 mL of 0.9% sodium chloride while pooling. Pooled CRYO must be administered within 4 hours of first entry and should be stored at room temperature until transfusion. Dosage varies with the patient's condition, weight, and level of the factor requiring replacement. This formula is shown in Fig. 14-11. If large volumes of CRYO are to be administered, ABO compatible units should be selected. CRYO does not necessitate crossmatching. Coagulation factor levels and other laboratory studies are performed to determine the effectiveness and the need for repeat doses.

> When thawing CRYO and FFP in a water bath, plastic overwraps prevent contamination of entry ports used for administration.

Cryoprecipitated AHF can also be pooled after separation from FFP at the collection facility. Units pooled by a closed system using a sterile collection device can be stored frozen for 1 year. After thawing, the pooled CRYO must be stored at 20° C to 24° C and used within 6 hours. If the CRYO was pooled in an open system, the product must be used within 4 hours. The number of units in the pool is indicated on the label, and the pooled product has a unique number. A record of the unit numbers contained in the pool must be maintained.

Fibrin Sealant from Cryoprecipitated Antihemophilic Factor

CRYO has also been used to prepare a topical hemostatic solution useful in controlling bleeding during surgery and various procedures. The solution contains 1 to 2 units of CRYO mixed with thrombin and is applied to the bleeding surface by layering, mixing, or spraying on the surgical field. Fibrinogen is converted to fibrin by the action of thrombin, which forms a clot to stop bleeding. Commercial products that are viral inactivated

$$\text{No. of factor VIII units} = \frac{\text{plasma volume} \times (\text{desired level \%} - \text{initial level \%})}{80 \text{ U/bag}}$$

Example: Plasma volume (PV, mL): 40 mL/kg × body weight (kg)
Quantity of factor VIII coagulant activity: stated on bottle
Factor VIII in CRYO: 80 U/bag

Patient: 70 kg
Initial factor VIII level: 2 units/dL: 2% activity
Desired factor VIII level: 50 units/dL: 50% activity

$$\text{No. of factor VIII units} = \frac{2800 \times (.50 - .02)}{80} = 16.8 \text{ bags of CRYO}$$

Fig. 14-11 Calculating the dose of CRYO concentrates. (From AABB/America's Blood Centers/American Red Cross, Armed Services Blood Program: *Circular of information for the use of human blood and blood components,* revised Dec 2009, Bethesda, MD, 2009.)

and have higher fibrinogen content are also available and have largely replaced the use of single CRYO units to prepare fibrin sealant.

APHERESIS GRANULOCYTES

Granulocytes are usually collected by apheresis techniques. Granulocyte transfusions are rarely used and limited to a small number of patients. This product contains leukocytes and platelets as well as 20 to 50 mL of red cells. The number of granulocytes in each product equals or is greater than 1.0×10^{10}. Granulocytes deteriorate rapidly on storage and should be administered within 24 hours of collection. They are maintained at 20° C to 24° C without agitation until transfused. A standard blood filter should be used, but not one that removes leukocytes.

A crossmatch is usually required before transfusion because of red cell contamination at greater than 2 mL.[4] Granulocyte support is usually continued until the granulocyte count increases and the infection is cured. Because patients undergoing this therapy are severely immunosuppressed, irradiation of the product to prevent GVHD is important.

The preparation and use of this product is uncommon as a result of the following[6]:
- More effective antibiotics
- Recombinant growth factor that stimulates the bone marrow to produce leukocytes
- Adverse reactions associated with granulocyte transfusions
- Granulocytes are limited to patients with the following conditions:
  - Neutropenia (generally $<0.5 \times 10^9$/L or 500/μL)
  - Documented infections, especially gram-negative bacteria and fungi
  - Lack of response to antibiotics

SECTION 3
DISTRIBUTION AND ADMINISTRATION

LABELING

The labeling of whole blood and its components is a process that includes a final review of records, quality control, donor testing, modifications, and the labels attached to the unit. **ISBT 128** labeling is an international standard of labeling that incorporates bar-coded labels that are computer-readable by blood centers and transfusion services around the world. The FDA approved the use of ISBT 128 in 2000, and AABB standards required that each accredited facility convert to ISBT 128 implementation by May 1, 2008. A

ISBT 128: ISBT recommendations regarding the uniform labeling of blood products for international bar code recognition by computers.

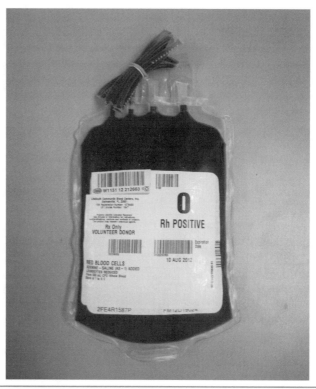

Fig. 14-12 Label requirements.
- Component name and unique identification that can be traced back to the blood donor.
- Manufacturer's name and registration number, license number if applicable.
- Expiration date and time if less than 72 hours.
- Amount of blood component and anticoagulant/preservative (within ± 10%).
- Test results of ABO and Rh type (D type may be omitted for Cryoprecipitated AHF). Selected tests such as CMV antigen or antibody identification can be indicated with a tie tag or label.
- Donor category: Paid, volunteer.
- Autologous units: "Autologous Use Only," name of the donor, blood group, hospital and identification number. Autologous units that have reactive infectious disease markers require a biohazard label.
- Statements regarding recipient identification, reference to the circular of information, infectious disease risk, and prescription requirement.

(Courtesy LifeSouth Community Blood Centers, Gainesville, FL.)

summary of current label requirements is included in Fig. 14-12. Progress and updates on the transition to ISBT 128 are available from the International Council on Commonality in Blood Banking Automation at www.iccbba.com.[3]

Labels on units are intended to provide sufficient information regarding the product without creating confusion. Standardization with regard to label placement, readability of bar codes by various computer systems, and product names is essential to prevent errors in transfusion and shipping. Required labels must be placed on the bag and cannot be substituted with tie tags (except for autologous blood labels). In addition to the standard label, specific requirements for other products are as follows:
- Irradiated components must have the name of the facility performing the irradiation.
- Pooled components must include the final volume, unique number assigned to the pool, and name of the facility preparing the pooled component.
- Autologous units must be labeled "For Autologous Use Only."

A facility receiving a unit of blood from another institution can place its own number on the unit; however, no more than two unique numeric or alphanumeric identification numbers should be visible on a blood component container. The original number must never be removed. The *Circular of Information* is referenced on the label as an important extension to component labels. This clear, concise guideline provides a description of each component, indications, and contraindications for use and information on dosage, administration, storage, side effects, and hazards. It is frequently updated and contains recent FDA guidelines.[8]

STORAGE AND TRANSPORTATION

Proper storage of blood components is important to maintain product potency and prevent bacterial growth. FDA and AABB guidelines define procedures for the calibration and maintenance of equipment designed for product storage, storage temperature limits, and monitoring parameters. Specifically, all refrigerators, freezers, and platelet incubators used for storing blood components must have the following:

- Recording devices to monitor the temperature at least every 4 hours
- Audible alarms to ensure a response 24 hours a day and an alarm set to signal the undesirable temperature *before* it is reached
- Alarm checks, performed on a regular basis
- Emergency procedures for power failure and alarm activation
- Emergency power backup systems; continuous power source for alarms
- Use of calibrated thermometers checked against referenced thermometers
- Written procedures for all the preceding

Appropriate storage temperatures for blood components are listed in Table 14-2. During storage, blood should be examined for evidence of hemolysis, abnormal coloring, or clots, any of which may indicate bacterial contamination.

Transportation of Blood Components

Whole blood or RBCs that are packaged for shipping must be maintained between 1° C and 10° C. Containers used for shipping must be validated periodically to ensure their effectiveness for shipping at wide ranges of outdoor temperatures (Fig. 14-13).[5]

Frozen units are shipped on dry ice. Because frozen products are brittle, they must be wrapped carefully. As dry ice evaporates, the extra space created allows the units to move about in the box and potentially break. Platelets must be maintained as close as possible to 20° C to 24° C during shipping. Discontinuation of the agitation of platelets during transportation should not exceed 24 hours.[4]

On receipt of a shipment of blood components, the temperature and appearance of the units must be observed and recorded (Table 14-5). Container closure and attached segments should also be inspected. Units that are received out of the designated

Fig. 14-13 Blood container for transporting blood products. (Courtesy LifeSouth Community Blood Centers, Gainesville, Fla.)

TABLE 14-5 Checklist for Receiving Blood
✓ Temperature acceptable for component
✓ Appearance: Clots, discoloration, hemolysis
✓ Container closure
✓ Attached segments intact: Red blood cells
✓ Expiration date and time
✓ Shipping list correct
✓ Intact labels

temperature range must be evaluated for their suitability for transfusion. The shipping facility should be notified if the product is unacceptable. Questionable units should be quarantined until a responsible person determines the disposition. Shipping records, including details of problems and the outcomes, must be maintained.[4]

Units that are issued to an unmonitored area, such as a patient's room, are usually not accepted back into inventory unless a time limit is set or the units have been transported in an insulated cooler or container.[12] Validation of the acceptable time for returning an unmonitored unit of blood must be set by each facility. Only 1 unit is typically issued at a time, unless the transfusion requirement is urgent.

Appropriate training of staff involved in the shipping and transportation of blood and blood components, in both the hospital and the blood center setting, is essential for the maintenance of quality products. Policies and procedures for all aspects of component packaging, inspection, record keeping, and monitoring must be understood and followed carefully.

ADMINISTRATION OF BLOOD COMPONENTS

This section summarizes important aspects of blood administration that pertain to the components described earlier. A more detailed discussion can be found in the *Technical Manual* and the *Blood Transfusion Therapy, Physician's Handbook,* both published by the AABB. Although laboratory personnel have limited involvement in blood administration, an understanding of the critical elements improves the communication between health care workers and the safety of the transfusion.

Requirements of safe blood administration include the following:
- *Positive identification* of the patient using two independent identifiers before transfusion is critical to avoid transfusion reactions that may be fatal.
- *A system to avoid and detect clerical errors* also contributes to avoiding serious reactions. Strict adherence to policies regarding identification numbers and mislabeled tubes should be followed.
- *Direct observation* of the patient should occur during the first 15 minutes after infusion begins and periodically until an appropriate time after the transfusion is completed.[4] Prompt intervention of a transfusion reaction is important in reducing its severity.
- *Only normal saline (0.9% USP)* should be administered with blood components. Hypotonic solutions such as 5% dextrose cause hemolysis in vitro. Ringer's lactate, which contains calcium, can initiate in vitro coagulation by reversing the action of citrate. The addition of medications to blood can cause hemolysis and mask adverse reactions.[8]
- *A 170- to 260-μm standard filter* must be used with all cellular and plasma components, even if leukocyte reduction of the product has been performed during preparation. The standard filter can be substituted with a bedside leukocyte reduction filter to prevent febrile reactions and HLA alloimmunization. They are specifically designed for either platelets or RBCs and cannot be interchanged.
- *Blood should be infused within 4 hours and before component expiration* because of the risk of bacterial growth. If the patient's condition requires blood infusion to extend past 4 hours, the unit should be divided and kept in the blood bank refrigerator until needed.[4]
- *Documentation and record keeping* are essential. AABB standards requires the following documentation with regard to a transfusion[4]:
  - Medical order for transfusion
  - Recipient consent
  - Name or type of component
  - Donor unit number or pool number
  - Date and time of transfusion
  - Pretransfusion and posttransfusion vital signs
  - Amount transfused
  - Identification of the transfusionist
  - Any adverse events possibly related to the transfusion

Adverse transfusion reactions can occur, regardless of how carefully the component was prepared, tested, crossmatched, and administered. If a transfusion reaction occurs, the transfusion must be discontinued immediately. The reporting of a reaction that occurs during or after administration is an important procedure that must be followed without deviation. Good communication between the transfusing personnel and the laboratory in the event of a reaction expedites its resolution and prevents further complications. Adverse consequences of transfusions are discussed in detail in Chapter 10.

CHAPTER SUMMARY

- The receipt, preparation, and issue of blood components is guided by current good manufacturing practice (cGMP) regulations published and enforced by the FDA.
- Each blood product is prepared and stored to optimize its purity and potency at the time of transfusion.
- Quality control parameters are set by the FDA and AABB (outlined in Table 14-4).
- The following table provides an outline of component indications to prevent adverse transfusion reactions (outlined in Chapter 10) and for selected patient therapy (discussed in Chapter 15).

Summary of Blood Component Therapy

Component	Indications	Comments
Whole blood	Increases red cell mass and plasma volume	Often available only for autologous units
Red Blood Cells (RBCs), Apheresis RBCs	Increase oxygen-carrying capacity in anemia, trauma, and surgery	Expiration varies with anticoagulant
Frozen/deglycerolized RBCs	Prolonged red cell storage for rare blood units and autologous storage	24-hour outdate following deglycerolization
Washed RBCs	Reduce plasma proteins to avoid allergic and anaphylactic reactions (IgA deficiency)	24-hour expiration following washing
Platelets and RBCs Leukocyte Reduced	Avoid febrile nonhemolytic reactions and prevent HLA alloimmunization, reduce CMV transmission	Prestorage filtration more effective in avoiding cytokines
Irradiated RBCs and Platelets	Prevent GVHD in immunocompromised patients, HLA-matched platelets or transfusions from a blood relative	Irradiation decreases shelf life of RBCs to 28 days
Platelets, Pooled Platelets	Bleeding caused by thrombocytopenia or thrombocytopathy	Pooling reduces expiration to 4 hours
Apheresis Platelets	Bleeding caused by thrombocytopenia or thrombocytopathy	May be HLA matched with recipient in cases of refractoriness
FFP, PF24	Replace stable and labile coagulation factors	Used in surgeries, trauma, and some factor deficiencies
Cryoprecipitated AHF (CRYO)	Contains fibrinogen, factors XIII and VIII, and von Willebrand's factor	Treatment of von Willebrand's disease, fibrinogen deficiency, and hemophilia A
Apheresis Granulocytes	Neutropenia with infection, unresponsive to antibiotics	Contains RBCs, must be ABO compatible

- Selection of ABO compatible red cells containing components and plasma is essential to prevent reactions and optimize component therapy and is summarized in the table that follows.[3]

Recipient ABO	Blood Component		
	Whole blood	RBCs	Plasma products (Platelets, FFP, PF24)
A	A	A, O	A, AB
B	B	B, O	B, AB
AB	AB	AB, A, B, O	AB
O	O	O	O, A, B, AB

ABO compatible CRYO is not required because of the small amount of plasma.
Compatibility testing is necessary for all products containing red cells, including granulocytes.
From ISBT-128. http://www.iccbba.org. Accessed February 2011.

CRITICAL THINKING EXERCISES

EXERCISE 14-1

Is it possible to prepare CRYO and FFP from the same blood unit? Explain your answer.

EXERCISE 14-2

A nonbleeding adult of average height and weight with chronic anemia is transfused with 2 units of RBCs. The pretransfusion hemoglobin is 7.0 g/dL. What is the expected post-transfusion hemoglobin? List several potential reasons for a failure of the patient's hemoglobin to increase after transfusion.

EXERCISE 14-3

A severely immunosuppressed adult patient has been transfused with 10 units of pooled platelets. The pretransfusion platelet count was 6000 μL. What is the expected platelet count 1 hour from transfusion? If the platelet count does not increase as expected, what are some potential causes?

EXERCISE 14-4

A unit of blood is released for a patient on the oncology floor. The nurse calls the blood bank 15 minutes later and reports that the patient has a visitor and does not want the transfusion until later that day. The nurse would like to hold the unit in the refrigerator on the floor because she is too busy to return it immediately. How do you respond?

EXERCISE 14-5

A 60-kg patient with hemophilia is going to surgery to have a small tumor removed. The physician requests enough Cryoprecipitated AHF to maintain the patient at 50% activity for surgery. The patient is currently at 15%. Determine how many units of Cryoprecipitated AHF will need to be pooled for surgery.

EXERCISE 14-6

1. A 70-lb child is scheduled for orthopedic surgery in 3 weeks. The physician requested that 2 units of autologous RBCs be drawn before surgery. Determine the amount to be drawn and the anticoagulant adjustment to collect RBCs from this child.
2. On the day of surgery, the patient becomes ill and surgery is postponed. Because of the tight operating room schedule, the surgery cannot take place for 2 months. Do the units need to be discarded and redrawn? Do any options exist?
3. The patient's older sister would like to be a donor for this patient. She meets the regular blood donor criteria and donates a unit of blood as a directed donor 1 week before the new surgery date. What procedure is required before this unit can be made available to her sibling? Will the expiration date change? If her sibling does not use the unit during surgery, can it be returned to regular inventory?

EXERCISE 14-7

1. A nurse is completing her shift in 1 hour and needs to start a transfusion and give the same patient an intravenous medication before she leaves. To expedite the process, she opts to give both through the Y-set she has prepared for the blood administration. She is not sure whether this is allowed, so she calls the blood bank before she picks up the blood. What should she be advised to do?

2. The nurse is in a hurry to start this transfusion and realizes that the intravenous solution she attached to the blood administration set is 2% dextrose instead of 0.9% saline. Can she proceed with this transfusion, or should she wait for 0.9% saline? Why?

STUDY QUESTIONS

For questions 1 through 7 match the clinical condition to the component that would have the best therapeutic value. Components may be used more than once.

Patient disease or condition	Component
1. TTP patient undergoing therapeutic apheresis	a. Factor VIII concentrate
2. Fibrinogen deficiency	b. Cryoprecipitated AHF
3. Thrombocytopenia	c. RBCs, washed
4. Refractory platelet response	d. Plasma, cryoprecipitate reduced
5. Hemophilia A	e. Platelets
6. Sickle cell disease	f. Apheresis platelets, HLA-matched
7. IgA-deficient patient with anti-IgA	g. RBCs

For questions 8 through 15 match the correct expiration times on the right with the appropriate blood component on the left. Expiration times can be used more than once.

Component	Expiration times
8. RBCs, AS-1 added	a. 35 days
9. Washed RBCs	b. 28 days
10. Irradiated RBCs	c. 3 days
11. RBCs collected in CPDA-1	d. 24 hours
12. Rejuvenated RBCs	e. 42 days
13. Frozen RBCs	f. 10 years
14. Deglycerolized RBCs	g. 21 days
15. RBCs collected in CPD	h. 1 year

16. The minimum amount of fibrinogen in 1 unit of Cryoprecipitated AHF is:
    a. 150 mg
    b. 250 mg
    c. 80 IU
    d. 1000 mg

17. Acute loss of less than 10% of blood volume usually necessitates:
    a. replacement with RBCs
    b. replacement with whole blood
    c. replacement with colloid solutions
    d. no replacement

18. Eight units of platelets were pooled without a sterile connecting device. The new expiration is:
    a. 2 hours
    b. 4 hours
    c. 6 hours
    d. 24 hours

19. In preparing platelets from a unit of whole blood, the correct order of centrifugation is:
    a. hard spin followed by hard spin
    b. light spin followed by light spin
    c. hard spin followed by light spin
    d. light spin followed by hard spin

20. RBCs that have been frozen are stored at which minimum temperature and maximum storage time?
    a. −65° C for 5 years
    b. −85° C for 10 years
    c. −65° C for 10 years
    d. −80° C for 10 years

21. Platelets collected by apheresis must contain a minimum of how many platelets to be acceptable?
    a. 5.5×10^{10}
    b. 3.3×10^{11}
    c. 5.0×10^{11}
    d. 3.0×10^{11}

22. Sterile connecting devices may be used for:
    a. connecting a leukocyte removal filter to RBCs
    b. preparing small aliquot transfusions for infants
    c. connecting platelets for pooling
    d. all of the above

23. Temperature limits for shipping RBCs are:
    a. 1° C to 6° C
    b. 1° C to 10° C
    c. 2° C to 8° C
    d. 20° C to 24° C

24. The pH and platelet count of 4 bags of platelets were tested at the end of the allowable storage period. Which of the following is an acceptable product?
    a. 5.5×10^{9} and pH of 6.5
    b. 6.0×10^{10} and pH of 7.0
    c. 4.2×10^{11} and pH of 5.9
    d. 3.0×10^{10} and pH of 6.2

25. Although ABO compatibility is preferred, ABO incompatibility is acceptable for which of the following components?
    a. PF24
    b. Cryoprecipitated AHF
    c. Apheresis Granulocytes
    d. Apheresis Platelets

REFERENCES

1. Food and Drug Administration: *Code of federal regulations, title 21 CFR parts 600-799*, Washington, DC, 2010, US Government Printing Office (revised annually).
2. Food and Drug Administration: *Code of federal regulations, title 21, CFR parts 210 and 211*, Washington, DC, 2010, US Government Printing Office (revised annually).
3. ISBT-128. http://www.iccbba.org. Accessed February, 2011.
4. Carson TH: *Standards for blood banks and transfusion services*, ed 27, Bethesda, MD, 2011, AABB.
5. Roback JD, editor: *Technical manual*, ed 17, Bethesda, MD, 2011, AABB.
6. King KE: *Blood transfusion therapy, a physician's handbook*, ed 10, Bethesda, MD, 2011, AABB.
7. Rejuvesol product insert, Braintree, MA, 1993, Cytosol Laboratories.
8. AABB/America's Blood Centers/American Red Cross, Armed Services Blood Program: *Circular of information for the use of human blood and blood components*, revised Dec 2009, Bethesda, MD, 2009.
9. Food and Drug Administration: *Guidance for industry: use of sterile connecting devices in blood bank practices (November 22, 2000)*, Rockville, MD, 2000, CBER Office of Communication, Outreach and Development.
10. Yazer MH, Cortese-Hassett A, Triulzi DJ: Coagulation factor levels in plasma frozen within 24 hours of phlebotomy over 5 days of storage at 1 to 6 C, *Transfusion* 48:2525, 2008.
11. Scott E, Puca K, Heraly J, et al: Evaluation and comparison of coagulation factor activity in fresh-frozen plasma and 24 hour plasma at thaw and after 120 hours of 1 to 6° C storage, *Transfusion* 49:1584, 2009.
12. Chenoweth A: Revisiting the 30-minute rule (again!): how to return and reissue blood components safely, *AABB News* 14(2):4-5, 2012.

Transfusion Therapy in Selected Patients

CHAPTER OUTLINE

LEARNING OBJECTIVES

On completion of this chapter, the reader should be able to:

1. Describe the pathophysiology of acute blood loss and massive transfusion therapy.
2. Discuss the transfusion requirements and causes of bleeding during cardiac surgery.
3. Describe the unique hematologic problems and transfusion therapy issues associated with neonates.
4. Discuss the pathophysiology and transfusion needs of patients with sickle cell disease, thalassemia, and autoimmune disease.
5. Explain the transfusion requirements of oncology patients.
6. Compare and contrast hematopoietic progenitor cells collected from bone marrow, peripheral blood, and cord

blood, and describe the transfusion support issues unique to these transplants.
7. List the acquired and congenital disorders of hemostasis and the appropriate transfusion support for each type of disorder.
8. Compare and contrast the various applications of therapeutic apheresis and the conditions and diseases associated with its use.
9. Discuss the transfusion issues unique to patients with chronic renal disease and how the use of erythropoietin affects the need for Red Blood Cell transfusions.
10. List several alternatives for transfusion of blood products and their application in patients with coagulation deficiencies, trauma patients, and oncology patients.

One of the benefits of blood component therapy is the ability to provide transfusion support for patients with many unique hematologic problems. For some patients, such as patients with sickle cell disease, the need for this support extends throughout their life. For others, it may be an urgent requirement resulting from surgery or trauma. By understanding the clinical conditions, laboratory professionals can appreciate the focus and urgency of laboratory testing and the value of the transfused blood components. Blood components, their therapeutic value, and the indications for their use were reviewed in Chapter 14. This chapter summarizes the pathophysiology of selected clinical conditions that commonly require transfusion support.

SECTION 1
TRANSFUSION PRACTICES

URGENT AND MASSIVE TRANSFUSION

Rapid blood loss, or **hemorrhage,** initiates a series of complicated physiologic responses that involve the nervous, hormonal, and circulatory systems. Acute blood loss of greater

Hemorrhage: bleeding through ruptured or unruptured blood vessel walls.

Fig. 15-1 Symptoms associated with hypovolemia and transfusion goals in treatment of trauma patients. (From Roback JD, editor: *Technical manual,* ed 17, Bethesda, MD, 2011, AABB.)

than 30% of the total blood volume may lead to hemorrhagic shock.[1] Characteristic signs and symptoms of hemorrhage that has progressed to hypovolemia are presented in Fig. 15-1. Severe hemorrhage affects electrolyte metabolism and oxygen transport, which ultimately increases the heart rate and the stress on internal organs. Prolonged hypotension and extensive tissue damage can result in cardiac and renal failure. Disseminated intravascular coagulation (DIC) is a pathologic activation of the coagulation cascade that may be caused by hemorrhage, which would further complicate the ability to control bleeding.

The most important goal in treating acute blood loss is the restoration of blood volume through the control of hemorrhage and replacement of intravascular volume to prevent shock. Infusing sufficient fluid volume to maintain adequate blood flow and blood pressure for tissue oxygenation is critical. Initial symptoms that occur with blood loss are the result of volume depletion, not depletion of red cells. Immediate volume restoration with crystalloid or colloid solutions is usually recommended.[2] The patient's vital signs, clinical situation, and hematocrit determine the requirement and urgency for Red Blood Cell (RBC) support. Fig. 15-1 lists priorities in acute blood loss.

RBC transfusions in trauma situations are usually urgent and of significant quantity. Massive transfusion is defined as the replacement of one or more blood volumes within 24 hours.[2] A blood volume is estimated at 5000 mL, which is about 10 units of whole blood in a 70-kg adult.

Adverse metabolic effects can occur from the transfusion of large quantities of stored blood over a short period. One blood volume exchanged within 3 to 4 hours can cause significant acute metabolic disturbances, such as citrate toxicity, hypothermia, and coagulation abnormalities. Coagulation abnormalities resulting in microvascular bleeding have been attributed to the dilution of platelets and coagulation factors occurring with two or three volume exchanges and the consumption of platelets and coagulation factors from extensive bleeding.[2] Hemostatic agents such as desmopressin, recombinant factor VIIa, and antifibrinolytics may also be administered to control bleeding.[2] Complications resulting from massive transfusion are summarized in Table 15-1.

Urgent transfusion requirements resulting from trauma or surgery sometimes necessitate the release of uncrossmatched blood, if insufficient time to obtain a sample for typing is available. This process of "emergency release" is discussed in Chapter 8. Group O RBCs should be transfused until the patient's type is known and should be D-negative for women with childbearing potential to avoid sensitization to the D antigen. Transfusion services are required to have guidelines related to releasing uncrossmatched blood components, type-specific RBCs, and changing blood types during massive transfusion.

> Massive transfusion is defined as the replacement of one or more blood volumes within 24 hours.

CARDIAC SURGERY

During cardiopulmonary bypass surgery, the patient's blood circulates through an oxygenating pump outside the patient's body. Extracorporeal circulation causes a decrease

TABLE 15-1   Complications in Massive Transfusion

PROBLEM	CAUSES	TREATMENTS
Microvascular hemorrhage	Dilution of coagulation factors and platelets Hypotension Consumption of coagulation factors Platelet consumption	Platelets Fresh Frozen Plasma to control defined deficiencies of coagulation factors Control hypotension
Citrate toxicity	Decrease in ionized calcium from anticoagulants in blood products	Slower infusion; calcium replacement if severe
Hypothermia	Rapid infusion of blood products	High-flow blood warmers

TABLE 15-2   Risk Factors for Bleeding during Cardiac Surgery

- Time on pump
- Age of patient
- Previous cardiac surgery
- Type of surgery: Valve replacement, CABG, or both
- Preoperative medications: Aspirin and anticoagulant
- Heparin effect
- Hypothermia decreases platelet function

From Despotis G, Eby C, Lubin DM: A review of transfusion risks and optimal management of perioperative bleeding with cardiac surgery, *Transfusion* 48:2S, 2008.
CABG, Coronary artery bypass graft.

in platelet function and numbers. Coagulation factors are also decreased because of hemodilution and the cell salvage instrument. Hypothermia, transfusion of shed blood, thrombin-mediated activation, and residual heparin also affect hemostasis.[3] Table 15-2 summarizes risk factors unique to cardiac surgery that increase the need for component support perioperatively and postoperatively.

During and after surgery, heparin causes the activated partial thromboplastin time to be prolonged. The thrombin time confirms heparin excess. Treatment with a protamine sulfate, rather than Fresh Frozen Plasma (FFP), corrects heparin excess.[2] FFP is usually indicated only for factor deficiency or massive transfusion from severe bleeding during cardiac surgery. The effects of preoperative warfarin therapy also contribute to postoperative blood loss and transfusion requirements.[4]

NEONATAL AND PEDIATRIC TRANSFUSION ISSUES

Neonatal and pediatric transfusion issues are significantly different from transfusion issues for adults because of the small size, hemoglobin changes, and erythropoietin response in early infancy. Ill neonates are more likely than hospitalized patients of any other age group to receive RBC transfusions.[5]

Fetal red cells contain hemoglobin F, which has a higher affinity or ability to bind oxygen. This affinity is important during the intrauterine period because it enhances oxygen transfer from maternal red cells to fetal red cells. The switch from fetal to adult hemoglobin begins at about 32 weeks' gestation.[1] For this reason, preterm infants have a higher level of fetal hemoglobin than infants born at term. The change from fetal to adult hemoglobin occurs during the first few weeks of life, and the process causes a condition called physiologic anemia of infancy. In a full-term infant of normal birth weight, this change is well tolerated; however, treatment is often necessary in an infant born prematurely with low birth weight.

In addition to the shift in hemoglobin, the need for frequent laboratory tests contributes to the need for transfusions. **Iatrogenic blood loss** is the most common indication of transfusion in a preterm infant with low birth weight. Newborns do not compensate for hypovolemia as well as adults do.

Erythropoietin in adults is released from the kidneys in response to diminished oxygen delivery. This growth factor triggers the bone marrow to increase RBC production and release more erythrocytes into the circulation. Erythropoietin production in an infant is believed to be triggered in the liver, which is less responsive to low levels of oxygen. The lower level of response to low oxygen levels (hypoxia) protects the infant from generating an excess of red cells (polycythemia) during fetal life but does not allow an effective response to anemia in the immature infant.

The response of a newborn to hypothermia is also different from an adult's response. The metabolic rate, hypoglycemia, and acidosis can cause the temporary cessation of breathing, or apnea. Apnea may lead to hypoxia, hypotension, and cardiac arrest. For this reason, a monitored blood warmer is often used to administer RBCs, especially for exchange transfusions.

The ability to metabolize citrate and potassium is more difficult for newborns because of their immature liver and kidneys. For this reason, washed or fresh red cells are often indicated for newborns. Because potassium increases when blood is irradiated, washing irradiated RBCs is also recommended. The transfusion of fresh blood to maximize the level of 2,3-diphosphoglycerate (2,3-DPG), which decreases during storage, is also important in newborns because of their limited ability to compensate for hypoxia.

In newborns, hemoglobin levels less than 13 g/dL indicate severe anemia during the first 24 hours of life.[1] RBC transfusions are usually given in small volumes prepared from multiple-pack systems that allow preparation of several aliquots from a single donor unit. Infants do not form red cell antibodies during the first 4 months; therefore crossmatching is not necessary. Antigen-negative blood must be provided if the mother or infant possesses a red cell alloantibody. ABO identical or ABO compatible blood that is D-negative or the same as the infant's can be released during the first 4 months.

Transfusion-transmitted cytomegalovirus (CMV) is a risk to preterm infants weighing less than 1200 g who are born to seronegative mothers or to mothers whose CMV status is unknown.[1] This risk is avoided by providing CMV antibody–negative blood to neonates. In addition, leukocyte reduction, using highly efficient leukocyte removal filters, is recommended because CMV resides within the white blood cell.[2]

Transfusion issues unique to infants are summarized in Table 15-3. Familiarity with these problems provides an understanding of the transfusion requirements for preterm newborns and infants.

TRANSPLANTATION

The transfusion service and blood bank provide support for transplantation of organs and hematopoietic progenitor cells (HPCs). This section describes the issues related to transplantation and transfusion requirements.

TABLE 15-3 Transfusion Issues Unique to Neonates
• Change from fetal to adult hemoglobin causing physiologic anemia of infancy
• Iatrogenic blood loss
• Decreased response of erythropoietin
• Low tolerance of hypothermia
• Greater risk of cytomegalovirus infection due to immature immune system
• Decreased ability to metabolize citrate and potassium
• Decreased ability to restore 2,3-DPG in older units

2,3-DPG, 2,3-Diphosphoglycerate.

Organ Transplants

Transfusion support for kidney, heart, and liver transplants is varied because of the nature of the organ. Liver transplantation can be associated with massive hemorrhage. Hemostatic problems are major complications of liver transplant because of the role the liver plays in the synthesis of factors and clearance of coagulation inhibitors. The preexisting liver disease also contributes to the excessive bleeding during the procedure. Average blood component requirements in an adult liver transplant procedure are 10 to 12 units each of RBCs, Plasma, and Platelets and up to 5 units of Cryoprecipitated Antihemophilic Factor (AHF).[2] Many transplant programs have preplanned algorithms for the use of specific combinations of blood components during the liver transplant surgery.[6] Intraoperative salvage instruments to reduce RBC usage are commonly used in liver transplant surgery. Cell salvage instruments are discussed in Chapter 12.

Heart and heart-lung transplants have similar product usage as cardiac surgery, outlined previously. Cardiopulmonary bypass can affect hemostasis secondary to hypothermia, heparin use, priming fluid used for bypass instrument, and duration of surgery. A ventricular assist device, which is a relatively new therapeutic option for patients with end-stage heart failure awaiting heart transplant, can also contribute to the need for transfusion support during implantation and after surgery.[7] Platelet and hemostatic defects may be caused by the surface of the device and flow characteristics. Transfusions should be limited to leukocyte-reduced components to avoid sensitization and increase complications caused by human leukocyte antigen (HLA) antibodies.

Graft survival is enhanced with HLA-matched donor-recipient combinations, particularly if the recipient is demonstrating HLA antibodies. Graft survival of renal transplants is also improved with living donors. ABO compatibility is critical to the success of vascularized grafts, such as livers, kidneys, and hearts, but it is not essential in tissue grafts, such as bone, heart valves, skin, and cornea.

In the 1970s, it was observed that kidney allografts had a higher rate of survival if patients were given blood transfusions before undergoing renal transplantation. In the 1980s, transfusion to induce tolerance in patients before kidney transplants was replaced by the use of cyclosporine for immunosupression.[3] Erythropoietin has also reduced the need for transfusion in patients with kidney disease. When RBCs are transfused, leukocyte-reduced blood products have decreased the alloimmunization to HLA antigens. When a potential kidney transplant recipient develops HLA antibodies, obtaining a compatible kidney becomes more challenging.

Table 15-4 summarizes average blood components transfused during transplant surgery.

Hematopoietic Progenitor Cell Transplantation

HPC transplants have become a common medical procedure performed in many tertiary care centers. They can be used for the treatment of malignant diseases, marrow failure, or immunodeficiency syndromes. Table 15-5 is a partial list of diseases treated with HPC transplants.[3] Hematopoietic cells contain stem cells that are capable of self-renewal. Progenitor cells that have the ability differentiate into committed blood cell lineages. Both

TABLE 15-4 Average Blood Components Transfused during Transplant Surgery

ORGAN	RBCs	APHERESIS PLATELETS	FFP	CRYOPRECIPITATED AHF
Kidney	<1	0	0	0
Heart	1-6	2.7	3.0	1.4
Liver (adult)	17.3	21.8	23.1	15.3
Liver (pediatric)	7.1	7.1	6.8	5.6
Lung	3.4	1.9	1.2	1.8

Data from McCullough J: *Transfusion medicine*, ed 2, Philadelphia, 2005, Elsevier.
RBCs, Red Blood Cells; *FFP*, Fresh Frozen Plasma, *AHF*, Antihemophilic Factor.

TABLE 15-5	Therapeutic Uses for Hematopoietic Progenitor Cell Transplantation
Congenital Immune Deficiencies	

Severe combined immunodeficiency disease
Wiskott-Aldrich syndrome
Aplastic anemia
Fanconi's anemia
Hemoglobinopathies
Thalassemia
Sickle cell disease

Malignancy

Acute leukemia
Non-Hodgkin's and Hodgkin's lymphoma
Myelodysplastic/myeloproliferative disorders
Multiple myeloma

Other

Paroxysmal nocturnal hemoglobinuria
Multiple sclerosis

From Roback JD, editor: *Technical manual*, ed 17, Bethesda, MD, 2011, AABB.

NMDP Transplants by Cell Source

Fig. 15-2 Trends in sources of transplants from the National Marrow Donor Program. (Courtesy National Marrow Donor Program, Minneapolis, Minn.)

cell lines are collectively termed hematopoietic progenitor cells. Progenitor cell transplants can be allogeneic (genetically unrelated), syngeneic (identical twin), or autologous (self). They can be derived from the following:

- Bone marrow—HPC(M)
- Peripheral blood: Mononuclear cell fraction separated by apheresis equipment—HPC(A)
- Umbilical cord blood—HPC(C)

The choices for stem cell sources are influenced by availability, optimal HLA matching, patient size, and donor safety. The trends in sources of HPCs transplanted are illustrated in Fig. 15-2. HPCs collected by apheresis, also referred to as peripheral progenitor cells, are the most common type of HPC at the present time. HPCs collected by apheresis are used for autologous, syngeneic, and allogeneic transplantation. Colony-stimulating factors can be given to donors to mobilize sufficient stem cells before apheresis. Collections by apheresis avoid the risk of general anesthesia needed for bone marrow harvest. HPCs derived from cord blood have been successfully used in pediatric patients and, to some extent, adults lacking an HLA-matched adult donor.[1] The decision to use HPC(M) over

HPC(A) is influenced by the type of disease, age of the patient, and risk status of the disease. Comparisons of outcomes related to HPC source consider the speed of engraftment, rate of chronic GVHD, disease relapse, and long-term graft survival. Retrospective reviews have suggested that improved overall survival may be obtained with HPCs collected from bone marrow for pediatric patients with aplastic anemia or acute leukemia.[1]

Autologous HPC transplantation is primarily used as a "rescue" in patients who have received myelodepletion therapy (chemotherapy or radiation or both). Patients receive hematopoietic growth factors before collection by leukapheresis, and the HPCs are stored frozen or nonfrozen for later infusion after chemotherapy.

HLA-matched related or unrelated donors provide the source of allogeneic HPCs. HLA class I and class II matching is necessary to reduce the risk of posttransplant graft-versus-host disease (GVHD) and to achieve successful engraftment. In addition, allogeneic HPCs provide a "graft-versus-leukemia" effect, in which the T cells in the graft attack residual tumor cells. These immune cells also attack the healthy tissues of the patient, often causing GVHD. Some studies have shown a decreased incidence of GVHD when transplanting HPCs derived from cord blood, despite the lower HLA-matching requirements of HPC(C).[8]

Before transplantation, transfusion support includes leukocyte-reduced blood products to avoid HLA alloimmunization, CMV infection, and febrile reactions.[6] After transplantation, patients usually require extensive platelet and RBC support for about 2 weeks. If the ABO types of the transplant recipient and donor are not matched, careful monitoring by the transfusion service is necessary, and additional RBC support may be necessary if hemolysis occurs.

Because of the immunosuppression of the patients undergoing transplants, the risk of GVHD is serious. Blood products received after transplant should be irradiated. The progenitor cell product must never be irradiated, however, because this would prevent engraftment.[6] CMV infection is another potential problem because of immunosuppression, which can be avoided with leukocyte-reduced or seronegative blood products. The progenitor cell product should never be administered through a leukocyte reduction filter.

Although HLA compatibility is crucial in the successful engraftment of myelosuppressed patients with HPCs, ABO compatibility is not essential. The early committed and uncommitted cells in these transplants do not possess A, B, and H antigens (ABH antigens). Approximately 40% to 50% of HPC transplants are ABO incompatible.[9] Delayed red cell engraftment may occur after a major ABO-incompatible transplant (e.g., group "A" HPC donor to group "O" recipient). Hemolysis can be observed after a minor ABO incompatible transplant (e.g., group "O" HPC donor to group "A" recipient). Red cell and plasma components transfused after transplant of ABO mismatched grafts must be compatible with the blood type of both the donor and the recipient. An example of the component selected for ABO incompatible HPC is given in Table 15-6. During the last phase of transplantation, when the forward and reverse typing is consistent with the donor's ABO group, components should be compatible with the donor's type. Chimerism or a dual cell population may occur if the recipient's hematopoietic cells survive and subsequently coexist with cells produced by the donor's transplanted HPCs.

THERAPEUTIC APHERESIS

Therapeutic apheresis involves the removal of abnormal cells, plasma, or plasma constituents from a patient's blood to achieve a clinical benefit. The replacement fluid varies with the condition and the portion that is removed. The goal may be to:
- Supply an essential substance that is absent
- Reduce the quantity of a particular antibody
- Modify mediators of inflammation
- Clear immune complexes
- Replace cellular elements

Photopheresis is a type of therapeutic apheresis where the buffy coat layer is collected and treated with 8-methoxypsoralen and exposed to ultraviolet (UV) light. The cells are reinfused after treatment. This therapeutic apheresis has been shown to prevent leukocyte

TABLE 15-6	Example of ABO Component Selection in ABO Unmatched Hematopoietic Progenitor Cell Transplants		

| | | ABO BLOOD GROUP SELECTION EXAMPLE IN ( ) | |
TYPE OF INCOMPATIBILITY	TRANSPLANT STAGE	RED BLOOD CELLS COMPATIBLE WITH:	PLASMA/PLATELETS/ CRYOPRECIPITATE COMPATIBLE WITH:
Major (Example: "A" donor to "O" recipient)	Pretransplant	Recipient (O)	Donor (A)
	Transplant	Recipient (O)	Donor (A)
	Recipient antibodies detected (anti-A and anti-B)	Recipient (O)	Donor (A)
	Recipient antibodies no longer detected	Donor (A)	Donor (A)
Minor (Example: "O" donor to "A" recipient)	Pretransplant	Donor (O)	Recipient (A)
	Transplant	Donor (O)	Recipient (A)
	Recipient antibodies detected (anti-A and anti-B)	Donor (O)	Recipient (A)
	Recipient antibodies no longer detected	Donor (O)	Donor (O)
Major and minor incompatibility (Example: "B" donor to "A" recipient)	Pretransplant	Group O	Group AB
	Transplant	Group O	Group AB
	Recipient antibodies detected (anti-A and anti-B)	Group O	Group AB
	Recipient antibodies no longer detected	Donor (B)	Donor (B)

Modified from Roback JD, editor: *Technical manual,* ed 17, Bethesda, MD, 2011, AABB.

replication and to induce apoptosis or cell death. The application of photopheresis is standard treatment for some forms of cutaneous T-cell lymphoma and Sézary syndrome and is under investigation for conditions such as autoimmune disease, solid-organ transplant rejection, and GVHD after HPC transplantation.[2]

Conditions treated with therapeutic apheresis are listed in Table 15-7. Replacement fluids include crystalloids, albumin, plasma protein fraction, plasma, cryoprecipitate reduced, or FFP in the case of a plasma exchange. When exchanges necessitate FFP or RBC support, large quantities are used; this requires adequate planning and communication with the transfusion service. A more comprehensive description of therapeutic apheresis is found in the AABB *Technical Manual.*

ONCOLOGY

A patient undergoing chemotherapy or radiation treatment for cancer relies on the transfusion service for many blood products. Cancers involve the unregulated, uncontrolled growth and division of a clone of cells from an organ or tissue. These clones of cells may divert the blood supply or crowd out the organ or neighboring organs, causing undesirable effects to the patient. Depending on where the abnormal cell originated, the cells, if left untreated, migrate and take hold in other organ systems in a process known as metastasis. The oncology patient in the hospital undergoes a combined treatment regimen of physical (radiation) and chemical therapies mostly targeting rapid cellular division. Most chemotherapeutic agents act by slowing down or inhibiting DNA replication or interfering with the DNA translation process to stop cell division.

Chemotherapeutic agents are not specific for the target cancer or clone of cells. Epithelial cells of the gastrointestinal tract and germinal epithelium of the hair follicles are also particularly affected. In the bone marrow, hematopoietic cells that differentiate into

TABLE 15-7	Indications for Therapeutic Apheresis	
PROCEDURE	**INDICATION**	**PURPOSE**
Plasmapheresis	Guillain-Barré syndrome	Remove pathologic autoantibody
	Myasthenia gravis	Remove HLA alloantibody
	Multiple sclerosis	Remove inhibitor of ADAMTS13
	Goodpasture's syndrome	and large vWF multimers;
	Antibody-mediated rejection	replace deficient enzyme
	(kidney)	Remove excessive protein or
	Desensitization before	immune complexes
	transplant	
	Thrombotic	
	thrombocytopenic purpura	
	Cryoglobulinemia	
	Hyperviscosity in monoclonal	
	gammopathies	
Cytapheresis	Sickle cell disease	Reduce hemoglobin S, replace
	Hyperleukocytosis	with hemoglobin A
	Babesiosis, malaria	Remove excessive leukocytes
		Reduce parasites
Photopheresis	Allograft rejection	Inhibit lymphocyte proliferation
	Cutaneous T-cell lymphoma,	and cause induction of
	Sézary syndrome	apoptosis
	Chronic graft-versus-host	
	disease	

From Roback JD, editor: *Technical manual,* ed 17, Bethesda, MD, 2011, AABB.
HLA, Human leukocyte antigen; *vWF,* von Willebrand's factor.

megakaryocytes, erythrocytes, and leukocytes are reduced. As treatment progresses, platelet, leukocyte, hemoglobin, and hematocrit levels decrease. The most common complications are bleeding, anemia, and infection. Careful monitoring of laboratory results and clinical conditions associated with bleeding and anemia is necessary to determine component therapy. Transfusion support with irradiated blood products after intensive chemotherapy and radiation therapy is common. In some patients, multiple platelet transfusions often cause refractoriness, or the inability to achieve therapeutic increments. When alloantibodies to HLA antigens cause refractoriness, HLA-matched platelets may become necessary. Colony-stimulating factors are becoming more widely used in preventing infection and bleeding risks associated with chemotherapy (Table 15-8).

CHRONIC RENAL DISEASE

Patients undergoing dialysis have many hematologic complications that necessitate transfusion therapy, usually in the form of RBC support. The high uremic content of the blood leads to altered red cell shapes; this prevents the red cells from traversing the spleen without being removed prematurely by macrophages, which results in hemolytic anemia. The act of dialysis itself causes a shearing of the red cells, which can contribute to hemolysis. These patients fail to produce sufficient levels of erythropoietin because of the nonfunctioning kidney; therefore an erythrocyte production problem adds to the anemic condition. Factors contributing to transfusion needs in dialysis patients are summarized on Table 15-9. Careful monitoring of hemoglobin and hematocrit levels that contribute to clinical symptoms determines transfusion therapy. The use of recombinant erythropoietin has significantly reduced the need for transfusion; however, in acute anemia, RBC transfusions are required. Transfusions are usually given while the patient is on dialysis equipment to reduce the need for an additional venipuncture. Leukocyte-poor RBCs are the preferred product to avoid the development of HLA antibodies, which increase the challenge of finding a compatible kidney.

TABLE 15-8   Alternatives to Transfusion

FACTOR	NAMES	USES
Erythropoietin	EPO rHuEPO (prepared by recombinant technology)	Chronic renal failure AZT treatment in HIV Cancer patients on chemotherapy
Colony-stimulating factors (CSFs)	Granulocyte CSF Granulocyte-macrophage CSF Recombinant interleukin-11	Decreased infection in patients undergoing chemotherapy Congenital agranulocytosis Acute leukemia Myelodysplastic syndrome Aplastic anemia in children Autologous and allogeneic bone marrow transplant Cancer patients with thrombocytopenia
DDAVP	Desmopressin	Promotes hemostasis by promoting release of vWF; used for hemophilia A, von Willebrand's disease, and some platelet function disorders

From King KE, editor: *Blood transfusion therapy, a physician's handbook,* ed 10, Bethesda, MD, 2011, AABB.
EPO, Erythropoietin; *rHuEPO,* human recombinant erythropoietin; *AZT,* azidothymidine; *HIV,* human immunodeficiency virus; *vWF,* von Willebrand's factor.

TABLE 15-9   Contributing Factors Associated with Anemia in Chronic Renal Disease

CAUSE	EFFECT
Elevated uremia	Altering of RBC shape, causing their premature removal
Dialysis procedure	Shearing of RBCs
Low erythropoietin level	Low RBC production

RBC, Red Blood Cell.

HEMOLYTIC UREMIC SYNDROME AND THROMBOTIC THROMBOCYTOPENIC PURPURA

Hemolytic uremic syndrome (HUS) and thrombotic thrombocytopenic purpura (TTP) are classified together because of the numerous overlaps in clinical symptoms.[10] Clinical symptoms include:

• Thrombocytopenia
• Microangiopathic hemolytic anemia
• Renal dysfunction
• Central nervous system involvement

In both of these disorders, damage to the vessel endothelium has activated and consumed platelets and coagulation proteins, causing microthrombi to become lodged in the kidney. TTP is caused by a deficiency or antibody to a protease (ADAMTS13) that cleaves von Willebrand's factor (vWF). Therapeutic plasma exchange removes the inhibitor and large-molecular-weight multimers, while simultaneously replacing the deficient enzyme.[1] HUS usually affects young children, often before their first year. It usually follows a severe viral infection, bacterial gastroenteritis, or treatment with certain cytotoxic drugs.

TABLE 15-10	Clinical Indications for Transfusion in Patients with Sickle Cell Disease

Acute anemia resulting from:
  Bleeding
  Infection
  Increased hemolysis
  Sequestration of cells in the spleen and liver
Prevention of:
  Stroke—reduce sickling, which blocks blood vessels
  Recurrent pain episodes owing to sickling in joints	

From Hillyer CD, Silverstein LF, Ness PM, et al: *Blood banking and transfusion medicine*, ed 2, Philadelphia, 2007, Elsevier.

Therapeutic plasma exchange is standard or acceptable supportive treatment for HUS caused by an autoantibody to factor H or complement factor deficiencies.[1]

ANEMIAS REQUIRING TRANSFUSION SUPPORT

Sickle Cell Anemia

Sickle cell disease (hemoglobin S) is one of the most prevalent hemoglobinopathies. The anomaly is a structural variant in the β-chain of the hemoglobin molecule. An amino acid substitution in the sixth position of the polypeptide chain (valine for glutamic acid) on the surface of the molecule alters the solubility of the hemoglobin molecule. The hemoglobin polymerizes under conditions of low oxygen, causing the characteristic sickling of the cell. Blockage of the microvasculature by these sickled cells causes "sickle cell crisis," which results in endothelial damage, thrombosis, and pain. The red cells have decreased life span, which causes symptomatic and compensated anemia. Serious complications include stroke, acute chest syndrome, and multiorgan failure.

Hemoglobin and hematocrit values can be low in sickle cell patients before they become symptomatic. Clinical symptoms associated with pulmonary or cardiac insufficiency indicate when RBC transfusions are necessary. In situations of severe pain and crisis, automated RBC exchange is often therapeutic. Indications for transfusion are summarized in Table 15-10.

Because a patient with sickle cell disease requires RBC support throughout most of his or her life, the potential for alloantibody production is high. Of chronically transfused patients with sickle cell disease, 25% to 30% develop red cell alloantibodies.[1] One reason for the high rate of alloantibodies is that the red cell antigens from the predominantly white donor populations are different from the antigens inherited in the black population. To avoid this problem, many hematologists consider partially phenotypically matched (D, C, c, E, e, and K) RBCs early in the treatment of sickle cell disease, which reduces the chance of potentially life-threatening hemolytic reactions. Encouraging support from black donors in areas where sickle cell disease is common is extremely beneficial for meeting the need for phenotypically matched RBCs. Antigen typing using molecular methods has become more common for transfusion support for sickle cell patients to ensure proper identification of variants or rare phenotypes in both patients and donors. Iron overload is a complication of repeated transfusions and can be treated with an oral iron chelator or avoiding iron accumulation with red cell exchange.

Thalassemia

Thalassemia is also an inherited syndrome characterized by deficient or abnormal hemoglobin structures. Thalassemia is caused by a deficiency in hemoglobin α-chain or β-chain production that ranges from mild to severe. Total absence of α-chain synthesis is fatal in utero, and absence of the β-chain is classified as thalassemia major. To compensate for the resulting anemia, hematopoietic tissue expands, resulting in bone deformities and liver and spleen enlargement. Transfusion in children is helpful to suppress ineffective erythropoiesis and avoid early complications of the disease.[3] Hemoglobin and hematocrit values are monitored to determine whether transfusion therapy is needed.

With both sickle cell disease and thalassemias, iron chelation therapy must accompany blood transfusions to prevent the iron overload these patients experience because of multiple transfusions.[11] The iron from normal red cell kinetics is neutralized, but the constant addition of cells of varying ages creates the iron excess that becomes stored and detrimental to many tissues.

Immune Hemolytic Anemias

The immune hemolytic anemias belong to a group of disorders characterized by decreased survival of the erythrocyte because of antibody coating of the red cell membrane. This sensitization causes the cell to be removed from the circulation much sooner than the average 120 days. These disorders are classified into three groups:

- *Autoimmune hemolytic anemia:* The antibody is reacting to a self-antigen on the red cell, which results in removal by the spleen and causes anemia. Based on serologic tests, this category is further divided into cold or warm autoantibodies.
- *Drug-induced hemolytic anemia:* Either the drug is adsorbed directly onto the membrane or the drug-antibody combination becomes adsorbed onto the red cell. Some medications can also induce the production of an autoantibody.
- *Alloimmune hemolytic anemia:* This occurs when RBC clearance from alloantibodies is produced against transfused RBCs or against fetal cells in hemolytic disease of the fetus and newborn.

Transfusion therapy in hemolytic anemia includes transfusions of RBCs depending on the extent of the anemia. In all cases, identification of the causative agent should be the first step in treatment. The severity of the anemia depends on the response by the bone marrow to keep up with increased destruction. In compensated anemia, the hemoglobin may be low; however, if no clinical symptoms are present, transfusions should be avoided.

Pretransfusion testing in patients with autoimmune hemolytic anemias caused by medications or disease can be challenging and time-consuming. The risk of an underlying alloantibody makes the serologic tests confusing and necessitates adsorption procedures to rule out the possibility of underlying alloantibodies. Laboratory investigations of warm and cold autoantibodies are outlined in Chapter 7.

HEMOSTATIC DISORDERS

Hemostatic disorders are characterized in two ways:
- A decrease in or lack of production of one or more of the coagulation proteins
- Normal production but an abnormal structure resulting in a nonfunctioning protein

The most common hereditary bleeding disorder is von Willebrand's disease.[6] Quantitative or qualitative abnormalities of vWF cause bleeding. vWF is necessary for platelets to adhere to endothelium. It is also needed for factor VII for correct functioning and maintenance of adequate levels. Other factor deficiencies are hemophilia A (factor VIII deficiency) and hemophilia B (factor IX deficiency). Factors VIII and IX are needed for the intrinsic pathway of fibrin formation. The clinical characteristics of coagulation deficiencies are prolonged bleeding, bleeding into joints, and subcutaneous bleeds. Most of the hemostatic disorders are treated with factor concentrates or DDAVP. Cryoprecipitated AHF is used only in urgent situations when the preferred concentrate is not available.[6] The administration of coagulation factor concentrate has the potential to cause the development of antibodies or "inhibitors" to one or more of the factors, which can lead to further bleeding episodes.

DIC is an acquired hemostasis disorder in which the patient develops microthrombi, which consume platelets and fibrinogen when the coagulation mechanism is turned on inappropriately, such as during surgery, massive blood loss, or after a snake or insect bite. Strands of fibrin trap platelets. Patients with DIC can spontaneously bleed or form a thrombus. The therapy, as with all other secondary manifestations, is to determine and treat the cause while stabilizing the patient.

SECTION 2
ALTERNATIVES TO TRANSFUSION

Blood is a limited resource and contains risks associated with transfusion-transmitted diseases and adverse reactions. For this reason, ongoing research exists to substitute blood products with safer, more effective, and more readily available products. Tables 15-8, 15-11, and 15-12 summarize three categories of these substitutes for blood, which include hematopoietic growth factors, blood derivatives, and volume expanders. More details regarding these products can be found in *Blood Transfusion Therapy, a Physician's Handbook,* published by the AABB.

Essential components or factors involved in the coagulation cascade, including factor VIII, factor IX, and antithrombin concentrate, are blood derivatives formulated to replace factor deficiencies and overcome the effects of inhibitors. The risk of transmitting viruses has been reduced with the use of heat and detergent treatment. Recombinant technology has eliminated the risk; however, these products are substantially more costly. The factor concentrates are sterile, stable, and lyophilized, which makes administration more convenient than administration of blood components. Each product differs in terms of purity and the method of treatment to inactivate potential viruses. The clotting factor per milligram of protein or specific activity differs and is indicated on the vial.

Volume expanders include crystalloids and colloids. These products are usually dispensed by the pharmacy rather than the transfusion service and are used with or in place of blood for hypovolemia.

Hematopoietic growth factors stimulate the bone marrow to produce erythrocytes, platelets, and leukocytes for patients with chronic anemia and various conditions, causing low cell counts. Their uses for patients undergoing chronic transfusions and renal dialysis and patients undergoing chemotherapy have been well documented.

TABLE 15-11 Alternatives to Transfusion: Factor Concentrates

DERIVATIVE	GENERAL INFORMATION	INDICATIONS
Factor VIIa	Recombinant (rFVIIa)	Bleeding or prophylaxis before surgery for hemophilia A or B Factor VII deficiency
Factor VIII	Produced by recombinant (rFVIII) or fractionation of pooled human plasma (AHF)	Hemophilia A von Willebrand's disease
Factor IX	Produced by recombinant and plasma-derived sources	Hemophilia B
Factor IX complex concentrate	Factor IX complex, also called vitamin K–dependent factors	Factor II, IX, and X deficiency Bypassing factor VIII inhibitors Warfarin overdose
Antithrombin concentrate	Inhibitor of coagulation; prepared from pooled plasma	Hereditary antithrombin deficiency
Protein C concentrate	Inhibitor of coagulation	Congenital protein C deficiency

From King KE, editor: *Blood transfusion therapy, a physician's handbook,* ed 10, Bethesda, MD, 2011, AABB.
AHF, Antihemophilic Factor.

TABLE 15-12 Alternatives to Transfusion: Volume Expanders

TYPE	NAME	CONTENT	USE
Crystalloids	Normal saline Lactated Ringer's solution	Na^+ and Cl^- ions in water K^+, Ca^{2+} ions, and lactate	Shock from hemorrhage and burns
Colloids	Hydroxyethyl starch (HES)	Synthetic polymer: amylopectin in saline	Prolonged intravascular volume expansion
	Dextran	Polymerized glucose in dextrose or saline	
	PPF: plasma protein fraction (5%)	83% albumin and 17% globulin	
	Albumin (25% or 5%)	96% albumin and 4% globulin	Also used as a replacement fluid for therapeutic plasma exchange

From King KE, editor: *Blood transfusion therapy, a physician's handbook*, ed 10, Bethesda, MD, 2011, AABB.

CHAPTER SUMMARY

Transfusion therapy provides patients with the correct component of critical value for many types of diseases and conditions. Transfusion support for selected patients discussed in this chapter is summarized in the following table.

Summary of Transfusion Support

Disease or condition	Problem	Transfusion therapy
Massive transfusion	Risk of hypovolemic shock	Crystalloids, colloids, plasma, RBCs
Cardiac surgery	Heparin; hypothermia; platelet destruction	RBCs, platelets, plasma
Premature infant	Iatrogenic blood loss; hemoglobin F; low erythropoietin response	Leukocyte-reduced, CMV-reduced-risk products, RBCs <7 days old
Liver transplant	Low levels of vitamin K–dependent factors; bleeding	RBCs, FFP, platelets, Cryoprecipitated AHF
Progenitor cell transplant	Immunosuppression; irradiation of bone marrow	Irradiated and leukocyte-reduced platelets and RBCs
Oncology	Chemotherapy and irradiation treatment reduce red cell and platelet production	Leukocyte-reduced Platelets and RBCs; colony-stimulating factors
Chronic renal disease	Unable to produce erythropoietin; red cell damage from dialysis and increases in uremia	Erythropoietin; leukocyte-reduced RBCs
TTP and HUS	Platelet and coagulation factors are consumed	Therapeutic apheresis, FFP, and RBCs
Sickle cell anemia	Chronic red cell destruction from sickling of cells	RBCs, phenotypically matched to avoid alloantibody production
Hemostatic disorders	Factor deficiencies: von Willebrand's disease, hemophilia A and B	Factor derivatives specific for factor that is lacking

RBC, Red Blood Cell; *CMV*, cytomegalovirus; *FFP*, Fresh Frozen Plasma; *AHF*, Antihemophilic Factor; *TTP*, thrombotic thrombocytopenic purpura; *HUS*, hemolytic uremic syndrome.

CRITICAL THINKING EXERCISES

EXERCISE 15-1

A trauma patient in the emergency department has received 6 units of group O D-negative RBCs by emergency release. A sample was obtained and sent to the blood bank, and the physician has requested 10 additional units of type-specific RBCs. What are some potential problems in determining an ABO/D type? At what point will the sample from this patient not reflect his own red cells?

EXERCISE 15-2

A 68-year-old man is undergoing a second cardiac surgery, this time to replace a valve. He has been in surgery 4 hours, and there has been a recent request for platelets, RBCs, and FFP. What are the potential problems that this patient may be undergoing, and what factors make this type of surgery a challenge?

EXERCISE 15-3

A 4-day-old premature infant has been using small aliquots of RBCs. The parents of the infant would like to donate blood for their child. Can they be potential donors? What special requirements are necessary for RBCs during the neonatal period? Are crossmatches required? Why is blood from first-degree relatives considered a risk, and what is required to make blood products from family members safer?

EXERCISE 15-4

A kidney dialysis center requested 2 leukocyte-reduced RBC units stat for a patient with a 7 g/dL hemoglobin. The center is an outpatient clinic, and three other stat orders for preoperative procedures need to be completed before the shift ends. The technologist fills the order but would like to know why the request did not come earlier. What are the unique transfusion needs of kidney dialysis patients, and why was this ordered as a stat? Does erythropoietin eliminate the need for all RBC transfusions for renal patients? What contributes to their anemia?

EXERCISE 15-5

The oncology unit has requested that platelets be available for a patient scheduled to undergo chemotherapy for breast cancer. The request for Leukocyte-Reduced Apheresis Platelets is common and often extends for a week or more every 2 to 3 days. Why is this product necessary, and what are potential problems associated with platelet transfusions with regard to antibodies?

EXERCISE 15-6

A sample from a 4-year-old sickle cell patient was sent to the blood bank with a request for 2 units of phenotypically matched RBCs. The patient needs to be typed, and a unit needs to be located. Why are closely matched RBCs important for this child? Will it be difficult to find RBCs for this patient?

STUDY QUESTIONS

1. Plasmapheresis has been reasonably effective in treating:
   a. TTP
   b. hemolytic disease of the newborn
   c. sickle cell disease
   d. renal disease

2. Finding compatible blood for patients with autoimmune disease is difficult because of the:
   a. potential of underlying alloantibodies
   b. positive DAT
   c. reactive eluate
   d. hemolysis in the serum

3. Infants do not require crossmatching during:
   a. the first 4 months
   b. the first 6 months
   c. the first year
   d. an indefinite period if a parent's blood is used

4. An example of a crystalloid solution used to treat hypovolemia is:
   a. PPF
   b. albumin
   c. Ringer's lactate
   d. HES solution

5. Hemophilia A patients are treated for bleeding with:
   a. Cryoprecipitated AHF
   b. FFP
   c. RBCs
   d. factor VIII

6. Common complications of chemotherapy include:
   a. bleeding
   b. infection
   c. anemia
   d. all of the above

7. In the adult, erythropoietin to stimulate red cell production is produced in the:
   a. bone marrow
   b. liver
   c. kidneys
   d. spleen

8. Transfusion of RBCs in the neonate may be needed to compensate for:
   a. iatrogenic blood loss
   b. hemoglobin F
   c. insufficient erythropoiesis
   d. physiologic anemia of infancy
   e. all of the above

9. ABO compatible organ transplants are *not* critical in which of the following transplants?
   a. kidneys
   b. liver
   c. heart
   d. bone marrow

10. The colony-stimulating factor to reduce infection while undergoing chemotherapy is one that stimulates:
    a. erythrocytes
    b. megakaryocytes
    c. granulocytes
    d. lymphocytes

REFERENCES

1. Roback JD, editor: *Technical manual*, ed 17, Bethesda, MD, 2011, AABB.
2. King KE, editor: *Blood transfusion therapy, a physician's handbook*, ed 10, Bethesda, MD, 2011, AABB.
3. Despotis G, Eby C, Lubin DM: A review of transfusion risks and optimal management of perioperative bleeding with cardiac surgery, *Transfusion* 48:2S, 2008.
4. Sobel M, NcNeill PM: Diagnosis and management of intraoperative and postoperative hemostatic defects. In Rossi EC, Simon TL, Moss GS, editors: *Principles of transfusion medicine*, Baltimore, 1991, Williams & Wilkins.
5. Strauss RG: Transfusion therapy in neonates, *Am J Dis Child* 145:904, 1991.
6. McCullough J: *Transfusion medicine*, ed 2, Philadelphia, 2005, Elsevier.
7. Livingston ER, et al: Increased activation of the coagulation and fibrinolytic systems leads to hemorrhagic complications during left ventricular assist implantation, *Circulation* 94 (9 Suppl):II227, 1996.
8. Laughlin MJ, Eapen M, Rubinstein P, et al: Outcomes after transplantation of cord blood or bone marrow from unrelated donors in adults with acute leukemia, *N Engl J Med* 351;2276, 2004.
9. Daniel-Johnson J, Schwartz J: How do I approach ABO-incompatible hematopoietic progenitor cell transplantation? *Transfusion* 51(6):1143, 2011.
10. Hillyer CD, Silverstein LF, Ness PM, et al: *Blood banking and transfusion medicine*, ed 2, Philadelphia, 2007, Elsevier.
11. AABB: Circular of information for the use of human blood and blood components, 2009. www.aabb.org.

Quality Assurance and Regulation of the Blood Industry and Safety Issues in the Blood Bank

16

CHAPTER OUTLINE

LEARNING OBJECTIVES

On completion of this chapter, the reader should be able to:

1. Define and list the elements of good manufacturing practices.
2. Describe regulatory agencies that govern activities in the blood bank and apply their regulations.
3. Apply voluntary agency compliance guidelines to the workplace.
4. Differentiate quality assurance (QA) from quality control (QC). Identify the responsibilities of the QA department.
5. Discuss the importance of job descriptions and personnel qualifications.
6. Compare and contrast proficiency and competency testing.
7. List the elements of and explain the importance of a well-written standard operating procedure (SOP).

8. Compare and contrast good record keeping with poor record keeping.
9. Describe the elements of a good training program.
10. Give examples of methods used to evaluate competency.
11. Define calibration, preventive maintenance, and QC requirements; discuss the importance to each in reporting accurate results.
12. Define and describe the purpose behind root-cause analysis in error management.
13. Define and apply universal and standard precautions.
14. Dispose of laboratory waste material properly.
15. List safety equipment and protective devices.
16. Recognize the need for accident reporting.
17. Encourage employee education in safety.
18. Conduct testing using safety principles.

The Food and Drug Administration (FDA) describes standards for quality and safety for transfusion services and blood banks through quality assurance (QA) programs and current Good Manufacturing Practices (cGMPs). Quality efforts and activities enhance efficiency and customer relations, satisfy regulatory requirements, and ultimately provide a safe blood product for transfusion. This chapter discusses the elements of a QA program as it applies to blood banks and transfusion services and the cGMPs that guide these efforts.

This chapter also provides an overview of a blood bank safety program. Safety is a concern for everyone. Employer and employee must understand their respective roles in the issues of compliance in blood banking safety. This understanding focuses on efforts to decrease infection risk and physical and chemical hazards in the workplace. The responsibility by law for employee safety ultimately resides with the employer or director of the laboratory. The employer has an obligation to provide a safe work environment by following the imposed standards of care. However, the individual employee must also assume responsibility for his or her health and safety and the safety of coworkers by following laboratory safety policies and procedures. When safety is endorsed and practiced by everyone in the blood bank, fewer errors and accidents occur.

SECTION 1
REGULATORY AND ACCREDITING AGENCIES FOR QUALITY AND SAFETY

The blood industry is monitored by many regulatory and accrediting agencies. Compliance with industry, federal, state, and local requirements is reviewed by these agencies. Although the rules are presented in different formats, they focus on ensuring product quality and donor and patient safety. Regulatory and accrediting agencies address similar issues regarding QA and quality improvement. The agencies differ in the degree of authority they have to enforce the standards. Compliance with standards set by governmental agencies, such as the FDA, Centers for Medicare and Medicaid Services (CMS), and state agencies, is enforceable by law. Accrediting agencies, such as the AABB, are considered industry associations, and compliance with their requirements is voluntary and evaluated by peer review.

FOOD AND DRUG ADMINISTRATION

The FDA enforces regulations to ensure the safety and efficacy of biologics, drugs, and devices, including blood and blood components and diagnostic reagents used or manufactured by blood establishments. The regulation of biologics products in the United States began when Congress passed the Biologics Control Act of 1902.[1] Provisions of the act include requirements for the licensing of manufacturers and products, labeling, facility inspections, suspension or revocation of licenses, and penalties for violation. Current implementation of the law is placed under the Public Health Service (PHS) Act 42 USC §262.[2]

The FDA is the agency that enforces the regulations of the PHS Act and the federal Food, Drug and Cosmetic Service Act.[3] Each inspection is designed to follow a unit of blood or a blood product from donor to patient. The inspection includes many elements of quality and safety: errors, accidents and fatalities, facilities, equipment, personnel, and disposal of infectious waste.

The FDA falls under the jurisdiction of the Department of Health and Human Services. Many industries fall within the jurisdiction of the FDA, including drugs, cosmetics, food, and blood. The agency is involved in three areas:
• Surveillance of facilities (inspections)
• Policy enforcement
• Establishment and issue of regulations

The FDA uses several tools to enforce its policy: regular unannounced inspections, warning letters, license suspension, license revocation, and injunction (consent decree). The last four tools are used only when the violations identified during an establishment inspection are considered serious enough to compromise public safety or when a persistent history of noncompliance with the organization exists.

TABLE 16-1	Elements of Quality Assurance

- Records and SOPs
- Personnel selection and training
- Validation, calibration, preventive maintenance, proficiency testing
- Supplier qualification
- Error management
- Process improvement
- Process control
- Label control
- Internal auditing

SOPs, Standard operating procedures.

AABB

The AABB is a voluntary accrediting agency. Its publications serve as guidelines for members seeking accreditation; these include the *Standards for Blood Banks and Transfusion Services,* the *Technical Manual,* and others. The AABB *Standards for Blood Banks and Transfusion Services* provides the basis for the inspection and accreditation of blood banks by a private, professional organization. Blood banks and transfusion services voluntarily comply with AABB inspection and accreditation. Accreditation is a high recognition of standards. AABB publications have served as principal guidelines for blood banks and transfusion services since 1958.

In recent years, the AABB has increased the emphasis on quality principles. The AABB has supported its members by designing documents that facilitate the implementation of QA programs, such as the *Quality Essentials.* Compliance with the AABB *Quality Essentials* became mandatory as of January 1, 1998, for organizations seeking accreditation. The *Quality Essentials* itemizes all the elements of QA appropriate for blood banks or transfusion services. The AABB *Quality Essentials* defined elements for the maintenance of a quality system within the blood bank or transfusion service. These quality essentials are listed in Table 16-1.

OTHER SAFETY REGULATIONS

Occupational Safety and Health Act

The Occupational Safety and Health Act was passed by Congress in 1970 "to assure safe and healthful working conditions for working men and women; by authorizing enforcement of the standards developed under the act; by assisting and encouraging the states in their efforts to assure safe and healthful working conditions; by providing for research, information, education, and training in the field of occupational safety and health; and for other purposes."[4] The act is enforced by the **Occupational Safety and Health Administration** (OSHA).

> **Occupational Safety and Health Administration:** agency responsible for ensuring safe and healthful working conditions.

Each year, updated regulations are published in the *Code of Federal Regulations* (CFR), and standards are enforced under OSHA by workplace inspections. Most clinical facilities are inspected following employee or consumer complaints. However, OSHA may choose under authority of the Occupational Safety and Health Act to inspect any facility at any time. Employers are responsible for informing employees of the OSHA standards and must post OSHA literature that informs employees of their rights and responsibilities.

States and territories operate their own job safety and health plans under OSHA. These standards are identical to, or as stringent as, the federal OSHA standards and must cover state and local government employees. In addition, state and local governments may impose additional requirements for safety.

Environmental Protection Agency

The Environmental Protection Agency (EPA) is involved in the assessment of medical waste as specified in the Medical Waste Tracking Act of 1988.[5] The act requires the EPA to determine types, numbers, and sizes of generators of medical waste in the United States.

The EPA examines the present or potential threat of medical waste to human health and the environment. Most medical waste regulations emanate from the individual states or local authorities and are variable because no national policy exists for the handling of medical waste.

SECTION 2
QUALITY ASSURANCE AND GOOD MANUFACTURING PRACTICES

QUALITY ASSURANCE

QA comprises the combined activities performed by an organization to ensure the quality of products and services they offer, which must include cGMPs. The basic components of a QA program are listed in Table 16-1. These activities must be planned and documented by written policies and procedures.

Quality Assurance Department
Responsibilities

> Internal quality audits evaluate the effectiveness of the quality system in the organization. Audits are systematic investigations to confirm the level of compliance with established SOPs.

Blood banks are required to establish QA departments that are separate from manufacturing and report to upper management. QA responsibilities include the following:
- Compliance with cGMPs
- Review and approval of all standard operating procedures (SOPs)
- Specifications and validation protocols
- Development, review, and approval of training programs
- Investigation of product recalls, errors, and complaints
- Coordination of internal quality auditing programs

GOOD MANUFACTURING PRACTICES

> QA is a comprehensive program monitoring the entire testing process. Quality control (QC) monitors the test system's components such as reagents and instrumentation. QC is part of the QA system.

Good manufacturing practices are performed in blood banks and transfusion services as part of QA and are legal requirements established by the FDA. These regulations itemize "what" needs to be done without necessarily specifying "how." In other words, each organization must determine the best way to implement all these practices. Table 16-2 describes the elements of cGMPs. cGMPs applicable to the blood industry are found in the *Code of Federal Regulations* (CFR), specifically Title 21, Part 606.[6] cGMPs are only a part of the overall QA program in any given facility.

COMPONENTS OF A QUALITY ASSURANCE PROGRAM

Records and Documents

According to the AABB *Standards for Blood Banks and Transfusion Services*, the facility shall have policies, processes, and procedures to ensure document identification, review,

---

TABLE 16-2   Elements of Good Manufacturing Practices

- Write SOPs
- Follow SOPs
- Record and document all work performed
- Qualify personnel by training and education
- Design and build proper facilities and equipment
- Clean by following a housekeeping schedule
- Validate equipment, personnel, and processes
- Perform preventive maintenance on facilities and equipment
- Control for quality
- Audit for compliance with all of the above

SOPs, Standard operating procedures.

TABLE 16-3	Retention of Donor and Blood Unit Records

Indefinite

Donors placed on permanent deferral and indefinite deferral lists

Minimum of 10 Years of Retention

Identification of individuals performing each significant step in collection, processing, compatibility testing, and distribution of blood and components

Final disposition of each unit of blood or blood component including recipient identification, if transfused

Unique identification of each unit

Consent of donors

Donor notification of significant abnormal findings

Comprehensive donor information including address, medical history, physical examination, and health history

Donor acknowledgment regarding educational materials and signed statement from donor confirming accuracy of information provided

ABO group and Rh type for all collections

Identification number and collecting facility for each unit in pooled components

Preparation of specific components

Allogeneic donor testing to detect unexpected antibodies to red cell antigens for donors with a history of transfusions or pregnancy

Interpretations of disease marker testing for allogeneic testing

Quarantine of units from prior collections when a repeat donor has a reactive disease marker screening test

Final review of records relating to testing and acceptability criteria

Review of donor records to ensure any units from an ineligible donor are quarantined

Transfusion service investigation of transfusion-transmitted disease report

Distribution or issue of units before completion of testing

Serologic confirmation of donor blood ABO/Rh typing

Signed statements from requesting physician in urgent release of blood before completion of compatibility testing or infectious disease testing

From Carson TH: *Standards for blood banks and transfusion services*, ed 27, Bethesda, MD, 2011, AABB.

approval, and retention.[7] Records are created and stored in accordance with the record retention policies. Examples of records include manual logs, worksheets, computer print-outs, temperature charts, CD-ROMs, DVDs, and photographs.

Document Control

Regulatory and accrediting agencies expect documentation to be thorough; well organized; appropriately stored; retrievable in a reasonable amount of time; and protected from unauthorized access, modification, and destruction.[8] **Document control** programs should specify and describe acceptable media to be used, types of documents to be kept, and record-retention intervals.[8] Alternative methods should be in place to handle situations when the automated systems become unavailable. Finally, all record systems, including control, handling, and disposal, must be described thoroughly in the facility's **standard operating procedures.**

Facility record-retention times are documented in the AABB *Standards for Blood Banks and Transfusion Services*, ed 27, Section 6, Reference Standards 6.2A and 6.2B.[7] Tables 16-3 and 16-4 describe some of the recommended retention times for blood donor and blood unit records and patient records.

Record Keeping

If it is not recorded, it never happened. The concept seems simple; however, poor record keeping is the most common violation identified by regulatory and accrediting agencies. Good documentation practices (GDP), whether manual or computerized, allow tracing of all products collected or transfused by an organization. A thorough record-keeping system recreates every step related to the production and distribution of a unit of blood

Document control: plan for the management of all documents in an organization that addresses the design, responsibility, storage, removal, and revision of all records, forms, and procedures.

Standard operating procedures: written procedures to help ensure the complete understanding of a process and to achieve consistency in performance from one individual to another.

TABLE 16-4	Retention of Patient Records

Indefinite

Difficulty in blood typing, clinically significant antibodies, significant adverse events to transfusions, and special transfusion requirements

Minimum of 10 Years of Retention

Source to final disposition of each unit of blood or blood component, if issued by the facility for transfusion

Test results and interpretations of patient's ABO group and Rh type

Patient testing for unexpected antibodies to red cell antigens

Additional testing to detect clinically significant antibodies

Pretransfusion testing for autologous transfusion

Test results and interpretations of serologic and computer crossmatch

Detection of ABO incompatibility when no clinically significant antibodies are detected

Two determinations of recipient's ABO group

Final check of transfusion service records at issue

Look-back to identify recipients who may have been infected with hepatitis C virus or HIV

Signed statements from requesting physician in urgent release of blood before completion of compatibility testing or infectious disease testing

Irradiation of cellular components

Minimum of 5 Years of Retention

Approval of medical director for transfusion of autologous blood to allogeneic recipient

Comparison of patient's previous test results for ABO group and Rh type in last 12 months, if comparison not performed electronically

Comparison of ABO group and Rh type during last 12 months with investigation and resolution of discrepancies

Recipient consent

Final inspection of blood and components before issue

Verification of patient identification before transfusion

Evaluation of suspected transfusion adverse event

Patient's medical record on transfusion

From Carson TH: *Standards for blood banks and transfusion services*, ed 27, Bethesda, MD, 2011, AABB. *HIV*, Human immunodeficiency virus.

Audit trail: record-keeping system that recreates every step in the manufacturing process.

and all its components. This concept is known as an **audit trail** and is important when investigating errors and accidents, as discussed later in this chapter.

Manual Record Guidelines

Good documentation practices for manual inputs are outlined in Table 16-5. Common record-keeping errors often encountered in laboratories are also listed. For example, error correction is a critical issue. The original data must not be obliterated or deleted when making a correction (Fig. 16-1). The identity of the person making the change also needs to be recorded. A standard practice is to cross off with a single line the item that is incorrect and write the correct data or information next to it, followed by the date and initials of the person making the correction. An additional recommendation is to state why the record was changed.

Computerized Record Guidelines

Never provide password information to another staff member. Never use another person's password to enter information into the computer.

A mechanism to trace back the original entry and the person making the correction is also necessary in computer systems.[8] There are processes and procedures to support the management of computer systems and routine backup of all critical data. Corrections to computer records must include the following information: the previous result, the new result, the date and time, and the name of the person changing the result. In the event of a system failure, a backup method for retrieval of computer records must be available. Backup data should be stored at an off-site location.

TABLE 16-5 Good Record Keeping versus Bad Record Keeping

GOOD RECORD KEEPING	BAD RECORD KEEPING
Use of indelible (permanent) blue or black ink	Use of correction fluid or white tape when making a correction
Blue ink is preferred	Use of pencil or nonpermanent ink
Recording data on appropriate form or log	Recording data on a piece of scratch paper or sticky notes
Recording date and initials of person making a correction	*Not* recording date or initials of person making a correction Recording data for someone else
Recording data immediately after performance of task	Recording data later or not immediately after performance of task
Not obliterating or deleting the original entry when making a correction	Obliterating or deleting original entry when making a correction
Indicating "broken," "closed," or "not in use" when appropriate	*Not* recording "broken," "closed," or "not in use" when appropriate
Not using "dittos"	Use of "dittos"

NOT ACCEPTABLE

Anti-A	Anti-B	Anti-D	A1 Cells	B Cells	Interpretation
0	0	3+	4+	4+	AB ~~positive~~ O positive

ACCEPTABLE

Anti-A	Anti-B	Anti-D	A1 Cells	B Cells	Interpretation
0	0	3+	4+	4+	~~AB~~ O positive Rm 9/1/99

Fig. 16-1 Correcting a manual record. A record is corrected by placing a single line through the error, recording the correct information next to the error, and placing initials of the person making the correction along with the date. A statement describing the reason for the correction is also recommended.

Standard Operating Procedures

SOPs describe how a particular task is to be accomplished. Established methods for performing and administering processes ensure the consistent quality of the final product or result. Internal and external auditors carefully assess noncompliance with written SOPs, one of the most serious violations that can be identified during an inspection.

SOPs are important training tools for new employees. These documents should be written using a standard format, as illustrated in Fig. 16-2. The Clinical and Laboratory Standards Institute publishes guidelines for the development of SOPs in document GP2-A5, *Laboratory Documents: Development and Control; Approved Guideline*, ed 5.[9] They need to be written following recommendations of reagent and equipment manufacturers and in compliance with other cGMPs and industry standards as appropriate. Effective procedures do not need to be wordy. If the documents are user-friendly, they are more likely to be used by staff. Well-written procedures include all the steps that ensure process control and contribute to the safety, purity, and potency of the blood product.

Facilities need to say what they do (write SOPs) and do what they say (follow SOPs).

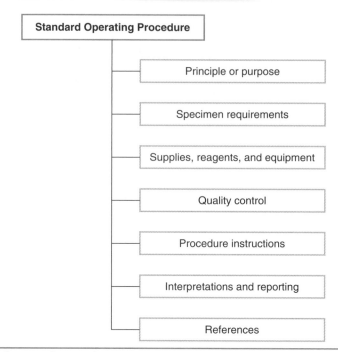

Fig. 16-2 Elements of a procedure. SOPs are written with a standardized format that is user-friendly.

Change Control

Change control: system to plan and implement changes in procedures, equipment, policies, and methods to increase effectiveness and prevent problems.

Change control is a general element of process control. Because the blood industry is in a constant state of change, blood banks and transfusion services need a process, known as change control, to develop or change existing processes or procedures. Blood banks and transfusion services are being challenged routinely by new technologies and new regulatory and accrediting requirements. In addition, facilities have to keep up with internal trends and business issues, such as mergers, acquisitions, employee turnover, expansion, and downsizing. These changes need to be controlled to prevent oversights that could affect multiple aspects of the organization. Manufacturing changes especially need to be well thought out and planned *before* implementation to guarantee their success and effectiveness. Similar to validation (discussed later in this chapter), change control needs the allocation of time, money, and manpower. However, the many benefits outweigh the cost.

The key in change control is the anticipation and prevention of problems.

Change control programs are used by manufacturing firms to ensure that nothing "falls through the cracks." For example, the addition of a new blood storage refrigerator would seem straightforward; however, the installation goes beyond the purchase and plug-in steps. Fig. 16-3 illustrates a change protocol for a new refrigerator that addresses critical steps in equipment installation to prevent potential problems.

Personnel Qualifications

Selection Criteria and Job Descriptions

Good employees are essential to the success of any organization. Hiring unqualified individuals can add significant expense to the organization and create a demoralizing environment for coworkers who have to accommodate poor performance. The selection process must be thorough, and minimal preestablished criteria should be identified. These criteria must be identified for each type of position in the organization and address the experience, background, skills, and credentials (e.g., degrees, licensure, and certification) deemed necessary to perform the job. The selection criteria are not stagnant. They should be revised as changes in job duties or tasks occur.

Job description documents should be developed for each type of position in the organization. These documents describe the tasks for which the employee is responsible and outline the areas of knowledge and skill that need to be acquired during training to

```
┌─────────────────────────┐
│   Change Control Plan for│
│        Refrigerator      │
└─────────────────────────┘
         │
         │   ┌────────────────────────────────────┐
         ├───│ Installation Qualification Protocol:│
         │   │   Refrigerator's specifications for │
         │   │ temperature, power supply, and alarms│
         │   └────────────────────────────────────┘
         │   ┌────────────────────────────────────┐
         ├───│  Validation Test Plan: Evaluation of│
         │   │     refrigerator's temperature and  │
         │   │    alarms before placed into service│
         │   └────────────────────────────────────┘
         │   ┌────────────────────────────────────┐
         ├───│ Initial Calibration and Quality Control:│
         │   │   Results of testing and alarm quality │
         │   │              control                │
         │   └────────────────────────────────────┘
         │   ┌────────────────────────────────────┐
         ├───│              SOPs:                  │
         │   │ Written for the operation, calibration,│
         │   │    quality control, and maintenance │
         │   └────────────────────────────────────┘
         │   ┌────────────────────────────────────┐
         ├───│   Staff Training: Operation and     │
         │   │     maintenance of refrigerator     │
         │   └────────────────────────────────────┘
         │   ┌────────────────────────────────────┐
         └───│    Refrigerator placed in use       │
             └────────────────────────────────────┘
```

Fig. 16-3   Change control plan for a new refrigerator.

perform the job. These documents also necessitate updating as appropriate to reflect all employee duties.

Training

Training is a critical aspect of compliance with cGMPs that necessitates a significant organization-wide commitment for success. Facilities that allocate time and resources for training and education benefit by reducing rework and inconsistency. In the development of a training program, the designation of trainers is important. Individuals selected as trainers should be able to convey information clearly, be respected by their peers, enjoy sharing expertise, and have a positive attitude toward building teams.

Training is provided during new employee orientation and is necessary whenever there are procedure changes or evidence of poor performance. Training activities usually include, but are not limited to, the following activities:

- Employee's review of SOP documents and associated materials
- Trainer's demonstration of task or procedure
- Employee's performance of task or procedure with the trainer's assistance
- Employee's demonstration of knowledge and application of the learned skill without the trainer's assistance

Good training programs allow the trainer to explain all functions and demonstrate the task before employee performance. Repetition of tasks in a "test" environment or with supervision is necessary before the trainee is allowed to perform the procedure independently. Throughout the training process, the employee must have ample opportunities to ask questions and receive explanations. Finally, training is not complete until it is documented, which typically takes place in the form of a checklist signed by the trainee, trainer, and supervisor.

Competency Assessment

Training is concluded only when documented evidence exists that the employee is able to demonstrate knowledge and application of the new skill. This demonstration is the purpose of **competency assessment.**

Initial competency assessment refers to the evaluation of the level of knowledge and skill an employee has gained during training to determine whether the individual is ready to perform a procedure. In addition, periodic competency assessment is used to determine

Competency assessment: evaluation of the employee's ability and knowledge to perform a procedure or skill.

whether the employee has maintained the level of knowledge and skill necessary to perform the job or task as described in the facility's SOP. The CMS and AABB, through the Clinical Laboratory Improvement Amendments of 1988, have established requirements of proof of competency for testing personnel twice during the first year of employment and annually thereafter.[8] Most regulatory and accrediting agencies require retraining for employees who fail to prove competency. The employee must not be allowed to perform the procedure (or procedures) until retraining is provided and subsequent competency assessment proves to be satisfactory.

In the case of unacceptable performance, corrective actions should be taken. Actions include retraining and documenting performance and competency assessment. The employee may not perform the tasks in which unacceptable performance was demonstrated.

Supplier Qualification

The quality of any given product is as good as the quality of the raw materials that go into its production. Supplier qualification has become a standard practice among many blood banks and transfusion services.[7] These facilities have established procedures to evaluate whether the quality of critical products and services received from suppliers meets preestablished criteria. Written agreements between blood banks and their suppliers are common practice. These documents, among many things, usually specify terms, including expectations between the involved parties. In some instances, facilities choose to audit their suppliers on an ongoing basis to determine the level of compliance with product specifications. This practice also should be included in written agreements. In addition, facilities should have procedures for inspecting and testing incoming materials (when applicable). These procedures should specify acceptable criteria and the course of action to be taken when they are not met.

Error Management

Root-Cause Analysis and Problem Solving

As part of a QA plan, facilities must have in place mechanisms for the detection and management of errors and their consequences. Errors, incidents, variances, and any nonconformance should be thoroughly documented and investigated. Employees must be actively involved in the problem-solving stages for the process to be successful. Once a problem is identified, an immediate response follows to correct the problem. The facility should initiate a **root-cause analysis** to identify what factors contributed to the occurrence of the problem. Once the cause is identified, a proposed plan for prevention should be drafted. After changes are made and the process is fine-tuned or adjusted, a subsequent review should be made to evaluate the effectiveness of the preventive corrective action. If the error recurs, another root-cause analysis is indicated. The adoption of this strategy ensures continuous quality improvement of all processes. Errors should be viewed as opportunities for improvement, and employees should be encouraged to report errors without concern for reprisal.

Errors can be identified internally by employees or externally by customers. Errors must be logged, and their frequencies must be tracked and monitored. Graphing incidences of occurrence and subsequent recurrences can provide QA departments with a comprehensive understanding of the reliability of a given process or individual and the effectiveness of a corrective action taken. Tracking can also help identify where quality efforts should be focused and which areas need to be addressed and corrected first.

Recalls

Recalls are usually issued by manufacturers in an attempt to remove products from the market that might compromise the safety of the recipient. They can be initiated voluntarily by the organization or at the request of the FDA. In some instances, recalls are issued months or years after the product has been transfused or has expired. In this case, the objective of the recall notification is to alert the client of possible hazards or adverse consequences the recipient might have incurred by receiving the product. Recalls are classified based on the degree of danger or hazard they impose.

Competency assessment may be performed by direct observation of performance, written tests, review of results and records, or using blind samples.

Blood products, test reagents, blood bags, and labels are examples of critical products.

Size, color, type of container, temperature, purity, and potency are examples of product specifications.

Root-cause analysis: investigation and subsequent identification of the factors that contributed to an error.

Errors are classified as incidents, deviations, complaints, and nonconformances.

Any error or accident that compromises the safety of a donor or patient requires reporting to the FDA.

Recalls: manufacturers' removal of products from the market that may compromise the safety of the recipient.

Validation

Validation is a process that establishes documented evidence providing a high degree of assurance that a specific process consistently produces a product that meets its preestablished quality and performance specifications. Even if regulatory and accrediting agencies did not make it necessary, validation is a good business practice. Procedures, equipment, personnel, new methods, and computer information systems must be proven reliable before being put into use. The best way to prove reliability is by stressing and challenging the process or system *before* it is implemented.

Validation: establishing that a specific process consistently produces a product that meets predetermined specifications.

Facilities and Equipment

The blood bank and transfusion service need to address the adequacy of the facility and equipment used in the facility for compliance to cGMPs. Figs. 16-4 and 16-5 summarize these activities.

Proficiency Testing

Proficiency testing is a required component of the QA program for testing laboratories. It is used to ensure that test methods and equipment are working as expected and that staff members are following procedures.[8] Proficiency surveys are prepared by accredited agencies that distribute samples for testing to requesting laboratories.

A common proficiency test is the CAP Survey, issued by the College of American Pathologists. Tests are run by routine testing personnel, using routine test equipment, during regular test runs, and in conformance with the facility's SOP. The results are recorded on standard forms and submitted to the agency within a given period. The test

Fig. 16-4   QA essentials for facilities.

Fig. 16-5   QA essentials for equipment.

results are evaluated and scored, and a report is returned to the institution for review. Corrective action is implemented and monitored for improvement when results are not acceptable. Proficiency tests can be used to prove competency; however, competency tests cannot replace proficiency testing.

Label Control

Many blood product recalls are due to mislabeling. If the incorrect label is placed on a unit of blood, the product is called misbranded. Similar to other recalls, mislabeling errors are not only time-consuming but also embarrassing. For this reason, blood banks, similar to pharmaceutical firms, have instituted label control programs. In many facilities, it is the responsibility of the QA department to inspect and approve all labels on receipt and before they are put into use, ensuring that all labels are in compliance with requirements. Labeling is a critical step in manufacturing and should be done in areas designed only for that purpose.

SECTION 3
SAFETY

STANDARD VERSUS UNIVERSAL PRECAUTIONS

Standard precautions: CDC term defining policies of treating all body substances as potentially infectious and applying safety measures to reduce possible exposure. Standard precautions incorporate universal precautions and body substance isolation together.

Universal precautions: OSHA term defining policies of treating all body substances as potentially infectious and applying safety measures to reduce possible exposure.

The concept of **standard precautions** was first introduced in 1987 by the Centers for Disease Control and Prevention (CDC) to decrease the occupational risks of blood-borne diseases, such as acquired immunodeficiency syndrome and hepatitis B virus (HBV), to health care workers.[10] In 1991, OSHA issued its final standard on occupational exposure to blood-borne pathogens, which mandated the use of **universal precautions.** Current universal precautions focus on treating all body substances as potentially harmful and applying appropriate safety measures to decrease possible exposure and infection. The use of protective measures is now based on the health care worker's contact with body fluids rather than on a patient's diagnosis. This concept, originally known as body-substance isolation, has been adapted and incorporated into the CDC two-tiered isolation guidelines as standard precautions (Table 16-6).[11]

BLOOD BANK SAFETY PROGRAM

The blood bank safety program must be a comprehensive program that includes policies and procedures of all regulatory bodies and any voluntary compliance accrediting agencies. In addition, any state and local laws must be taken into consideration. Most important, the safety program must be one that employees and employers endorse. Adherence to the safety program reduces any occupational hazards of the workplace and maintains a safe environment. The program should incorporate the OSHA regulations as outlined in Table 16-7.

The director or administrator of the blood bank must appoint an individual or individuals responsible for the program. A written safety program that itemizes the requirements must be available to all blood bank personnel. The document should enumerate

TABLE 16-6	Centers for Disease Control and Prevention Standard Precautions Isolation Guidelines
TIER I	**TIER II**
Blood, all body fluids, secretions, and excretions regardless of patient diagnosis or evidence of visible blood	Airborne, droplet, and contact from patients of documented or suspected infection of highly transmissible or epidemiologic pathogens for which additional precautions are necessary

From Centers for Disease Control and Prevention: *Guidelines for isolation precautions in hospitals,* (CDC) 59(214):55552, Washington, DC, 1995, US Government Printing Office.

TABLE 16-7	Occupational Safety and Health Administration Regulations for Protection from Blood-Borne Pathogens Requirements

Employers must:
- Provide a hazard-free workplace
- Educate and train staff
- Evaluate all procedures for potential exposure risks
- Evaluate each employment position for potential exposure risks
- Implement labeling procedures and post signs
- Apply universal precautions for handling all body substances
- Provide personal protective equipment, such as gloves or other barriers, without cost to the employee
- Make HBV vaccine prophylaxis available to all staff who have occupational exposure, unless previously vaccinated or immune, and provide hepatitis B immune globulin treatment for percutaneous injury at no cost to the employee

HBV, Hepatitis B virus.

current safety policies, which need to be cross-referenced in each preanalytical, analytical, and postanalytical procedure in the laboratory. Safety program administrators need to consider not only the technical staff but also potential risks for donors, ancillary personnel, volunteers, and visitors.

Physical Space, Safety Equipment, Protective Devices, and Warning Signs

Physical Space

The physical design of the blood bank and organization of tasks can reduce many potential hazards. Ready access to eyewashes, showers, and hand washing is essential.

Laboratory Attire

Most tasks in the blood bank can be safely performed while wearing laboratory attire that protects the worker from common infectious hazards. A fluid-resistant laboratory coat, gown, or apron, whether disposable or made of cotton material, is recommended. Laboratory coats should be large enough to close completely in front, or aprons may be worn over long-sleeved uniforms. These personal barrier protection garments should be changed immediately if they are contaminated with blood or toxic substances. All outerwear worn during the performance of blood banking tasks should be considered contaminated. Such garments should not be worn outside the laboratory into public areas. If nondisposable protective garments are used, they must be removed and stored in a suitable container and laundered in a manner that ensures decontamination. To contain the risk of infectious materials, home laundering is prohibited because unpredictable methods of transportation and handling can spread contamination, and laundering techniques might not be effective.

Safety facts:
- Hair should be secured away from the face and off the shoulders.
- Jewelry should be kept to a minimum, and rings that could perforate gloves should not be worn.
- Open-toed shoes are not permitted in areas where blood exposure exists.
- Cosmetics should not be applied in the laboratory.

Personal Protective Equipment, Eyewashes, and Showers

Safety glasses, face shields or masks, splash barriers, and goggles are devices categorized as personal protective equipment (Fig. 16-6). Safety glasses or goggles should be worn when splashes are likely to occur during a task. Masks are better because they protect the mouth, nose, and eyes. Face shields are made of shatterproof plastic and wrap around the face, offering greater protection. Permanently mounted splash barriers over the bench area are preferred when task performance risks splashing or aerosol contamination. Opening tubes of blood and using corrosive liquids warrant this protection for the employee. The shields should be cleansed and decontaminated on a regular basis.

If a splash does occur, the blood bank should have the availability of a shower and an eyewash device. An eyewash device should be capable of providing a gentle stream or spray of aerated water for an extended period of time. Safety showers are for treating immediate first-aid needs of personnel contaminated with hazardous materials and for extinguishing clothing fires. Procedures and indications for use must be posted, and routine maintenance checks must be performed.

Fig. 16-6 Personal protective equipment. Gloves, gown, and face shield used while working with liquid nitrogen frozen red blood cell samples. (Courtesy Micro Typing Systems, Inc., Pompano Beach, FL.)

Biological Safety Cabinets

Biological safety cabinets (BSCs) are containment devices that facilitate safe handling of infectious materials and reduce the risk to personnel and the laboratory environment. Procedures that expose opened tubes of blood or units known to be positive for hepatitis B surface antigen or human immunodeficiency virus (HIV) are examples of blood bank procedures in which a BSC may be useful.

Employees need training in the operation of the BSC for maximum protection. The effectiveness of the BSC is a function of directional airflow inward and downward through a high-efficiency filter. Disruption of the airflow prevents maximum efficiency and usefulness of the cabinet.

Gloves and Hand Washing

Blood bank personnel should wear gloves as a protective barrier when handling any blood or blood products. OSHA does not require the routine use of gloves by phlebotomists working with healthy, prescreened donors or, if gloves are worn, the changing of unsoiled gloves between donors. Guidelines recommend the use of gloves for the phlebotomy of autologous donors or patients (e.g., therapeutic apheresis procedures). However, all employees likely to be exposed to blood should follow good practice by wearing gloves as another measure of precaution because even prescreened "healthy" donors may have had contact with an infectious agent and may be unaware of the contact. A prudent part of the safety procedure of the blood bank includes the policy that all employees must wear gloves when tasks are likely to involve exposure to blood. Gloves used in a contaminated area should not be worn to a "clean" area or when using or touching telephones, doorknobs, or computer terminals.

Even when gloves are worn, hand washing remains the most effective defense in infection control and safety. Blood-borne pathogens generally do not penetrate intact skin, and hand washing prevents their transfer to mucous membranes, such as nasal passages or broken skin areas. Hand washing also reduces the transmission of infectious agents to others. Hands should be washed after the removal of gloves in the following situations: following task completion; before leaving a work area; before, between, and after seeing patients; and immediately after contact with blood.

Warning Signs

Many regulatory agencies have designed warning signs and posted them in the laboratory for identification of hazardous materials or areas. OSHA emphasizes the importance of

> **Safety fact:**
> • Blood bank personnel should wear gloves as a protective barrier when handling any blood or blood products.

BIOHAZARD

Fig. 16-7 Biohazard symbol.

alerting personnel to potential danger with labels and signs. Biohazard warning labels, signs, and containers are fluorescent orange or red with lettering or symbols in a contrasting color (Fig. 16-7). Signs are intended to alert workers and others to take necessary precautions.

Decontamination

All laboratory surfaces and reusable equipment should routinely be cleaned and decontaminated daily and as needed while performing tasks and as spills occur. EPA-approved disinfectant solutions are published by the agency.[12] An economic and effective disinfectant is a fresh solution of 1:10 dilution of sodium hypochlorite (bleach), which can be used for general disinfection or for spills.

Chemical Storage and Hazards

The blood bank houses chemicals that may be of significant hazard. Chemical hazards are most often classified by their corrosiveness, ignitability, reactivity, and toxicity. Containment of chemicals is based on the nature of these hazards. The Hazard Communications Standard (29 CFR 1910.1200) created a "right to know" procedure for the worker who handles or is exposed to hazardous chemicals. Manufacturers, importers, or distributors of all toxic substances are required to supply Material Safety Data Sheets (MSDS). MSDS are required by OSHA and contain information including the chemical names, hazards, and personal protective equipment to be used and the spill clean-up details. MSDS must be made readily available in the workplace to all employees.

Radiation Safety

Few laboratory tests incorporate radionuclides. However, the blood bank uses gamma irradiators for the irradiation of blood components. Employee safety needs to be emphasized with proper training in the use of the equipment, personal protective equipment, and exposure monitoring.

   Blood irradiators vary in the amount of radiation scatter and leakage. The Nuclear Regulatory Commission requires training for all personnel using irradiators and records indicating exposure. Although monitors may not be required for some equipment, leak detection is necessary.

Biohazardous Wastes

Blood bank safety programs must include policies for handling all waste materials from areas where waste is contaminated with blood or body fluids. All laboratory personnel should be trained in a waste management program that protects staff members and meets

Safety fact:
- All laboratory surfaces and reusable equipment should routinely be cleaned and decontaminated daily and as needed while performing tasks and as spills occur.

federal, state, and local regulatory requirements. Untrained personnel should not come in contact with or be responsible for biohazardous waste materials.

Correct identification of material is important to segregate potentially infectious waste from mainstream waste and to control cost and volume of infectious waste. Proper handling ensures that medical waste marked as biohazardous materials is placed in designated containers. Containers should be leakproof. Incineration and decontamination by autoclaving are currently recommended for disposing of blood samples and blood products.

Storage and Transportation of Blood and Blood Components

Storage

Storage of blood and blood components for transfusion should be separate from reagents, specimens, and any other unrelated materials. Ideally, a separate refrigerator should be used; however, if one is not available, areas within the refrigerator must be segregated to reduce spills or accidents. Refrigerators should be large enough to accommodate the anticipated blood storage need.

> **Safety fact:**
> • Food or drink should not be allowed in the blood storage or testing areas.

Transportation

Blood and blood components transferred within an institution for transfusion purposes do not require packaging and labeling as for shipping. Specimens should be transported in a plastic bag to prevent spills or leakage. To avoid contamination, paperwork should not be placed in the bag.

Any shipping of diagnostic materials or etiologic agents to or from the laboratory must follow the regulations of the Department of Transportation and the U.S. Postal Service. Blood banks should contact the carrier for correct packaging and label identification requirements.

Personal Injury and Reporting

In the event an employee or other person is injured or possible injury or infection exists, an accident report should be initiated. These reports are required by worker's compensation, OSHA, and other regulatory and accrediting bodies. An accident report should be initiated in *all* accidents and injuries involving employees or other persons. Routine investigation of a minor incident and follow-up to correct the risk may thwart a major accident later. Personnel should be encouraged to report all incidents no matter how insignificant they may seem because accident reporting is an essential part of maintaining a safe working environment. Each incident should be treated with a thorough investigation in a nonthreatening manner to the employee.

Employee Education

Employee education not only makes good sense, but it is a mandate of OSHA and other regulatory and accrediting agencies. The blood bank safety program should be reviewed with new employees during their orientation and training before independent work is permitted. All employees whose tasks carry risk of infectious exposure should annually review the safety program as a condition of OSHA. The supervisor or responsible safety officer should document all employee participation in this education, and performance evaluations should include the employee's adherence to the safety policies and procedures of the blood bank.

CHAPTER SUMMARY

• The blood industry is regulated by multiple regulatory and accrediting agencies. All these entities require compliance with QA and quality improvement concepts. However, only regulatory agencies have the lawful authority to enforce their requirements.
• cGMPs are the minimum federal requirements that guarantee the safety, potency, purity, and quality of blood products.
• cGMPs are only a part of the QA program.

- QA encompasses all other planned activities that, when executed, ensure the quality of the products or services offered. These include record keeping and SOPs, personnel selection and training, validation, supplier qualification, calibration, preventive maintenance, proficiency testing, error management, process improvement, process control, label control, and internal auditing.
- Safety concerns everyone. Employer and employee must understand their respective roles in the issues of compliance in blood banking safety. This understanding centers on the need to decrease infection risk and physical and chemical hazards in the workplace.
- The responsibility by law for employee safety ultimately resides with the employer or director of the laboratory. The employer has an obligation to provide a safe work environment by following the imposed standards of care.
- Individual employees must assume responsibility for their own health and safety and the safety of coworkers by following laboratory safety policies and procedures.
- When safety is endorsed and practiced by everyone in the blood bank, fewer errors and accidents occur.

CRITICAL THINKING EXERCISES

EXERCISE 16-1

PEC is a successful and modern blood donor center located in the northeastern region of the United States. Its management style has always stood out among other blood centers in the United States because of its modern and progressive views. The blood center is well known for embracing changes in manufacturing with a positive approach by appropriately planning and allocating resources to ensure things are done the right way. However, in the last few years, both employees and customers have noticed a steady decline in control and quality. The number of manufacturing errors and product and service complaints reported by customers has drastically increased. PEC has tripled in size in the last 3 years, following the acquisition of several small blood banks in the state. Changes have occurred quickly to accommodate this growth, and thorough planning before the implementation of these changes has not always been possible. Among many of its growing pains, PEC employees finally realized that their blood bank computer system was outdated and unable to handle the workload volume increase in the last few years.

Management at PEC selected EJO, Inc., as the new software vendor. Although EJO's experience, reputation, expertise, and client support were well known, its new blood banking software was not. However, the cost of implementing this new software fit well within the approved fiscal budget. With full management support, validation and training efforts began early in the year with a proposed "live" date for September of that year. By June, multiple "bugs" had been identified during system testing. EJO's technical support was excellent, but with so many problems to be addressed and corrected, management was getting anxious. They wanted the new system to go "live" before their next FDA inspection. September came and went, and the system was not ready for implementation. Finally, in March of the following year, parallel testing was completed. Because of time constraints, not all functions were tested, in particular, functions pertaining to the issue of products. Management was aware but decided to go ahead with implementation of the system.

In April, the new system at PEC was implemented with no major problems. Everything was okay until 3 months later, when the distribution supervisor noticed that the system had allowed the release of human T-cell lymphotropic virus (HTLV) I/II repeatedly reactive donor units. The PEC QA department was immediately notified, and recall procedures were initiated. By that time, 35 donor units and all their parts had been released.

1. What did PEC fail to do? What were the consequences?
2. What are some of the factors that contributed to the release of unacceptable units?
3. What can be done to prevent this situation from happening again?

EXERCISE 16-2

AKC Blood Center collects more than 600 platelet apheresis products each month. Platelet counts for donors and these products are determined using KB1, a state-of-the-art automated hematology instrument. This piece of equipment, similar to many others, requires extensive QC and preventive maintenance by the manufacturer. During the last 4 days, Fred, the medical technologist assigned to run the instrument, has failed to notice that the low-level control has consistently fallen below the mean. Fred has been too busy trying to train new personnel in the department and has had no time to plot his results on the QC chart, which is a departmental procedure requirement. If he performed this task, he would have noticed the obvious shift.

Today the new trainee, Fran, is running platelet counts with Fred's assistance. Once again the low-level control falls below the mean, but this time it is outside the manufacturer's range altogether. Fran notices the value is being flagged by KB1 and notifies Fred of the problem. Fred is too busy on the phone handling an irate call from a client hospital and tells Fran to "keep running it until it falls in. You know, sometimes it takes a while for controls to come in."
1. If you were Fred's supervisor, what would you do?
2. What is the root cause of the problem?
3. What can be done to prevent this from happening again?
4. What can be said about Fred's results since he started using the instrument?

EXERCISE 16-3

The transfusion services department at PSB Medical Center has always been happy with the level of service offered by YR Blood Center. However, during the last 3 months, they have noticed quite a few platelet units with visible agglutinants. If you worked for the QA unit at YR Blood Center and were told to investigate this problem, what areas would you investigate to identify the root cause of the problem?

EXERCISE 16-4

Prepare a list of all the things that need to be done before the implementation of a new component centrifuge.

EXERCISE 16-5

Identify the consequences of the following cGMP violations:
1. *Not* taking daily temperature reading for a blood refrigerator
2. Extending test incubation times beyond what the SOP states
3. Overloading a refrigerator beyond its capacity
4. Cutting an employee's training short
5. Running proficiency samples over and over until the sample is used up
6. Using expired reagents
7. Reporting test results when controls are out of range
8. Not performing preventive maintenance on an instrument as required by the manufacturer

STUDY QUESTIONS

1. Which of the following is *not* a basic component of a QA program?
   a. calibration
   b. preventive maintenance
   c. viral marker testing
   d. record keeping

2. Manual records can be corrected as long as:
   a. the original entry is neither obliterated nor deleted
   b. the person making the correction dates and initials the change
   c. the item to be corrected is crossed off with a single line
   d. all of the above

3. All of the following statements are true about SOPs *except* that they are:
   a. step-by-step instructions
   b. used to monitor accuracy and precision
   c. written in compliance with cGMPs
   d. written in compliance with manufacturer's recommendations

4. What is the purpose of competency assessment?
   a. identify employees in need of retraining
   b. evaluate an individual's level of knowledge during a job interview
   c. identify employees who need to be fired
   d. all of the above

5. All of the following statements are *true* regarding internal audits *except* that they:
   a. help identify problems early
   b. ensure continuous quality improvement efforts
   c. are used solely for the purpose of identifying "troublemakers"
   d. are one of the many responsibilities of the QA unit

6. Employees are the core of an organization, and therefore they:
   a. must be trained
   b. must report errors without fear of reprisal
   c. are a key part of problem solving
   d. all of the above

7. cGMPs applicable to the blood industry can be found in the:
   a. AABB *Standards for Blood Banks and Transfusion Services*
   b. SOP manual
   c. FDA *Code of Federal Regulations*
   d. QA manual

8. Early identification of problems by evaluating the compliance with established SOP is the purpose of:
   a. internal audits   c. root-cause analysis
   b. accident reports   d. FDA inspections

For questions 9 through 11, match the following descriptions with the appropriate organization:

Description	Organization
9. government agency that regulates blood banks	a. AABB
10. voluntary peer review organization	b. FDA
11. agency responsible for safety	c. OSHA

12. Ultimately the responsibility for a safety program in the laboratory belongs to:
    a. CDC   c. OSHA
    b. the employer or laboratory director   d. the employee

13. The *Technical Manual* often used for principal guidelines in the blood bank is a publication of:
    a. CAP   c. AABB
    b. TJC   d. OSHA

14. All blood banks as mandated by law must have a:
    a. water fountain   c. BSC
    b. written laboratory safety program   d. foot-operated hand wash

15. Goggles, face shields, and splash barriers are:
    a. personal protective equipment
    b. not necessary unless working with HIV-positive or HBV-positive specimens
    c. mandated at all times when working with blood specimens and blood products
    d. provided by the employee if needed

16. The policy of treating all body substances as potentially harmful, regardless of the patient diagnosis, is known as:
    a. OSHA Exposure Program
    b. isolation guidelines
    c. AABB safety policy
    d. universal precautions

17. The most effective defense for infection control and safety is wearing gloves and:
    a. goggles
    b. laboratory coats
    c. posting warning signs
    d. hand washing

18. One of the most economical disinfectants to use is a:
    a. 1:10 fresh solution of sodium hypochlorite (bleach)
    b. 1:5 solution of household Lysol
    c. 1:15 solution of sodium hydroxide
    d. detergent and water mixture

19. The reporting of an accident or injury should occur when any:
    a. injury may result in a fatality
    b. injury involves possible infection with HIV or HBV
    c. accident involves nonemployees or jeopardizes a patient
    d. accident or injury occurs

20. One of the best ways to protect employees and keep a safe laboratory environment is to provide employees with:
    a. health insurance
    b. safety education
    c. rest breaks
    d. fluid-repellent laboratory coats

REFERENCES

1. The coroner's verdict in the St. Louis tetanus cases, 1901 New York Medical Journal 74, *JAMA* 37:1255, 1902.
2. Public Health Service Act of 1944, Public Law 42 USC 262, 1944.
3. Food, Drug and Cosmetic Act of 1938, Public Law 21 USC 321, 1938.
4. Occupational Safety and Health Act of 1970, Public Law 29 USC 651, 1970.
5. US Environmental Protection Agency: *Medical waste tracking act, 40 USC 6992,* Washington, DC, 1988, US Government Printing Office.
6. Food and Drug Administration: *Code of federal regulations, 21 CFR 600-799,* Washington, DC, 2011, US Government Printing Office. Revised April 2011.
7. Carson TH: *Standards for blood banks and transfusion services,* ed 27, Bethesda, MD, 2011, AABB.
8. Roback JD, editor: *Technical manual,* ed 17, Bethesda, MD, 2011, AABB.
9. Clinical and Laboratory Standards Institute: *Laboratory documents: development and control; approved guideline,* ed 5, GP2-A5, Wayne, PA, 2006, CLSI.
10. Centers for Disease Control and Prevention: Recommendations for preventing HIV transmission in health care settings, *MMWR Morb Mortal Wkly Rep* 36(2S):1, 1987.
11. Centers for Disease Control and Prevention: *Guidelines for isolation precautions in hospitals,* (CDC) 59(214):55552, Washington, DC, 1995, US Government Printing Office.
12. Centers for Disease Control and Prevention: Regulatory framework for disinfectants and sterilants, *MMWR Morb Mortal Wkly Rep* 52:62, 2003.

Answers to Study Questions

Chapter 1
1. d
2. a
3. b
4. c
5. d
6. a
7. b
8. a
9. c
10. a
11. c
12. e
13. d
14. c
15. c
16. a
17. b
18. b
19. c
20. c
21. d
22. c
23. b
24. c
25. c

Chapter 2
1. a
2. b
3. a
4. c
5. d
6. c
7. b
8. c
9. a
10. b
11. d
12. a
13. b
14. a
15. c

Chapter 3
1. d
2. b
3. d
4. b
5. a
6. a
7. c
8. d
9. c
10. c
11. a
12. d
13. d
14. c
15. c
16. c
17. c
18. a
19. c

Chapter 4
1. c
2. d
3. a
4. d
5. a
6. d
7. c
8. b
9. c
10. b
11. c
12. d
13. a
14. d
15. c
16. a
17. b
18. d
19. c
20. b

Chapter 5
1. d
2. a
3. d
4. a
5. a
6. b
7. b
8. d
9. d
10. a
11. a
12. b
13. a
14. c
15. a
16. a
17. b
18. d
19. a
20. b

Chapter 6
1. c
2. c
3. a
4. a
5. d, e, and g
6. d
7. d
8. c
9. d
10. c
11. a
12. d
13. a
14. c
15. d
16. a
17. c
18. c
19. b
20. d

21. c
22. b
23. b
24. b
25. d

Chapter 7
1. a
2. c
3. d
4. d
5. a
6. c
7. c
8. c
9. b
10. d
11. a
12. c
13. c
14. d
15. c

Chapter 8
1. b
2. c
3. c
4. d
5. a
6. b
7. c
8. c
9. b
10. d
11. a
12. c
13. d
14. c
15. c
16. f
17. f
18. f
19. f

20. f
21. f
22. t
23. f
24. f
25. t

Chapter 9
1. a
2. c
3. c
4. b
5. d
6. d
7. c
8. b
9. a
10. d
11. t
12. t
13. t
14. f
15. t
16. t
17. t
18. t
19. f

Chapter 10
1. a
2. c
3. d
4. b
5. d
6. c
7. d
8. a
9. c
10. c
11. a
12. b
13. d
14. a
15. b

16. a
17. b
18. b
19. a
20. c
21. d
22. d

Chapter 11
1. c
2. b
3. c
4. c
5. d
6. c
7. a
8. a
9. a
10. c
11. d
12. a
13. b
14. d
15. c
16. c
17. b
18. a
19. c
20. b
21. a
22. a
23. a
24. b
25. c

Chapter 12
1. TD
2. A
3. A
4. TD
5. PD
6. TD
7. A
8. A

9. PD
10. PD
11. PD
12. PD
13. d
14. b
15. d
16. t
17. f
18. f
19. t
20. f

Chapter 13
1. d
2. d
3. e
4. b
5. a
6. b
7. d
8. b
9. a
10. c

Chapter 14
1. d
2. b
3. e
4. f
5. a
6. g
7. c
8. e
9. d
10. b
11. a
12. c
13. f
14. d
15. g
16. a
17. c
18. b

19. d
20. c
21. d
22. d
23. b
24. b
25. b

Chapter 15
1. a
2. a
3. a
4. c
5. d
6. d
7. c
8. e
9. d
10. c

Chapter 16
1. c
2. d
3. b
4. a
5. c
6. d
7. c
8. a
9. b
10. a
11. c
12. b
13. c
14. b
15. a
16. d
17. d
18. a
19. d
20. b

Glossary

AABB formerly known as the American Association of Blood Banks; professional organization that accredits and provides educational and technical guidance in the field of cellular therapy, blood collection and safety, and transfusion medicine

ABO antibodies anti-A, anti-B, and anti-A,B; patients possess the ABO antibody to the ABO antigen lacking on their red cells (e.g., group A individuals possess anti-B)

ABO discrepancy occurs when ABO phenotyping of red cells does not agree with expected serum testing results for the particular ABO phenotype

acanthocytosis presence of abnormal red cells with spurlike projections in the circulating blood

accuracy degree to which a measurement represents the true value of the attribute being measured

acquired agammaglobulinemia absence of gamma globulin and antibodies associated with malignant diseases such as leukemia, myeloma, or lymphoma

acquired B phenotype group A_1 individual with diseases of the lower gastrointestinal tract, cancers of the colon and rectum, intestinal obstruction, or gram-negative septicemia who acquires reactivity with anti-B reagents in ABO red cell testing and appears as group AB

acquired hypogammaglobulinemia lower than normal levels of gamma globulin in the blood associated with malignant diseases (chronic leukemias and myeloma) and immunosuppressive therapy

acquired immunity results when immunologic memory and specificity develop in response to the antigen and involves cell-mediated and humoral responses

acute hemolytic transfusion reaction complication of transfusion associated with intravascular hemolysis, characterized by rapid onset with symptoms of fever, chills, hemoglobinemia, and hypotension; major complications include irreversible shock, renal failure, and disseminated intravascular coagulation

acute reaction reaction occurring within 24 hours of transfusion

adsorption immunohematologic technique that uses red cells (known antigens) to remove red cell antibodies from a solution (plasma or antisera); for example, group A red cells can remove anti-A from solution

affinity strength of the binding between a single antibody and an epitope of an antigen

affinity maturation process of somatic mutations in the immunoglobulin gene causing the formation of variations in the affinity of the antibody to the antigen; B cells with the highest affinity are "selected" for the best fit, and the resulting antibody is stronger

agglutination visible clumping of particulate antigens caused by interaction with a specific antibody

agglutinogen an older term referring to a group of antigens or factors that are agglutinated by antisera

alleged father man accused of being the biological father; the putative father

allele different forms of a gene present a particular chromosomal locus

alloantibodies antibodies with specificities other than self; stimulated by transfusion or pregnancy

allogeneic cells or tissue from a genetically different individual

allogeneic adsorption use of blood from a genetically different individual, such as reagent or donor cells that have been phenotyped for common red cell antigens to remove alloantibodies and autoantibodies

allogeneic donation donation for use by the general patient population

alternative pathway activation of complement that is initiated by foreign cell-surface constituents

amniocentesis process of withdrawal of amniotic fluid by aspiration for the purpose of analysis

amorphic describes a gene that does not express a detectable product

amplicon amplified target sequence of DNA produced by PCR

anamnestic response secondary immune response

anaphylatoxins complement split products (C3a, C4a, and C5a) that mediate degranulation of mast cells and basophils, which results in smooth muscle contraction and increased vascular permeability

antenatal (prenatal) time period before birth

antepartum period of time between conception and onset of labor, used with reference to the mother

antibody glycoprotein (immunoglobulin) that recognizes a particular epitope on an antigen and facilitates clearance of that antigen

antibody identification the process of determining the identity of a red cell antibody detected in the antibody screen by reacting serum with commercial panel cells or other reagent red cells

antibody potentiators reagents or methods that enhance or speed up the antibody-antigen reaction

antibody screen test test to determine the presence of alloantibodies

antigen foreign molecules that bind specifically to an antibody or a T-cell receptor

antigenic determinants sites on an antigen that are recognized and bound by a particular antibody or T-cell receptor (also called epitope)

antigen-presenting cells cells that process and present antigenic peptides in association with Class II major histocompatibility complex molecules and activate T cells

antigram profile of antigen typings of each donor used in the manufacturing of commercially supplied screening and panel cells

antithetical opposite antigens encoded at the same locus

apheresis method of blood collection where whole blood is removed from a donor or patient and separated into components; one or more of the components are retained, and the remainder is returned to the donor or patient

apheresis donation donation of a specific component of the blood; parts of the whole blood that are not retained are returned to the donor

apheresis platelets apheresis procedure in which the platelets are removed from a donor, and the remaining red cells and plasma are returned

audit trail record-keeping system that recreates every step in the manufacturing process

audits systematic investigations to determine whether policies and procedures are being performed and supported properly

autoadsorption attachment of the patient's antibodies to the patient's own red cells and subsequent removal from the serum

autoantibodies antibodies to self-antigens

autocontrol testing a person's serum with his or her own red cells to determine whether an autoantibody is present

autoimmune hemolytic anemia immune destruction of autologous or self–red cells

autologous pertaining to self (e.g., cells or tissue from self)

autologous donation donation by a donor reserved for the donor's later use

autosomes chromosomes other than the sex chromosomes

avidity overall strength of reaction between several epitopes and antibodies; depends on the affinity of the antibody, valency, and noncovalent attractive forces

B lymphocytes (B cell) lymphocytes that mature in the bone marrow, differentiate into plasma cells when stimulated by an antigen, and produce antibodies

B(A) phenotype group B individual who acquires reactivity with anti-A reagents in ABO red cell testing; in these individuals, the B gene transfers trace amounts of the immunodominant sugar for the A antigen and the immunodominant sugar for the B antigen

biphasic hemolysin antibody, such as the Donath-Landsteiner antibody, that requires a period of cold and warm incubations to bind complement with resulting hemolysis

bivalent having a combining power of two

blocked D D antigen phenotype may be falsely negative if the cells are heavily coated with anti-D; usually associated with D-positive cord blood and maternal anti-D

blood group systems groups of antigens on the red cell membrane that share related serologic properties and genetic patterns of inheritance

blood warmer medical device that prewarms donor blood to 37° C before transfusion

Bombay phenotype rare phenotype of an individual who genetically has inherited *h* allele in homozygous manner; individual's red cells lack H and ABO antigens

bradykinin potent vasodilator of the kinin family

calibration process of standardizing an instrument against a known value

carbohydrates simple sugars, such as monosaccharides and starches (polysaccharides)

cell separation technique used to separate transfused cells from autologous or patient cells

cellular immunity adaptive immunity in which T lymphocytes recognize and react with the antigen through direct cell-to-cell interaction

change control system to plan and implement changes in procedures, equipment, policies, and methods to increase effectiveness and prevent problems

chemokines group of cytokines involved in the activation of white blood cells during migration across the endothelium

chemotactic movement of cells in the direction of the antigenic stimulus

chimerism mixture of donor and recipient cell populations following hematopoietic stem cell transplants

chromosomes structures within the nucleus that contain DNA

chronic granulomatous disease inherited disorder in which the phagocytic white blood cells are able to engulf but not kill certain microorganisms

cis two or more genes on the same chromosome of a homologous pair

classical pathway activation of complement that is initiated by antigen-antibody complexes

Clinical Laboratory Improvement Act act enacted to ensure that laboratory tests are consistently reliable and of high quality

clinical significance antibodies capable of causing decreased survival of transfused cells as in a transfusion reaction; have been associated with hemolytic disease of the fetus and newborn

clinically insignificant antibody that does not shorten the survival of transfused red cells or has been associated with hemolytic disease of the fetus and newborn

clone family of cells or organisms having genetically identical constitution

closed system collection of blood in a sterile blood container

cluster of differentiation (CD marker) cell membrane molecule used to differentiate human leukocyte subpopulations; determined by specific monoclonal antibodies

Code of Federal Regulations publication from the Food and Drug Administration outlining the legal requirements of blood banking facilities

codominant equal expression of two different inherited alleles

cold alloantibodies red cell antibodies specific for other human red cell antigens that typically react at or below room temperature

cold autoantibodies red cell antibodies specific for autologous antigens that typically react at or below room temperature

cold hemagglutinin disease autoimmune hemolytic anemia produced by an autoantibody that reacts best in colder temperatures (<37° C)

colony-stimulating factors cytokines that promote the expansion and differentiation of bone marrow stem cells and progenitor cells

compatibility testing all steps in the identification and testing of a potential transfusion recipient and donor blood before transfusion in an attempt to provide a blood product that survives in vivo and provides its therapeutic effect in the recipient

competency assessment evaluation of the employee's ability and knowledge to perform a procedure or skill

competitive ELISA (EIA) enzyme-linked immunosorbent assay technique used to determine the presence or quantity of an antigen or antibody; in this test, a lower absorbance indicates detection of the marker

complement system group of serum proteins that participate in an enzymatic cascade, ultimately generating the membrane attack complex that causes lysis of cellular elements

components parts of whole blood that are separated into therapeutic units usually by centrifugation; consist of RBCs, plasma, Cryoprecipitated Antihemophilic Factor, and platelets

compound antigens distinct antigen produced when two other antigens are encoded by the same gene

congenital agammaglobulinemia genetic disease characterized by the absence of gamma globulin and antibodies in the blood

congenital hypogammaglobulinemia genetic disease characterized by reduced levels of gamma globulin in the blood

constant regions nonvariable portions of the heavy and light chains of an immunoglobulin

cord blood whole blood obtained from the umbilical vein or artery of the fetus

corrected count increment relative increase in platelet count adjusted for the number of platelets transfused and the size of the patient

CPRA calculated panel reactive antibodies; estimates the percentage of donors that would be incompatible with the candidate, based on the candidate's antibodies to HLA antigens

crossing over exchange of genetic material during meiosis between paired chromosomes

crossmatch compatibility testing procedure in which donor RBCs are combined with the patient's serum to determine the serologic compatibility between donor and patient

cryoprecipitated AHF blood component recovered from a controlled thaw of Fresh Frozen Plasma; the cold-insoluble precipitate is rich in coagulation factor VIII, von Willebrand's factor, factor XIII, and fibrinogen

cryoprotective solution added to protect against cell damage that occurs at or below freezing temperatures

current good manufacturing practices (cGMPs) methods used in, and the facilities or controls used for, the manufacture, processing, packing, or holding of a drug (including a blood product) to ensure that it meets safety, purity, and potency standards

cytokines secreted proteins that regulate the activity of other cells by binding to specific receptors; they can increase or decrease cell proliferation, antibody production, and inflammation reactions

deacetylating removal of the acetyl group (CH_3CO^-)

delayed reaction reaction occurring more than 24 hours after transfusion

diastolic pressure filling of the heart chamber; the second sound heard while taking a blood pressure

differential adsorption adsorption or attachment of antibodies in the serum to specific known antigens, usually to different aliquots of red cells

differential DAT immunohematologic test that uses monospecific anti-IgG and monospecific anti-C3d/anti-C3b reagents to determine the cause of a positive DAT with polyspecific antiglobulin reagents

direct antiglobulin test test used to detect antibody bound to red cells in vivo

direct exclusion exclusion of paternity when a child has a trait that neither parent demonstrates

directed donation donation reserved for use by a specific patient

DNA probe short sequence of DNA complementary to the area being identified; it is attached to a marker (usually fluorescent) that can be read by an instrument such as a flow cytometer

document control plan for the management of all documents in an organization that addresses the design, responsibility, storage, removal, and revision of all records, forms, and procedures

Dolichos biflorus plant lectin with specificity for the A_1 antigen

dominant gene product expressed over another gene

dosage effect stronger agglutination when a red cell antigen is expressed from homozygous genes

eluate antibody removed from red cells to be used for antibody identification

elution process that dissociates antigen-antibody complexes on red cells; freed IgG antibody is tested for specificity

enhancement media reagents that enhance or speed up the antibody-antigen reaction

epitopes single antigenic determinants; functionally, the parts of the antigen that combine with the antibody

erythroblastosis fetalis also called hemolytic disease of the fetus and newborn

extravascular hemolysis red cell destruction within phagocytes or removal of red cells from circulation by phagocytic cells residing in the reticuloendothelial system (liver and spleen), usually by IgG opsonization

false-negative result test result that incorrectly indicates a negative reaction (lack of agglutination); an antigen-antibody reaction has occurred but is not demonstrated

false-positive result test result that incorrectly indicates a positive reaction (presence of agglutination or hemolysis); no antigen-antibody reaction occurred

fetomaternal hemorrhage escape of fetal cells into the maternal circulation, usually occurring at the time of delivery

Food and Drug Administration U.S. agency responsible for the regulation of the blood banking industry and other manufacturers of products consumed by humans

fresh frozen plasma blood component prepared from whole blood that contains only the plasma portion of whole blood and is frozen after separation to retain labile factors

gene segment of DNA that encodes a particular protein

genetic loci sites of a gene on a chromosome

genotype actual genetic makeup; determined by family studies or molecular tests

glycolipids compounds containing carbohydrate and lipid molecules

glycophorin glycoprotein that projects through the red cell membrane and carries many blood group antigens

glycoproteins compounds containing carbohydrate and protein molecules

glycosyltransferase enzyme that catalyzes the transfer of glycosyl groups (simple carbohydrate units) in biochemical reactions

graft-versus-host disease (GVHD) a disease caused by the reaction of mature T cells in the graft or transfused cells against alloantigens on host cells

granulocyte concentrates blood component collected by cytapheresis; contain a minimum of 1.0×10^{10} granulocytes

group A with acquired B antigen group A_1 individual with disease of the lower gastrointestinal tract, cancer of the colon and rectum, intestinal obstruction, or gram-negative septicemia who acquires reactivity with anti-B reagents in ABO red cell testing and appears as group AB

haplotype set of linked genes inherited together because of their close proximity on a chromosome

hapten small-molecular-weight particle that requires a carrier molecule to be recognized by the immune system

haptoglobin plasma protein that binds free hemoglobin and carries the molecule to the hepatocytes for further catabolism

heavy chains larger polypeptide of an antibody molecule composed of a variable and constant region; five major classes of heavy chains determine the isotype of an antibody

hematopoietic progenitor cells (HPCs) stem cells committed to a blood cell lineage that are collected from marrow, peripheral blood, and cord blood and used to treat certain malignant diseases and congenital immune deficiencies

hematopoietic progenitor cell transplant replacement of hematopoietic stem cells derived from allogeneic bone marrow, peripheral stem cells, or cord blood to treat certain leukemias, immunodeficiencies, and hemoglobinopathies

hemolysis lysis or rupture of erythrocytes

hemolytic disease of the fetus and newborn (HDFN) disease caused by destruction of fetal or neonatal red cells by maternal antibodies

hemorrhage bleeding through ruptured or unruptured blood vessel walls

hemotherapy treatment of a disease or condition by the use of blood or blood derivatives

heterozygous two alleles for a given trait are different

hinge region portion of the immunoglobulin heavy chains between the Fc and Fab region; provides flexibility to the molecule to allow two antigen-binding sites to function independently

histamine compound that causes constriction of bronchial smooth muscle, dilation of capillaries, and decrease in blood pressure

homozygous two alleles for a given trait are identical

humoral immunity adaptive immunity in which B lymphocytes and plasma cells produce specific antibodies that recognize and react with an antigen

hybridization attachment of a complementary sequence of DNA by complementary base pair sequences

hybridoma hybrid cell formed by the fusion of a myeloma cell and an antibody-producing cell; used in the production of monoclonal antibodies

hydatid cyst fluid fluid obtained from a cyst of the dog tapeworm

hydrops fetalis edema in the fetus

iatrogenic blood loss blood loss caused by treatment (e.g., collection of samples for testing)

icterus pertaining to or resembling jaundice

idiotope variable part of an antibody or T-cell receptor; antigen binding site

immediate-spin interpretation of agglutination reactions immediately after centrifugation and without incubation

immediate-spin phases source antigen and source antibody used in immunohematologic testing are combined, immediately centrifuged, and observed for agglutination

immune complex complex of one or more antibody molecules bound to an antigen

immune-mediated reaction reactions involving antigen-antibody complexes, cytokine release, or complement activation

immunodominant sugar sugar molecule responsible for specificity

immunogen antigen in its role of eliciting an immune response

immunogenicity ability of an antigen to stimulate an immune response

immunoglobulins antibodies; glycoproteins secreted by plasma cells that bind to specific epitopes on antigenic substances

immunohematology study of blood group antigens and antibodies

incompatible crossmatches occur when agglutination or hemolysis is observed in the crossmatch of donor red cells and patient serum, indicating a serologic incompatibility

in vitro reaction in an artificial environment, such as in a test tube, microplate, or column

in vivo reaction within the body

independent assortment random behavior of genes on separate chromosomes during meiosis that results in a mixture of genetic material in the offspring

independent segregation passing of one gene from each parent to the offspring

indirect antiglobulin test test used to detect antibody bound to red cells in vitro

indirect ELISA (EIA) enzyme-linked immunosorbent assay technique used to determine the presence or quantity of an antibody, also called EIA

indirect exclusion failure to find an expected marker in a child when the alleged father is apparently homozygous for the gene

intravascular hemolysis destruction of red cells and release of hemoglobin within the vascular compartment through immune or nonimmune mechanisms; antibodies of the ABO system can cause this type of hemolysis (e.g., IgM activation of complement)

ISBT 128 International Society of Blood Transfusion recommendations regarding the uniform labeling of blood products for international bar code recognition by computers

ischemia decreased supply of oxygenated blood to an organ or body part

isotype one of five types of immunoglobulins determined by the heavy chain: IgM, IgG, IgA, IgE, and IgD

kappa chains one of the two types of light chains that make up an immunoglobulin

kinins group of proteins associated with contraction of smooth muscle, vascular permeability, and vasodilation

labile factors factors V and VIII, which are coagulation factors that deteriorate on storage

lambda chains one of the two types of light chains that make up an immunoglobulin

Landsteiner's rule rule stating that normal, healthy individuals possess ABO antibodies to the ABO blood group antigens absent from their red cells

lattice formation combination of antibody and a multivalent antigen to form crosslinks and result in visible agglutination

lecithin/sphingomyelin ratio ratio of lecithin to sphingomyelin that indicates lung maturity

lectins plant extracts useful as blood banking reagents; they bind to carbohydrate portions of certain red cell antigens and agglutinate the red cells

light chains smaller polypeptide of an antibody molecule composed of a variable and constant region; two major types of light chains exist in humans (kappa and lambda)

Liley graph graph used to predict severity of hemolytic disease of the fetus and newborn during pregnancy by evaluation of the amniotic fluid

linkage disequilibrium occurrence of a set of genes inherited together more often than would be expected by chance

linked when two genes are inherited together by being very close on a chromosome

lipids fatty acids and glycerol compounds

LIS interface laboratory information system interface for reporting results from the computer

look-back identification of persons who have received seronegative or untested blood from a donor subsequently found to be positive for disease markers

lymphocytes leukocytes that mediate humoral or cell-mediated immunity

major histocompatibility complex (MHC) group of genes located on chromosome 6 that determine the expression of the HLA and complement proteins

medical directors designated physicians responsible for the medical and technical policies of the blood bank

meiosis cell division in gametes that results in half the number of chromosomes present in somatic cells

membrane attack complex C5 to C9 proteins of the complement system that mediate cell lysis in the target cell

memory B cell B cell produced following the first exposure that remains in the circulation and can recognize and respond to an antigen faster

mitosis cell division in somatic cells that results in the same number of chromosomes

mixed field agglutination pattern in which a population of the red cells has agglutinated and the remainder of the red cells are unagglutinated

mixed lymphocyte culture (MLC) in vitro reaction of T cells from one individual against MHC antigens on leukocytes from another individual. The technique measures the response of HLA class II differences between donor and recipient cells usually through radioactive measurements of DNA synthesis; this test was historically used for compatibility and D (class II) antigen typing.

monoclonal antibody made from single clones of B cells that secrete antibodies of the same specificity

mononuclear phagocyte system system of mononuclear phagocytic cells, associated with the liver, spleen, and lymph nodes, that clears microbes and damaged cells

monospecific antihuman globulin reagents reagents prepared by separating the specificities of the polyspecific antihuman globulin reagents into individual sources of anti-IgG and anti-C3d/anti-C3b

multiple myeloma malignant neoplasm of the bone marrow characterized by abnormal proteins in the plasma and urine

naïve lymphocyte lymphocyte that has not previously encountered the antigen that matches its specific receptor

neonatal time period within the first 28 days after birth

neonatal alloimmune thrombocytopenia antibody destruction of a newborn's platelets caused by antibodies formed from prior pregnancies and directed to paternal antigens

neutralization blocking antibody sites, causing a negative reaction

non–immune-mediated reaction reactions that may be due to the component transfused, the patient's underlying condition, or the method of infusion

non–red blood cell stimulated immunologic stimulus for antibody production is unrelated to a red cell antigen

nonsecretor individual who inherits the genotype *sese* and does not express H soluble substance in secretions

nucleotide phosphate, sugar, and base that constitute the basic monomer of the nucleic acids DNA and RNA

null phenotypes absences of a particular blood group system from the red cell membrane

obligatory gene gene that should be inherited from the father to prove paternity

Occupational Safety and Health Administration (OSHA) U.S. agency responsible for ensuring safe and healthful working conditions

oligosaccharide chain chemical compound formed by a small number of simple carbohydrate molecules

one-stage enzyme technique antibody identification technique that requires the addition of the enzyme to the cell and serum mixture

open system collection or exposure to air through an open port that would shorten the expiration because of potential bacterial contamination

opsonin substance (antibody or complement protein) that binds to an antigen and enhances phagocytosis

p value probability value; value that provides a confidence limit for a particular event

parenterally by routes other than the digestive tract, including needle stick and transfusion

paroxysmal cold hemoglobinuria rare autoimmune disorder characterized by hemolysis and hematuria associated with exposure to cold

partial D D antigen that is missing part of its typical antigenic structure

passively transfused when an antibody is transferred to the recipient from the plasma portion of a blood product during transfusion

perinatal period extends from 28 weeks of gestation to 28 days following delivery

perinatally exposure before, during, or after the time of birth

phagocytic cells cells that engulf microorganisms, other cells, and foreign particles; include neutrophils, macrophages, and monocytes

phenotype observable expression of inherited traits

phototherapy treatment of elevated bilirubin or other conditions with ultraviolet light rays

plasma cell antibody-producing B cell that has reached the end of its differentiating pathway

platelet concentrates platelets obtained from a whole blood donation; contain a minimum of 5.5×10^{10} platelets

plateletpheresis collection of platelets by apheresis

polyagglutination property of the cells that causes them to be agglutinated by naturally occurring antibodies found in most human sera; agglutination occurs regardless of blood type

polyclonal antiserum made from several different clones of B cells that secrete antibodies of different specificities

polymorphic genetic system that expresses several possible alleles at specific loci on a chromosome

posttransfusion purpura antibody destruction of platelets after transfusion

postzone excess antigen causing a false-negative reaction

potency strength of an antigen-antibody reaction; or the effectiveness of a blood component

potentiators reagents added to the serum-cell mixture to enhance antibody uptake during the incubation phase of the indirect antiglobulin test

prenatal (antenatal) time period before birth

preventive maintenance maintenance that maximizes the duration of the equipment or facility, decreases "downtime," and avoids unnecessary costly repairs

prewarming technique patient serum and test cells are prewarmed separately before combining to prevent reactions of cold antibodies binding at room temperature and activating complement

primary immune response immune response induced by initial exposure to the antigen

proficiency testing surveys performed to ensure that a laboratory's test methods and equipment are working as expected

proteolytic enzymes enzymes that denature certain proteins

prozone excess antibody causing a false-negative reaction

Punnett square square used to display the frequencies of different genotypes and phenotypes among the offspring of a cross

Rabbit Erythrocyte Stroma (RESt) red cell membranes from rabbits used for adsorption of IgM antibodies

random-access system devices or workstations are used for multiple occurrences of a given laboratory operation within the automated procedure

reaction phase observation of agglutination at certain temperatures, after incubation, or after the addition of antihuman globulin

recalls manufacturers' removal of products from the market that may compromise the safety of the recipient

receptors molecules on the cell surface that have a high affinity for a particular ligand

recessive trait expressed only when inherited by both parents

recipient patient receiving a transfusion

red cell stroma red cell membrane that remains after hemolysis

refractoriness unresponsiveness to platelet transfusions caused by HLA-specific or platelet-specific antibodies or platelet destruction from fever or sepsis; responsiveness is measured by posttransfusion platelet counts

refractory unresponsive to platelet transfusions (*see* refractoriness)

regulator gene gene inherited at another locus or chromosome that affects the expression of another gene

respiratory distress syndrome inability to maintain stable pulmonary alveolar structures, caused by low levels of surfactant, lecithin, and other pulmonary lipids in premature infants

reticulocytosis increase in the number of reticulocytes in the circulating blood

Rh immune globulin (RhIG) commercially available immune serum globulin (gamma globulin) consisting of purified, high-titered anti-D from immunized donors that is given to prevent the formation of anti-D by D-negative individuals; also known as RhoGAM

root-cause analysis investigation and subsequent identification of the factors that contributed to an error

rule of three confirming the presence of an antibody by demonstrating three cells that are positive and three that are negative

rule out to eliminate the possibility that an antibody exists in the serum based on its nonreactivity with a particular antigen

saline replacement technique test to distinguish rouleaux and true agglutination

sandwich ELISA (EIA) enzyme-linked immunosorbent assay technique used to determine the presence or quantity of an antigen

secondary immune response immune response induced following a second exposure to the antigen, which activates the memory lymphocytes for a quicker response

secretor individual who inherits *Se* allele and expresses soluble forms of H antigens in secretions

segment sealed piece of integral tubing from the donor unit bag that contains a small aliquot of donor blood; used in the preparation of red cell suspensions for crossmatching

selected cells cells chosen from another panel to confirm or eliminate the possibility of an antibody

sensitization binding of antibody or complement components to a red cell

sensitized immunoglobulin or complement attached to the cells from the immune system (in vivo) or from a test procedure (in vitro)

serotonin potent vasoconstrictor liberated by platelets

serum-to-cell ratio ratio of antigen on the red cell to antibody in the serum

sialic acid constituents of the sugars attached to proteins on red cells that lend a negative charge to the red cell membrane

specificity unique recognition of an antigenic determinant and its corresponding antibody molecule

standard operating procedures written procedures to help ensure the complete understanding of a process and to achieve consistency in performance from one individual to another

standard precautions term from U.S. Centers for Disease Control and Prevention defining policies of treating all body substances as potentially infectious and applying safety measures to reduce possible exposure; standard precautions incorporate universal precautions and body substance isolation together

Standards for Blood Banks and Transfusion Services publication of the AABB that outlines the minimal standards of practice in areas relating to transfusion medicine

sulfhydryl reagents reagents that disrupt the disulfide bonds between cysteine amino acid residues in proteins; DTT, 2-ME, and AET function as sulfhydryl reagents

supernatant fluid above cells or particles after centrifugation

suppressor genes genes that suppress the expression of another gene

surrogate markers disease markers such as antibodies or elevations in enzymes that can be used as indicators for other potential infectious diseases; often used when direct testing is not available

syntenic genetic term referring to genes closely situated on the same chromosome without being linked

systolic pressure contraction of the heart; the first sound heard while taking a blood pressure

T cytotoxic cells subset of T lymphocytes responsible for the destruction of cells that have become infected by viruses or other intracellular pathogen

T helper cells subset of T lymphocytes that activates macrophages in cell-mediated responses and stimulates B cells to produce antibodies

T lymphocyte (T cell) lymphocytes that mature in the thymus and produce cytokines to activate the immune cells including the B cell

Technical Manual publication of the AABB that provides a reference to current acceptable practices in blood banking

thalassemia inherited disorder causing anemia because of a defective production rate of either α-hemoglobin or β-hemoglobin polypeptide

therapeutic apheresis removal of blood from a patient and retention of the portion that might be contributing to a pathologic condition; the remainder is returned along with a replacement fluid such as colloid or Fresh Frozen Plasma

throughput productivity of a machine, procedure, process, or system over a unit period

titers extent to which an antibody may be diluted before it loses its ability to agglutinate with antigen

Tn-polyagglutinable red cells type of polyagglutination that occurs from a mutation in the hematopoietic tissue, characterized by mixed-field reactions in agglutination testing

trans genes inherited on opposite chromosomes of a homologous pair

transferase class of enzymes that catalyzes the transfer of a chemical group from one molecule to another

transfusion reaction undesirable response by a patient to the infusion of blood or blood products

two-stage enzyme technique treatment of red cells with an enzyme before the addition of serum

Ulex europaeus plant lectin with specificity for the H antigen

unacceptable antigens antigens that the potential graft recipient is reacting against; antibodies to these antigens could reduce graft survival

universal donors group O donors for RBC transfusions; these RBCs may be transfused to any ABO phenotype because the cells lack both A and B antigens

universal precautions term from Occupational Safety and Health Administration defining policies of treating all body substances as potentially infectious and applying safety measures to reduce possible exposure

universal recipients group AB recipients may receive transfusions of RBCs from any ABO phenotype; these recipients lack circulating ABO antibodies in plasma

valency number of epitopes per molecule of antigen

validation establishing that a specific process consistently produces a product that meets predetermined specifications

variable regions amino-terminal portions of immunoglobulins and T-cell receptor chains that are highly variable and responsible for the antigenic specificity of these molecules

vasoactive amines products such as histamines released by basophils, mast cells, and platelets that act on the endothelium and smooth muscle of the local vasculature

Waldenström's macroglobulinemia overproduction of IgM by the clones of a plasma B cell in response to an antigenic signal; increased viscosity of blood is observed

weak D weak form of the D antigen that requires the indirect antiglobulin test for its detection

Wharton's jelly gelatinous tissue contaminant in cord blood samples that may interfere in immunohematologic tests

whole blood blood collected from a donor before separation into its components

zeta potential electrostatic potential measured between the red cell membrane and the slipping plane of the same cell

zone of equivalence number of binding sites of multivalent antigen and antibody are approximately equal

Index

Page numbers followed by "f" indicate figures, "t" indicate tables, and "b" indicate boxes.

Hypothermia, response of newborn to, 332
Hypovolemia, symptoms of, 329-330, 330f

I

I blood group system, 142, 142t, 152t
  autoanti-I, 143
  I antigens, 143, 143f
    biochemistry of, 143, 143f
    characteristics of, 143
    structure of, 143f
IAT. *See* Indirect antiglobulin test.
Icterus
  defined, 239
  in transfusion reaction, 239
ID-MTS Gel Test procedure, 220, 222-223, 222f
Identification, patient
  for blood products, 199
  in compatibility testing, 195, 195f
Idiotope
  defined, 5
  and heavy chains, 5
IgG antibodies, 12
  characteristics of, 6f, 6t, 7
  in immune response, 8, 9f
  subclasses of, 7
  weak, 171, 172f
IgG molecule
  basic structure of, 3, 4f
  and zeta potential, 16-17, 16f
IgM antibodies
  characteristics of, 6-7, 6f, 6t
  in immune response, 8, 9f
IgM molecules, and zeta potential, 16-17, 16f
Ii Blood Group Collection 207, 143
Immediate-spin agglutination, 6, 15
Immediate-spin crossmatch, in massive transfusion, 201
Immediate-spin phases, 35
Immune complex, 8
Immune response
  comparison of polyclonal and monoclonal, 33, 33f
  primary, 7-8, 9f
  secondary, 8, 9f
Immunization, during pregnancy, 12
Immunogen, 3
Immunogenicity
  of D antigen, 112
  defined, 112
  factors contributing to, 4t
Immunoglobulin (Ig)
  defined, 4
  use of term, 3-4
  variable region of, 5, 5f
Immunoglobulin (Ig) class, 127-128
Immunoglobulin (Ig) molecule, 5
Immunohematology, 2
  antigen-antibody reactions
    in vitro, 14-18
    in vivo, 12-14
  antigens of interest in, 59
  automation in, 208-211
  molecular genetics of, 60
Immunohematology reference laboratory, 170

Immunohematology testing, 29-31, 29f-30f
  examples of, 29, 30f
  routine procedures, 30-31, 31t
  sources of antibody for, 30, 30t
  sources of antigen for, 29-30, 30t
Immunosuppression, and risk of GVHD, 335
In vitro, 14
In vivo, 12
Incubation time, in agglutination, 15
Independent assortment, law of, 63-64, 63f
Independent segregation
  defined, 63
  Mendel's law of, 63-64
Indirect antiglobulin test (IAT)
  in antibody screen, 159
  applications of, 43, 43t
  for D antigen, 112-114, 114t, 115f
  defined, 41
  distinguished from DAT, 41-42, 44t
  procedure, 43, 43f, 44t
  SPRCAs for, 215, 216f
Indirect exclusion, in relationship testing, 69
Infants. *See also* Newborns.
  crossmatching of, 202-204
  iatrogenic blood loss in, 332
Infections, potential transfusion-transmitted, 273, 273t
Infectious diseases, in health history interview, 272-274, 273t
Infectious hepatitis, 292-293. *See also* Hepatitis.
Informed consent, in donor screening, 276
Infusion rate, for administration of blood components, 324
Inheritance patterns, 62
  codominant, 62
  dominant, 62
  recessive, 62
International Council on Commonality in Blood Banking Automation, 321-322
International Society of Blood Transfusion (ISBT)
  and Hemovigilance Model, 227
  blood group system numbers used by, 127-128
  blood group system symbols of, 127-128
  blood group systems defined by, 127
  ISBT 128 labeling of, 321-322
  on Rh blood system, 107-108
  standardized numeric terminology of, 109t, 111
  terminology of, 305
  Working Party on Terminology for Red Cell Antigens of, 78
Intraoperative cell recovery instrument, 280, 280f
Intrauterine transfusions
  for HDFN, 258-259
  interpreting test results with, 255
Inventory requirements, 309

Investigation, transfusion reaction
  initiating, 238-241
  instructions to medical staff, 238, 239f
  laboratory testing in, 240-241, 240t
  postreaction work-up, 239, 239f
  records and reporting of, 241
Ionic bonding, 8-10, 10t
Ionic strength, in agglutination, 15t, 16
Irradiated blood products, in TA-GVHD, 235-236, 236t
Irradiation, of RBCs, 315-316
ISBT. *See* International Society of Blood Transfusion.
Ischemia
  defined, 229
  in AHTR, 229
Isotype
  defined, 5
  distinguishing, 5

J

Jaundice, in HDFN, 247
JMH blood group system, 151t
The Joint Commission, 191

K

K_0 phenotype, 130-131
Kappa chains, 3-5
KEL gene, 131
Kell blood group system, 129, 129t, 152t
  antibodies of, 131-132, 138t
  antigens of
    biochemistry of, 129-130
    frequencies for, 127, 130t
    immunogenicity of, 130, 132
    K_0 or Kell$_{null}$ phenotype, 130-131
    terminology for, 129
    treated with papain or ficin, 130
  common frequencies in, 131t
  common phenotypes in, 131t
  discovery of, 129
  genetics of, 131, 131t
  inheritance of, 63-64, 63f
  and Kx antigen, 132
  phenotypes, 132, 133t
Kell$_{null}$ phenotype, 130-131
Kernicterus, in HDFN, 247, 248f
Kidd blood group system, 63, 136, 136t, 152t
  antibodies of, 137-138, 138t
  antigens of
    biochemistry of, 136-137
    characteristics of, 136
  common frequencies in, 136, 137t
  common phenotypes in, 136, 137t
  genetics of, 137
Kidney transplant, transfusion support in, 333
Kinins
  defined, 229
  in AHTR, 229
Kleihauer-Betke acid elution, 258, 258f
Knops blood group system, 151t
Kx antigen, and Kell blood group system, 132
Kx blood group system, 129, 131-133
  Kx antigen, 132
  and McLeod phenotype, 132